Calculating and Reporting Healthcare Statistics

Fifth Edition

Revised Reprint

Loretta A. Horton, MEd, RHIA, FAHIMA

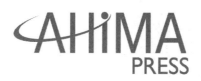

AHIMA
PRESS

ISBN: 978-1-58426-595-5
AHIMA Product No.: AB120717

AHIMA Staff:
Jessica Block, MA, Project Editor
Chelsea Brotherton, MA, Assistant Editor
Elizabeth Ranno, Vice President of Product and Planning
Pamela Woolf, Director of Publications

Cover image: © aleksandarvelasevic, iStock

For more information, including updates, about AHIMA Press publications, visit http://www.ahima.org/education/press.

American Health Information Management Association
233 North Michigan Avenue, 21st Floor
Chicago, Illinois 60601-5809
ahima.org

Table of Contents

About the Author . . . . **ix**

Acknowledgments . . . . **xi**

About the Online Resources . . . . **xiii**

Chapter 1   Introduction to Health Statistics **1**

Statistics 2
   Reasons for Studying Statistics 2
   Importance of Data 3
Descriptive Statistics versus Inferential Statistics 3
   Sources of Healthcare Statistics 4
Users of Health Statistics 6

Chapter 2   Mathematics Review **13**

Fractions 13
   Quotient 15
   Decimals 15
Rounding Numbers 15
   Rounding to the Nearest Ten 15
   Rounding to the Nearest Hundred 15
   Rounding to the Nearest Thousand 16
   Rounding Decimals 16
Percentage 18
   Changing a Fraction to a Percentage 18
   Changing a Decimal to a Percentage 18
   Changing a Percentage to a Fraction 19
   Changing a Percentage to a Decimal 19
Ratio 21
   Calculating Ratio 21
   Proportion 22

Rate...23
Averages 25

Chapter 3   Patient Census 31

Inpatient Census...32
 Complete Master Census...32
 Daily Inpatient Census...34
 Inpatient Service Days...35
Total Inpatient Service Days...36
Calculation of Inpatient Service Days................................37
 Patients Admitted and Discharged on the Same Day 40
 Recapitulation of Census Data 41
Average Daily Inpatient Census.......................................45
 Average Daily Newborn Census.......................................46
 Average Daily Inpatient Census for a Patient Care Unit 47

Chapter 4   Percentage of Occupancy 53

Percentage of Occupancy 54
 Inpatient Bed Count..54
 Labor Room Beds and Newborn Bassinets..............................54
 Emergency Services Department Beds 55
 Bed Count Days 55
 Inpatient Bed Occupancy Ratio/Percentage...........................56
 Change in Bed Count..59
 Newborn Bassinet Occupancy Ratio/Percentage........................61
Bed Turnover Rate..64

Chapter 5   Length of Stay 71

Length of Stay...71
 Discharge Days 72
 Calculating Length of Stay in an Outpatient Setting................74
 Total Length of Stay...76
 Average Length of Stay 78
 Average Newborn Length of Stay.....................................79
Leave of Absence Days..80

Chapter 6   Death (Mortality) Rates 91

Guidelines for Calculating Death Rates...............................92
 Gross (Hospital) Death Rate 93
 Net Death Rate 95
 Postoperative Death Rate 97

Anesthesia Death Rate 100
Maternal Death Rate 102
Newborn Death Rate 106
Fetal Death Rate 109
Cancer Mortality Rate 112

Chapter 7   Hospital Autopsies and Autopsy Rates. 121

Autopsy Rates 122
Gross Autopsy Rate 122
Net Autopsy Rate 123
Hospital Autopsies 127
Adjusted Hospital Autopsy Rate 128
Newborn Autopsy Rate 132
Fetal Autopsy Rate 133

Chapter 8   Morbidity and Other Miscellaneous Rates. 145

Morbidity Rates 146
Infection Rate 146
Postoperative Infection Rate 150
Complication Rate 153
Cesarean Section Rate 155
Consultation Rates 158
Other Rates 161

**Chapter 9   Statistics Computed within the Health Information
            Management Department 173**

Health Information Statistics 174
Employee Compensation and Unit Labor Costs 174
Unit Costs for Release of Information 177
Other Labor Unit Costs 179
Productivity 185
Staffing Levels 186
Budgets 193
Operational Budget 193
Capital Budget 194
Verification of Statistical Reports 197
Computerized Discharge Reports 197
Computerized Financial Statistical Reports 200
Computerized Readmission Rate Reports 200
Case-Mix Index Report 200
Physician Reports 204
Spreadsheets 208

Chapter 10   Descriptive Statistics in Healthcare. 213

Concepts in Descriptive Statistics 214
   Frequency Distribution 214
   Rank. 215
   Quartile 215
   Decile 216
   Percentile 216
   Measures of Central Tendency 220
   Median 222
   Median Used to Describe Length of Stay 223
   Mode. 224
   Measures of Variation 227
   Variability 228
   Range 228
   Variance 229
   Standard Deviation. 231
   Other Curves. 234
   Correlation. 236

Chapter 11   Presentation of Data. 245

Types of Data 245
   Categorical Data. 246
   Numerical Data. 248
Data Display 249
   Tables 249
   Graphs 257
Preparing Reports 275

Chapter 12   Basic Research Principles. 283

Basic Research Principles. 284
Types of Research 284
   Research Methodology 284
The Research Process 286
   Defining the Problem. 286
   Reviewing the Literature. 287
   Designing the Research and Collecting the Data 287
   Analyzing the Data. 295
   Drawing Conclusions 296
Data Interpretation Issues 296
   Misleading Presentation of Numbers. 297
   Ignoring the Baseline 297
   Selection Bias 297
   Graphical Misrepresentations. 297
   Sabotage. 298
   Importance of Data Validation. 298
   Introduction to Institutional Review Boards 298

Privacy Considerations in Clinical and Biomedical Research 300
Ethical Guidelines in Statistics 303

Chapter 13   Inferential Statistics in Healthcare 309

Inferential Statistics 310
Standard Error of the Mean and Confidence Intervals 310
The Null Hypothesis 312
Type I Error 314
Type II Error 314
The *t* Test 314
ANOVA 316
Chi-Square 317

Chapter 14   Data Analytics 321

Introduction to Data Analytics 321
Types of Healthcare Data 322
Types of Data Analytics 323
Descriptive Analytics 323
Predictive Analytics 323
Data Mining 324
Predictive Modeling 324
Real-time Analytics 325
Prescriptive Analytics 325
Using Data Analytics for Decision-Making 325
Information Governance 327

References 331
Appendix A   Formulas 335
Appendix B   Glossary of Healthcare Services and Statistical Terms 343
Appendix C   Answers to Odd-Numbered Chapter Exercises 363
Index 417

Online Resources
Exercise worksheets

About the Author

Loretta A. Horton, MEd, RHIA, FAHIMA, received a medical record technician certificate from Research Hospital and Medical Center and a bachelor's degree in psychology from Rockhurst College, both in Kansas City, MO; a health information administration post-baccalaureate certificate from Stephens College in Columbia, MO; and a master's degree in education, with an emphasis in curriculum and instruction, from Wichita State University in Wichita, KS. She also has completed graduate work in sociology at the University of Nebraska in Omaha.

Horton has served as co-chair of the Allied Health Department and coordinator of the health information technology program at Hutchinson Community College in Hutchinson, KS. Previously, she worked in a variety of health information settings, including acute care and mental health, and has consulted in the fields of long-term care, intellectual disability, home health, hospice, and prisons. Horton has been an instructor in the health information administration program at the College of St. Mary in Omaha, NE, and a marketing and training coordinator for 3M in Salt Lake City, UT.

Horton has contributed chapters in AHIMA's foundational textbooks, *Health Information Management: An Applied Approach* and *Health Information Management: Concepts, Principles, and Practice.*

Horton has been an active member of the Kansas Health Information Management Association receiving the Motivator award in 2002, the Achievement award in 2006, the Champion award in 2009, and the Outstanding Member award in 2015. She has been active in the American Health Information Management Association, serving on the Item Writing Task Force for the Council on Certification, Council on Accreditation, and Scholarship Committee and Associate Education Consortium. She is a Fellow in the American Health Information Management Association.

Horton currently lives in Hutchinson, KS, with her husband, Bill, who is also a health information professional. She has two daughters, Merritt and Maura, and three grandchildren, Noah, Harriett, and Amelia.

Acknowledgments

Loretta Horton gives a special word of thanks to Susan White, PhD, CHDA for her review of the text and insightful comments. Also, a word of thanks to the AHIMA Publications staff whose professional work helped to make this textbook a reality. A special thanks to Bill Horton and Christopher Lau, who helped with a review of the textbook.

AHIMA Press and Loretta Horton also thank Donna Estes, MPM, RHIT, CPHQ, Connie Renda, MA, RHIA, CHDA, and Ray Hylock, PhD, for their technical review of this edition.

About the Online Resources

To access the online student resources, go to http://www.ahimapress.org/horton5955 and download the zip file. When you attempt to open the file, you will be prompted to enter the case-sensitive password. Enter ahi5955maHorton.

CHAPTER 1

Introduction to Health Statistics

Learning Objectives

At the conclusion of this chapter, you should be able to

- Explain what statistics are and identify reasons to study healthcare statistics
- Identify the sources of data
- Compare and contrast between data and information, validity and reliability, descriptive and inferential statistics, primary and secondary data sources
- Identify the users of healthcare statistics

Key Terms

Agency for Healthcare
  Research and Quality
  (AHRQ)
Ambulatory care facility
Census
Centers for Disease Control
  and Prevention (CDC)
Centers for Medicare and
  Medicaid Services (CMS)

Descriptive statistics
Encounter
Home health (HH)
Hospice
Inferential statistics
Inpatient
Inpatient census
Managed care organization
  (MCO)

Nursing facility
Outpatient
Primary data source
Secondary data source
Visit
Vital statistics
World Health Organization
  (WHO)

The term statistics has two meanings. First, it is a number computed from a larger group of numbers, which collectively constitute a sample of data—for instance, the average number of days that patients stay in the hospital overnight. Second, statistics is more broadly defined as a branch of mathematics concerned with collecting, organizing, summarizing, and analyzing data.

Statistics

Originally, the term *statistics* referred to the collection of data about and for the "state." The word comes from the Italian word *stato*, meaning "state." One need only think of our own government and its statistics-collecting organizations, such as the Bureau of Labor Statistics, the Centers for Disease Control and Prevention (CDC), and the Centers for Medicare and Medicaid Services (CMS), for examples.

Health statistics provide information about the health of people and their use of healthcare services. Examples of healthcare statistics include average longevity; birth rates; death rates; incidence of a particular disease in a county, state, the United States as a whole, or the world; and the frequency of usage of a particular type of service within a healthcare organization.

Reasons for Studying Statistics

Statistics is really about decision making, which is required in every area of our lives. To do that, we must have some information. In healthcare settings, information is often incomplete. As a result, we must learn to estimate the characteristics of a complete population using statistics.

Most organizations keep statistics in order to make decisions about their business. For example, an organization may use statistics to determine its markets, that is, to identify who is buying its product or using its services and how it can increase the availability and variety of products and services. Healthcare organizations use statistics to determine the use and cost of services as well as outcomes of patients.

Healthcare Operations Needs

In the healthcare industry, there are compelling reasons to collect and analyze data. For example, statistics kept on activities in the healthcare facility indicate why patients come to the facility and the costs of taking care of them. Patient care statistics and studies on performance can show the quality of care provided. Many accrediting agencies require a data analysis system as part of accreditation, and many third-party payers require facilities to collect performance data. Administrators also may use statistics for prioritizing needed services and to point to areas where efficiency and effectiveness might be increased. For example, the laboratory data on appointments may show that most outpatients come in for blood work early in the day, so the lab may add more staff in the morning hours. Additionally, healthcare facilities are interested in the types of patients they have with respect to their diagnoses in order to maintain the optimum physician specialty and other professional staff mix they need to treat their patients.

Public Health Needs

Government also needs to maintain statistics on and about the population in order to provide services. For example, the CDC, a division of the Department of Health and Human Services (HHS), is recognized as the lead agency responsible for protecting the health of the United States' population by providing credible information to help individuals make the right healthcare decisions and promoting quality of life through the prevention and control of disease, injury, and disability. They use health statistics, such as birth and death statistics, to understand the conditions of life and health in our country.

The **CMS** is the division of the HHS that is responsible for developing healthcare policy in the United States and for administering the Medicare program and the federal portion of the

Medicaid program. They also publish information on death rates among Medicare patients, specific ethnic groups, and patients in particular diagnosis categories. Researchers use this information for their studies, which will lead to improvement in patient care and services. Keeping track of death statistics "is one of the best investments to reduce premature mortality worldwide as it is one of the most robust ways to measure accurately the effectiveness of investments aimed at reducing child and adult mortality" (Prabhat 2012).

The **Agency for Healthcare Research and Quality (AHRQ)**, part of the HHS, tries to make healthcare safer; of higher quality; and more accessible, equitable, and affordable. For example, the AHRQ publishes research-based fact sheets for patients and consumers on a variety of issues, such as patient safety and reducing errors when a patient is in the hospital. It also works within the HHS and with other partners to make sure that the information is understood and used. The AHRQ conducts research on the elderly, children, and various healthcare conditions to provide information to consumers and other HHS agencies so they may meet their objectives. For example, their publication on how to reduce Medicaid readmissions is intended to help hospitals by providing tools to identify causes of readmissions and aid in the development of prevention strategies.

The **World Health Organization (WHO)**, an international organization founded by the United Nations (UN), is the directing and coordinating authority on international health within the UN's system. The WHO provides leadership on critical health matters and works to support countries to ensure all their citizens have accessible and safe healthcare and helps prevent the spread of communicable diseases, especially vaccine-preventable diseases. They support good health through the continuum of life and are working toward reducing quality of life disparities among countries. The WHO supports healthcare research in maternal, child, and adolescent health; malaria; tuberculosis; HIV; Ebola and other global healthcare issues (WHO 2016). For example, in 1988, the WHO helped launch the Global Polio Eradication Initiative to help protect all children from polio. As a result of this immunization initiative, the number of polio cases has dropped by 99%. Today, only two counties remain polio-endemic, meaning that the disease is regularly found in the population. The WHO continues to work with these two countries to ensure that polio will be stopped.

Importance of Data

To obtain the knowledge they need to make decisions, organizations first must have data. Data are raw facts and figures that can pertain to a measurement that an organization is interested in. Information is derived from facts for the purpose of making decisions. The data used in the statistics must be valid and reliable. Validity answers the question of whether one measured what one intended to measure, and reliability means that there is some consistency of results. For example, if a supervisor is checking the coding work of a new employee, the codes assigned should be the same for the supervisor as they were for the employee (that is, consistent) in order for the results to be reliable.

Descriptive Statistics versus Inferential Statistics

The primary focus of descriptive statistics is to organize and describe the features of data in a study. **Descriptive statistics** describe what the data show about the characteristics of a group or population; in other words, they tell us information about a particular population. For example, it might be necessary to know the average age of patients or which service is used most in a given facility. **Inferential statistics**, on the other hand, help make inferences or guesses about a larger group of data by drawing conclusions from a small group of data. The smaller group of data is often called a *sample*, which is a portion of the larger group or population. The results obtained from the sample, if gathered carefully, are assumed to be typical of the entire population. Both types of statistics are used to describe data.

Sources of Healthcare Statistics

Healthcare data are derived from both primary and secondary data sources. Statistics usually come from a primary data source, also known as firsthand documents.

Primary Data Sources

In healthcare, **primary data source** refers to the record that was developed by healthcare professionals in the process of providing care or services to a patient. Medical records are one of the most important primary sources of health statistics because they contain a systematic record of a patient's medical history and care.

The patient's medical record will contain administrative data, such as admission and discharge dates, patient data, billing data. Notes from physicians, such as physician orders and progress notes, operative reports, history and physical examination, and a discharge summary, will be included. Nurses' documentation includes their notes and assessments on admission and throughout the hospital stay and medication records. Reports from clinical departments in the facility, such as laboratory and blood bank, radiology, pharmacy, rehabilitation services, and dietary services, may also be included in the medical records.

Hospital departments also keep statistics on the activities they perform for patients. For example, the laboratory department may keep data on the number of lab tests performed. The radiology department may keep track of the number of chest and hip x-rays. The physical therapy department may use statistical data, such as the number of patient visits, to decide whether to hire additional physical therapists or add physical therapist assistants to their staff. These reports may be used in turn by the managers of the departments for productivity reports and combined with other departments to produce a report of activity for the entire facility. The administration of a hospital might ask staff to keep data on the number of patients transferred to another hospital for procedures the facility does not offer in order to determine the need for that service at the facility.

Another example of a primary source of data is vital statistics. The National Vital Statistics System (NVSS) is part of the National Center for Health Statistics (NCHS) of the CDC. These data are provided to the NCHS throughout the 50 states; Washington, DC; New York City; and the five inhabited territories of the United States, Puerto Rico, the Virgin Islands, Guam, American Samoa, and the Commonwealth of the Northern Mariana Islands. **Vital statistics** refers to a special group of statistics that record important events in our lives, such as birth, marriage, death, divorce, and fetal death. Healthcare facilities are interested in births and deaths, fetal deaths, and induced terminations of pregnancy; facilities generally are responsible for completing certificates for births, fetal deaths, abortions, and occasionally, death certificates. All states have laws that require this data. The certificates are reported to the individual state registrars and maintained permanently. State vital statistics registrars compile the data and report them to the NCHS (2015).

Censuses

Another primary source of health data is the census. A **census** is defined as a count of a particular population. The US government conducts a population census, that is, a count of the people residing in the United States and their location. The US Constitution requires that a population census be taken decennially, that is, every 10 years, mainly to determine the number of congressional representatives in the states.

Over the years, Congress has authorized gathering more information about each person. The census now is used in many ways. For instance, the amount of government money given to school districts is based partly on the number of children in a particular district. Congress also has requested that other types of censuses be taken periodically. These include a census of the types of businesses and industries in the United States, for example, farms and fisheries, construction, foreign trade, manufacturing, and energy companies. Aggregated census data, or data that have been clustered together, are available to the public. Healthcare researchers use the US census when they want to determine statistics about the population at large. For example if researchers want to show the number of maternal deaths in a population, they must know information about the population at large, which the US census provides.

Healthcare facilities also have a census, which is the count of patients present at a specific time and in a particular place. A hospital patient, or **inpatient**, is a patient who is provided with room, board, and continuous general nursing services in an area of an acute-care facility where patients generally stay at least overnight. In hospitals, this is referred to as the **inpatient census**. The hospital census is a source of primary data. Ambulatory care facilities also may keep a census. An **ambulatory care facility** is one that provides preventive or corrective healthcare services on a nonresident basis in a provider's office, clinic setting, or hospital outpatient setting. This figure usually represents the number of **visits** or encounters during a specified period, usually one day. A visit is a single encounter with a healthcare professional that includes all the services supplied during the encounter. An **encounter** is defined as the direct personal contact between a patient and a physician or other person authorized by state licensure and, if applicable, by medical staff bylaws to order or furnish healthcare services for the diagnosis or treatment of the patient.

Secondary Data Sources

Secondary data sources are data derived from primary sources and may be collected by someone other than the primary user. Secondary data sources are facility specific. For example, the disease and operation index is a secondary source of data. The disease index is a listing of patients discharged with a particular diagnosis code, and an operation index is similar to the disease index, but the patients are listed by the operation or procedure code. All the data in the index comes from a primary data source, the medical record. Registries are also considered secondary data sources. A registry is a listing of patients who share a common characteristic. For example, data from patients' medical records may be used to create a cancer or trauma registry. This is a listing of patients in the facility who have been diagnosed with cancer and will include their treatment information as well as follow-up information.

The NCHS has developed standard certificates and procedures that states and territories must use to help facilitate the consistent collection of data. The standard certificates represent the minimum basic data set necessary for the collection and publication of comparable national, state, and local vital statistics data. The standard forms are revised about every 10 to 15 years, and the latest adoption to the 2003 revisions of the US Standards Certificate of Live Birth were completed in 2015.

At the time of this writing, the NCHS is working on the development of an e-Vital Standards Initiative that will provide support for the development of vital statistics standards to enable an exchange of data regarding births and deaths from a healthcare facility's electronic health record system directly to the state registrar and then to the NCHS.

Data from the states and territories provide important information for use in medical research and are extremely valuable in estimating population growth in particular areas of the country and essential in planning and evaluating maternal and child health programs. The NCHS prepares and publishes national statistics based on vital statistics data because they are important in the fields of social welfare and public health. Because of their many uses, the data on these certificates must be complete and accurate.

Real-World Example: A public health department uses census data to determine the demographics of its county. These include population, age, education, marital status, household income, poverty, employment, and number of uninsured. They also use data from the CDC to determine mental health prevalence, physical activity rates, tobacco use, obesity, and substance abuse. The state department of health also provides data on sexually transmitted infections and communicable diseases, number of births, number of premature births, number of teen pregnancies, mortality rates, and causes of deaths. When they put all this data together, they get a picture of the health needs of the community as well as the socioeconomic factors that are contributing to these needs and can provide education for the community as needed (Slavenburg 2016).

Exercise 1.1

Identify the following as either a primary or a secondary data source:

Type of Healthcare Data	Type of Data Source
1. Productivity reports pulled from patient visit report	
2. Tumor registry	
3. State vital statistics	
4. Hospital census	
5. Hospital disease index	
6. Patient health record	
7. Health insurance data pulled from national census	

Users of Health Statistics

All healthcare entities and third-party payers collect and use statistics. Following are examples of individuals and organizations that collect statistics and how they use statistics:

- **Healthcare administration:** Inpatient facilities use health statistics to help address staffing issues and to determine the types of services to provide. For example, if the number of patients in the intensive care unit is increasing, the hospital administration may want to consider adding beds and staff to meet the growing need. Conversely, if a request is made to the hospital administration for new facilities and equipment that cannot be substantiated by the statistics, it is unlikely the request will be granted. Quality management departments in healthcare facilities collect data to determine how the facility is performing in regard to patient care and to how it can improve their patient care services. Administrators also use statistics to determine if they have the correct mix of medical specialties to treat the citizens in their communities.

- **Healthcare department managers:** Individual department managers in healthcare organizations use statistics to implement their department goals. For example, a manager needs to know if he or she is staying within budget. If not, the manager will need to investigate.

- **Cancer registries:** A cancer registry may be maintained by a separate department or may be a function of the health information department. States may also have a state cancer registry that is responsible for collecting data about cancer. A cancer registry collects data about the diagnosis, treatment, and follow-up of cancer patients. These statistics are important in tracking cancer survival rates. Facilities may choose to undergo accreditation through the American College of Surgeons Commission on Cancer (2014). This is an evaluation by an independent team to determine whether the facility's cancer registry meets their standards, which guide treatment and ensure patient-centered care. Statistics must show the facility is providing high-quality care and follow-up to its cancer patients. Physicians and researchers conduct research studies to learn about the biology of cancer and investigate new treatments and tests and learn how to prevent cancers from occurring.

- **Nursing facilities:** Long-term care (LTC) facilities may use statistics to determine the types of payers their patients have. These statistics also are helpful in demonstrating to the public the types of patients being cared for and the quality of care given. For example, a LTC facility will collect data on the number of patients who are incontinent. This will tell the facility if protocols need to be established for patients in order to help them void. The American Health Care Association, a non-profit association of LTC associations, publishes statistics on the trends in nursing home care.

- **Home health (HH):** HH agencies provide care to elderly, disabled, and convalescent patients in their homes. This is also called home care. These agencies keep statistics to determine the types of services used by their patients and their outcomes. For example, a HH agency would need to know the number of nursing visits, HH aide visits, physical therapy treatments, and patients using various types of equipment, such as oxygen machines or other respiratory aids. Additionally, agencies will report patient outcomes, such as the number of patients who have improved, the number of patients who were compliant with taking their medications, or the number of patients who had to be readmitted to a hospital.

- **Hospice:** Hospice programs provide interdisciplinary programs of palliative care and supportive services that address the physical, spiritual, social, and economic needs of terminally ill patients and their families. These services may be given in either the home or an inpatient setting. A hospice needs to know types of illnesses in order to match the appropriate caregiver with each patient.

- **Mental health facilities:** These may be inpatient or outpatient facilities. These facilities use health statistics to determine whether they are providing the proper services for patients in the community. Because the economic burden of psychiatric illness is great, the CDC collects data about mental illness and its impact on the country.

- **Drug and alcohol facilities:** These programs may be inpatient, ambulatory, or a combination of the two. Statistics are important in this area to show the success rates of these facilities' clients. The National Institute of Drug Abuse and the National Institute on Alcohol Abuse and Alcoholism are centers in the National Institutes of Health that each collect statistics to conduct research.

- **Outpatient facilities:** These include physician clinics, surgery centers, emergency centers, and the like. Outpatient facilities often use statistics to determine whether they are providing the proper level of care to the community.

- **Managed care organizations (MCOs):** An **MCO** is a type of healthcare organization that delivers medical care and manages all aspects of care or payment for care by limiting providers of care, discounting payment to providers of care, or limiting access to care. MCOs use statistics to determine whether they are providing the correct level of care at the best cost. Additionally, MCOs contract with healthcare facilities to provide specific services to their members at a particular cost. The MCO pays the agreed-upon amount each time a member uses the service. Typically, the MCO receives a discounted rate, and this results in individual members of the MCO paying less out of pocket.

- **Healthcare researchers:** Researchers depend on healthcare statistics to conduct research and help develop solutions to healthcare problems. Some examples include research in managed care, health law and regulations, mergers and acquisitions of healthcare facilities, physician practice issues, different types of illness and risk factors, telehealth issues, pharmaceutical research, drug and alcohol research, and so on. Healthcare statistics can also help researchers understand our quality of life.

- **Accreditation agencies:** These organizations use healthcare statistics to determine the most common diagnoses and procedures and whether the resources are available to treat patients with those diagnoses.

- **Federal government:** The US government collects data for public health issues. For example, the CDC reports data on births, deaths, birth defects, cancer, and HIV/AIDS, just to name a few of the categories of data. CMS uses data collected by quality improvement organizations for its quality improvement projects. Legislators and other policymakers use healthcare statistics when working on new laws, conducting program oversight, and considering the amount of the budget that should be allotted to federal health agencies.

Tip: Health information management (HIM) practitioners must remember that, first and foremost, statistics must be gathered and formulated, or expressed in systematic terms or concepts, before they even exist. HIM practitioners are usually the individuals who gather and formulate this data.

Because HIM practitioners have a broad knowledge of healthcare facilities as well as immediate access to a wide range of clinical data, they are in the best position to collect, prepare, analyze, and interpret healthcare data. HIM practitioners must learn acceptable terminology, definitions, and computational methodology if they are to provide the basic and most frequently used health statistics. One important point to remember is that health statistics are dependent upon accurate reporting by those individuals responsible for the task.

Chapter 1   Matching Quiz

Match the definition with the term.

Definitions:

a. A type of healthcare organization that delivers medical care and manages all aspects of the care or the payment for care by limiting providers of care, discounting payment to providers of care, or limiting access to care

b. A comprehensive term for LTC facilities that provide nursing care and related services for residents requiring medical, nursing, or rehabilitative care

c. The direct personal contact between a patient and a physician or other person authorized by state licensure law and, if applicable, by medical staff bylaws to order or furnish healthcare services for the diagnosis or treatment of the patient

d. A group of federal agencies that oversees health promotion and disease control and prevention activities in the United States

e. An interdisciplinary program of palliative care and supportive services that addresses the physical, spiritual, social, and economic needs of terminally ill patients and their families

f. Data related to births, deaths, marriages, and fetal deaths

g. An umbrella term that refers to the medical and nonmedical services provided to patients and their families in their places of residence

h. Record developed by healthcare professionals in the process of providing patient care

i. The UN's specialized agency created to ensure the attainment or the highest possible levels of health by all peoples

j. Data derived from the primary patient record, such as an index or database

Terms:

1. _____ Secondary data source
2. _____ Nursing facility
3. _____ Hospice
4. _____ Vital statistics
5. _____ MCO

6. _____ Encounter
7. _____ CDC
8. _____ The WHO
9. _____ Home health
10. _____ Primary data source

Chapter 1   Review

Select the best answer to the following questions:

1. The CDC is the lead agency that _____.
   a. Accredits and licenses acute hospital facilities in the United States
   b. Is responsible for providing vital statistics to various agencies, such as the NCHS
   c. Develops and updates ICD-10 for the world
   d. Is responsible for protecting the health of the people of the United States

2. The type of statistics that makes inferences or a best guess about a larger group of data by drawing conclusions from a smaller group of data is called _____.
   a. Descriptive statistics
   b. Inferential statistics
   c. Generalized statistics
   d. Mathematical statistics

3. Which of the following is considered to be a primary source of data?
   a. Inpatient census
   b. Vital statistics collected by the NCHS
   c. Health record
   d. a, b, and c
   e. b and c only

4. The division of the HHS that is responsible for developing healthcare policy in the United States is the _____.
   a. CDC
   b. CMS
   c. AHRQ
   d. WHO

5. A secondary data source includes _____.
   a. Vital statistics
   b. The medical record
   c. The physician's index
   d. A videotape of a counseling session

6. Which user of statistics has the primary job of supporting terminally ill patients and their families?
   a. Home health agencies
   b. Nursing facilities
   c. Hospice
   d. MCOs

7. The NCHS keeps statistics on _____.
   a. The licensing information on all healthcare providers in the 50 states
   b. Cancer and other deadly diseases in the 50 states and the US-owned territories
   c. Vital statistics, such as births, deaths, and fetal deaths, in North America
   d. Vital statistics, such as births, deaths, and fetal deaths, in the 50 states and the US-owned territories

8. Which of the following is *not* a primary source of statistics?
   a. Health record
   b. Vital statistics
   c. Hospital census
   d. Disease and operation index

9. In order to be useful, the figures used in statistics must be _____.
   a. Fair and exact
   b. Valid and reliable
   c. Honest and justified
   d. Simple and clear

10. To be reliable, statistical data must _____.
    a. Have some consistency
    b. Be applicable to what is being measured
    c. Be collected from one source only
    d. Have multiple meanings

11. A healthcare organization that delivers medical care and manages all aspects of the care or the payment for care by limiting providers of care, discounting payment to providers of care, or limiting access to care is called a(n) _____.
    a. Long-term care facility
    b. MCO
    c. Hospital
    d. Hospice agency

12. Facilities may choose to pursue accreditation for their cancer registries with the _____.
    a. American College of Physicians
    b. American Cancer Society
    c. American College of Surgeons
    d. National Institutes of Health

13. The type of patient who receives care in a hospital-based clinic or department is called a(n) _____.
    a. Inpatient
    b. Outpatient
    c. Hospice patient
    d. MCO patient

14. The number of inpatients present in a healthcare facility at any given time is called a(n) _____.
    a. Survey
    b. Census
    c. Sample
    d. Enumeration

15. An international organization founded by the UN that is the directing and coordinating authority on international heath is called the _____.
    a. CDC
    b. AHRQ
    c. NCHS
    d. WHO

CHAPTER 2

Mathematics Review

Learning Objectives

At the conclusion of this chapter, you should be able to

- Differentiate and apply the terms fraction, quotient, decimal, ratio, proportion, rate, and percentage
- Compare and contrast the difference between a numerator and denominator
- Round whole numbers and decimals
- Convert fractions and decimals to percentages
- Compute the average of a group of numbers

Key Terms

Average	Numerator	Rate
Decimal	Percentage	Ratio
Denominator	Proportion	Rounding
Fraction	Quotient	Whole number

Numbers may be expressed in a variety of ways for use in calculating statistics. As discussed in the previous chapter, data are needed to help healthcare organizations make decisions. The following sections explain and review fractions, quotients, decimals, proportions, how to round numbers, percentages, ratios, rates, and averages. We will use these statistics in subsequent chapters.

Fractions

A **fraction** is one or more parts of the whole. Figure 2.1 shows two circles; the first circle is split into two equal parts, and the second shows one part of the circle larger than the other part. The

Figure 2.1. Fractions of a circle

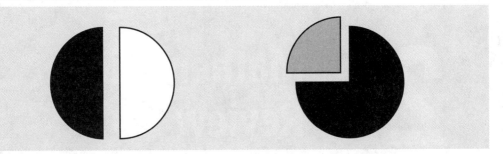

fraction of the first circle is $\frac{1}{2}$; the fraction of the second circle (in darker color) is $\frac{3}{4}$. The top number is called the **numerator** and the bottom number is called the **denominator**. The denominator tells us how many parts a whole is broken into. For example, if we have a fraction of $\frac{4}{6}$, the denominator is 6. That indicates there are six equal parts that make up the whole. The numerator tells us how many parts there are of the whole. In the fraction $\frac{4}{6}$, there are 4 out of the total 6 parts.

Example: Of the 40 patients with diabetes seen last month in a physician's clinic, 20 were Caucasian, 10 were African-American, and 10 were Asian-American. The following fractions show the number of patients of each race compared with the total number of patients who visited the clinic: Caucasian, $\frac{20}{40}$; African-American, $\frac{10}{40}$; and Asian-American, $\frac{10}{40}$. Fractions should be converted to their simplest form. Each fraction can be converted by dividing both top (numerator) and bottom (denominator) by a common factor. In this example, both the numerator and the denominator can be divided by 10: Caucasians, $\frac{2}{4}$; African-American, $\frac{1}{4}$; and Asian-American, $\frac{1}{4}$. The first fraction can be further simplified with the common factor of 2; thus, $\frac{2}{4}$ can be expressed as $\frac{1}{2}$.

Exercise 2.1

Find the simplest form of each of the following fractions:

1. $\dfrac{20}{40}$

2. $\dfrac{4}{6}$

3. $\dfrac{12}{54}$

4. $\dfrac{8}{12}$

5. $\dfrac{16}{28}$

Quotient

A **quotient** is the number obtained by dividing the numerator of a fraction by the denominator. This number may be expressed in **decimals**.

> **Example:** The 14 members of your health information class decide to participate in your college's information day. The booth is going to be open for 21 hours over a three-day period. To find out how many hours each student would need to attend to the booth, you would divide the numerator (21 hours) by the denominator (14 students). This calculation gives a quotient of 1.5. Thus, each student would have to attend the booth for 1.5 hours.

Decimals

Decimal fractions are simply referred to as decimals. The notation indicates a value that is less than one. In 14.37, for example, the digits to the right of the decimal point (3 and 7) are called decimal digits. The decimal point is used to separate the fraction (.37) of a **whole number** from the whole number itself (14). The decimal point is not ordinarily used in whole numbers (for example, 14.0) unless the healthcare facility has a particular reason for doing so.

> **Tip:** The decimal .5 is usually written as 0.5 in order to call attention to the decimal point.

Rounding Numbers

Rounding is a process of approximating a number. Numbers may be rounded to the nearest 10, 100, and so on. In healthcare facilities, rounding is commonly used when expressing data because staff must manage both parts of a whole, as in length of stay, and the whole, as in the number of patients or census.

Rounding to the Nearest Ten

Rounding to the nearest ten means that any number between multiples of ten (10, 20, 30, 40, and so on) is rounded to the multiple it is closest to. For example, 31 falls between 30 and 40 but is closer to 30, so it is rounded to 30. Numbers ending with 6, 7, 8, or 9 are closer to the ten above it. For example, 37 is closer to 40, so it is rounded to 40. When a number is exactly between the two multiples of ten, the rule of thumb is to round up. For example, 35 would be rounded up to 40.

Rounding to the Nearest Hundred

Rounding to the nearest hundred refers to rounding numbers that fall between multiples of 100. When rounding to the nearest hundred, look at the last two digits. If the last two digits are 49 or less, round down. For example, 327 falls between 300 and 400 but is closer to 300. Thus, the 27 indicates that 327 should be rounded down to 300. On the other hand, any last two digits that are 50 and above should be rounded up. For example, the 76 in 376 indicates that 376 should be rounded up to 400. When the last two numbers are exactly between two multiples of 100, the rule of thumb is to round up; 350 would be rounded to 400.

Rounding to the Nearest Thousand

When rounding to the nearest thousand, look at the last three digits. If the last three digits are 499 or less, then the number is rounded down. For example, in the number 7,337, the 337 indicates that 7,337 should be rounded down to 7,000. The number 7,868 falls between 7,800 and 7,900. In this case, the 868 indicates that 7,868 should be rounded up to 8,000. Just as in the previous examples, if the last three numbers are exactly between two multiples of 1,000, the rule of thumb is to round up; 7,500 would be rounded up to 8,000.

Rounding Decimals

Most healthcare statistics are reported as decimals, and each healthcare facility has its own policy on the number of decimal places to be used in computing and reporting percentages. The principles that apply to rounding whole numbers also apply to rounding decimals. To round to the nearest whole number, look at the first digit to the right of the decimal point (tenths place); if the number is 5 or more, the whole number should be rounded up; if the number is less than 5, the whole number should be left as it is. Thus, the whole number in 14.4 should remain at 14; however, 14.5 should be rounded up to 15.

To round to the nearest tenth, perform the same procedure, but use the hundredths digit rather than the tenths. The hundredths is the second digit to the right of the decimal point. For example, 14.46 would be rounded up one to 14.5 because the 6 (hundredths place) in .46 is greater than 5. In the case of 14.13, the 3 in .13 is less than 5, so the .1 is kept rather than rounding up. To round to the nearest hundredths, the calculation must be carried out to three decimal places (the thousandths place) and then rounded. For example, 14.657 would be rounded up to 14.66 because the 7 in .657 is greater than 5. In the case of 14.654, the 4 in .654 is less than 5; therefore, the decimal is rounded down to 14.65.

Remember to only round once. For example, 93.46 would be rounded to 93.5. It would not then be rounded to 94.0.

Exercise 2.2

Find the quotient in the following fractions. Round to two decimal places.

1. $\dfrac{2}{5}$

2. $\dfrac{3}{4}$

3. $\dfrac{7}{8}$

4. $\dfrac{107}{98}$

5. $\dfrac{54}{65}$

Exercise 2.3

Round the following numbers to the nearest 10.

1. 42
2. 338
3. 217
4. 6,989
5. 8,532

Round the following numbers to the nearest hundred.

6. 156
7. 321
8. 3,807
9. 4,357
10. 8,175

Round to the nearest whole number.

11. 38.1
12. 55.6
13. 14.7
14. 625.2
15. 100.5

Round to one decimal place.

16. 19.76
17. 34.62
18. 172.87
19. 99.98
20. 125.96

Round to two decimal places.

21. 8.36801

22. 14.5264

23. 0.87642

24. 27.99999

25. 15.90176

Percentage

The ratio of a part to the whole is often expressed as a **percentage**. A percentage is a fraction expressed in hundredths. Percent means "per 100." There is a specific way to write this. For example, 0.34 would be written as $\frac{34}{100}$ and is equal to 34 percent.

Percentages are a useful way to make fair comparisons. For example, if 20 patients died in hospital A last month and 50 patients died in hospital B during the same period, one might conclude that it would be better to use the services at hospital A because hospital A had fewer deaths. However, that conclusion would be wrong if hospital A had 100 discharges during the month and hospital B had 500 discharges for the same period.

Hospital A: 20/100 = 20%
Hospital B: 50/500 = 10%

Not all percentages are converted to whole numbers. For example:

$$\frac{1}{8} = 0.125 = 12.5\%$$

Changing a Fraction to a Percentage

To change a fraction to a percentage, divide the numerator by the denominator and multiply by 100. For example, to change $\frac{1}{2}$ to a percentage, divide 1 by 2 and multiply by 100. The calculation is as follows:

$$\frac{1}{2} = 0.5 \times 100 = 50\%$$

Changing a Decimal to a Percentage

To change a decimal to a percentage, simply multiply the decimal by 100. The calculation changes the position of the decimal point. For example:

$$0.29 \times 100 = 29\%$$

Changing a Percentage to a Fraction

To convert a percentage to a fraction, eliminate the percent sign and multiply the number by $\frac{1}{100}$. A simpler version of this is to place the number in the numerator and 100 in the denominator. For example:

$$5\% \text{ would be } 5 \times \frac{1}{100} = \frac{5}{100}$$

$$15\% \text{ would be } 5 \times \frac{1}{100} = \frac{15}{100}$$

Fractions are usually converted to their simplest form. In the example of 5 percent, both 5 and 100 can be divided by 5, which would result in a fraction of $\frac{1}{20}$. In the example 15 percent, again, both 15 and 100 are divisible by 5, resulting in a fraction of $\frac{3}{20}$.

Changing a Percentage to a Decimal

To convert a percentage to a decimal, eliminate the percent sign and place a decimal point two places to the left. If the percentage is only one digit, place a 0 in front of it and place the decimal point in front of the 0. For example:

76 percent would be 0.76
4 percent would be 0.04
104 percent would be 1.04

Exercise 2.4

Complete the following conversions.

Fractions to percentages (round to one decimal place):

1. $\frac{5}{8}$

2. $\frac{3}{5}$

3. $\frac{2}{4}$

4. $\frac{7}{12}$

5. $\frac{3}{15}$

Decimals to percentages (round to one decimal place):

6. 0.28

7. 0.07

8. 0.125

9. 0.429

10. 0.998

Percentages to fractions:

11. 42%

12. 58%

13. 78%

14. 75%

15. 20%

Percentages to decimals:

16. 12%

17. 27%

18. 0.5%

19. 7.5%

20. 3.4%

21. A family practitioner in your local physician's clinic saw 150 adults in one week for their annual physical examinations. 67 received the flu vaccine.

Express the rate of the flu vaccine administration in percent. Round to one decimal place.

22. The physician practice you work for needs a new paper shredder. They want a cross-cut shredder that can cut 20 sheets at a time. It must be strong enough to destroy staples and small paper clips with a waste bin of at least eight gallons. You did some investigation and secured five offers from different companies. The shredders are all of equal quality. Using the information here, which company is giving you the best deal?

	List Price	Discount	Cost of Two-Year Replacement Warranty	Shipping and Handling	TOTAL COST
Company A	$600.00	20%	$20.00	Free $00.00	
Company B	$625.00	30%	$25.00	$25.00	
Company C	$551.00	15%	$18.00	$33.00	
Company D	$584.00	25%	$25.00	$30.00	
Company E	$579.00	20%	$20.00	Local $00.00	

Exercise 2.5

Using the information found in the scenario below, complete the following tables.

Forty patients were seen in the Hematology/Oncology Clinic last Tuesday. Twenty patients had sickle-cell anemia, twelve patients had hemophilia, six patients had Ewing's sarcoma, and two patients had Wilms's tumor.
   Express in fractions, decimals (round to two places), and percentages the number of patients with each condition compared with the number of patients who visited the clinic last Tuesday. Remember to convert each fraction to its simplest form.

Sickle-Cell	Hemophilia	Ewing's Sarcoma	Wilms's Tumor

	Fraction	Decimal	Percentage
Sickle cell			
Hemophilia			
Ewing's			
Wilms's			

Ratio

A **ratio** expresses the relationship of one quantity to another. It is a mathematical parameter used to relate the number of cases, diseases, patients, or outcomes in the healthcare environment to the size of the source population in which they occur.

Calculating Ratio

To calculate a ratio, one quantity is divided by another. The number can be greater than 1 or less than 1. For example, if seven men and five women were in a group, the ratio of men to women would be $\frac{7}{5}$. This ratio also may be written as 7:5 and verbalized as 7 to 5. The numbers 7 and 5 have no common factors, so this ratio cannot be simplified. However, if the group consisted of 6 men and 10 women, for example, the ratio would be 6:10. Because the numbers in this ratio have a common factor of 2, the ratio can be simplified by dividing each number by 2, which simplifies the ratio to 3:5. Simplification is done in the same manner as in the section on fractions. This is converted by dividing both the top and bottom numbers by a common factor. In this example, both numbers can be divided by 2.

$$\text{Ratio} = \frac{x}{y} = \frac{6}{10} = \frac{\dfrac{6}{2} = 3}{\dfrac{10}{2} = 5}$$

or

$$\text{Ratio} = \frac{y}{x} = \frac{10}{6} = \frac{\dfrac{10}{2} = 5}{\dfrac{6}{2} = 3}$$

Exercise 2.6

Express the following ratios in their simplest form.

1. $8:96$

2. $3:15$

3. $8:16$

4. $12:72$

5. $5:7$

6. A group of 15 men and 20 women have diabetes. Express the ratio of men with diabetes to women with diabetes. Calculate it to its simplest form.

7. Your college bookstore reported that of the 1,000 books sold during enrollment, 320 were health information management (HIM) books. Express the ratio of HIM books to the total number of books sold. Calculate to its simplest form.

8. There are 12 instructors in your HIM program. Five of these are male instructors, the rest are female. Express the ratio of male instructors to female instructors. Calculate it to its simplest form.

9. Of the 12 instructors in the previous example, three have a master's degree and the rest have a bachelor's degree. Express the ratio of bachelor's degree prepared instructors to master's degree prepared instructors. Calculate to its simplest form.

10. Community Hospital reported sixteen births this past month. Four were male. What is the ratio of male births to female births? Calculate to its simplest form.

Proportion

A **proportion** is a type of ratio in which x is a portion of the whole $(x + y)$. In a proportion, the numerator is always included in the denominator. For example, if two women out of a group of 10 over the age of 50 have had breast cancer, where $x = 2$ (women who have had breast cancer) and $y = 8$ (women who have not had breast cancer), the calculation would be 2 divided by 10. The proportion of women who have had breast cancer is 0.2.

$$\frac{x}{(x + y)} = \frac{2}{(2 + 8)} = 0.2$$

Exercise 2.7

1. A school district wants to know the proportion of students who have deferrals for mandated vaccines. District School #1 has 237 students. Of the 237 students, 225 students are up to date on their vaccines. There are 12 students with deferrals. What is the proportion of students with deferrals who have not been vaccinated? Round to two decimal places.

2. At Community Clinic, 50 patients were seen in one day. Of those, six have Type II diabetes mellitus. What is the proportion of people in the group that have diabetes? Express as a decimal and round to two decimal places.

3. At Community Clinic, Dr. Clark treats only diabetic patients. He has 650 active patients. Of those, 458 have attended his specialized training session for newly diagnosed diabetes. What proportion of Dr. Clark's patients have undergone his training? Express as a decimal and round to two decimal places.

4. At Community Clinic, Dr. Simpson, an interventional cardiologist, saw 270 patients last quarter. Of those, he performed stent procedures on 182 patients. What is the proportion of Dr. Simpson's patients who have had stent procedures? Express as a decimal and round to two decimal places.

5. Dr. Rutan, an internist at Community Clinic, asked that 14 of the 35 patients he saw last week get their x-rays and lab work completed the day before their appointments. What is the proportion of Dr. Rutan's patients who had preliminary work completed prior to their appointments? Express as a decimal and round to two decimal places.

Rate

A **rate** is a ratio in which there is a distinct relationship between the numerator and denominator and the denominator often implies a large base population. A measure of time is often an intrinsic part of the denominator. Healthcare facilities calculate many types of rates in order to determine how the facilities are performing.

> **Tip:** Misplaced decimal points can result in mathematical errors. All calculations should be checked for sensible answers. For example, a hospital death rate of 25 percent should seem unreasonable because it indicates that one of every four patients treated at this hospital died. Why would anyone want to be treated at a hospital that had a 25 percent death rate? Thus, the decimal placement in this calculation should be checked. The correct death rate for this hospital may be 2.5 percent or 0.25 percent, which would be more realistic.

The term *rate* is often used loosely to refer to rate, proportion, percentage, and ratio. Indeed, many books and organizations use these terms interchangeably. For this reason, it is important to be aware of how any measure being reported has actually been defined and calculated.

Calculating Rate

The basic rule of thumb for calculating rate is to indicate the number of times something *actually* happened in relation to the number of times it *could have* happened (actual/potential). For example, let's say you have been eating out often in the past few weeks. To calculate the rate of meals you have eaten out in one week, divide the number of meals that you ate out (for example, 13) by the number of meals you could have eaten out (21). The rate is $\frac{13}{21}$, or 61.9 percent. The formula for determining rate is as follows:

$$Rate = \frac{Part}{Base}, \text{ or } R = \frac{P}{B}$$

Figure 2.2 shows the equations for calculating ratio, proportion, percentage, and rate.

Table 2.1 shows a sample computerized statistical report provided by the information systems (IS) department of an acute-care facility and illustrates how the department uses percentages.

> **Tip:** Everyone has heard this saying about computers: "garbage in, garbage out," or "GIGO." Computers are great for many things, including performing statistical calculations, but they must be programmed accurately to calculate correctly. Even the function of rounding needs to be validated. For example, it is not unheard of for an IS manager to ask a HIM professional for the formula for the death rate because the computer system crashed and all new formulas and specifications had to be reprogrammed.

Figure 2.2.   Review of equations for calculating ratio, proportion, percentage, and rate

The following list of equation differentiates among ratio, proportion, percentage, and rate, where $x = 5$ men and $y = 3$ women.

Ratio: $\dfrac{x}{y} = \dfrac{5}{3}$

Proportion: $\dfrac{x}{(x+y)} = \dfrac{5}{(5+3)}$

Percentage: $\left[\dfrac{x}{(x+y)}\right] \times 100 = \left[\dfrac{5}{(5+3)}\right] \times 100$

Rate: $R = \dfrac{Part}{Base}, \text{ or } R = \dfrac{P}{B}$

Table 2.1. Administrator's semiannual reference report

Administrator's Semiannual Reference Report Admissions by Day of Week 7/1/20XX–12/31/20XX		
Day	**Number of Patients**	**Percent of Patients**
Sunday	1,283	18.7
Monday	577	8.4
Tuesday	1,126	16.4
Wednesday	1,301	18.9
Thursday	1,240	18.0
Friday	702	10.2
Saturday	645	9.4
Total	**6,874**	**100.0**

Averages

An **average** is the value obtained by dividing the sum of a set of numbers by the number of values. Average is generally referred to as the arithmetic mean to distinguish it from the mode or median. (This is covered in more detail in chapter 10.)

The symbol $\overline{X}$ (pronounced "ex bar") is used to represent the mean in this formula.

$$\frac{Sum\ of\ all\ the\ values}{Number\ of\ all\ the\ values\ involved} = \overline{X}$$

Example: Let's say that you have taken six medical terminology tests. Your scores are 82, 78, 94, 56, 91, and 85. Adding together the scores gives you a total score of 486. Now, divide this by 6 (the number of tests you have taken). This equals 81. This means that your average score on the medical terminology tests is 81.

Exercise 2.8

1. Community Hospital reported the following birth weights for babies born January 30, 20XX: 6.9 lbs, 3.7 lbs, 7.7 lbs, 6.6 lbs, 7.3 lbs, 5.5 lbs, 9.9 lbs, 7.0 lbs, 5.5 lbs, and 7.7 lbs. What was the average birth weight for the day? Round to two decimal places.

2. A patient's temperature for five days after surgery taken at 7:00 a.m. each morning was recorded as 101.7, 100.4, 98.9, 100.2, and 98.6. What was the patient's average temperature after surgery? Round to two decimal places.

3. A patient's blood sugar was recorded for seven days at 8:00 a.m. and recorded as the following: 164, 155, 172, 145, 138, 136, and 142. What was the patient's average blood sugar at 8:00 a.m.? Round to a whole number.

4. A patient's systolic blood pressure was recorded from February 1 through February 7 at 6:30 a.m. each morning as the following:

February 1	130
February 2	135
February 3	132
February 4	126
February 5	120
February 6	122
February 7	124

What was the patient's average systolic blood pressure at 6:30 a.m.? Round to a whole number.

5. There are five health record analysts in the HIM department where you are working. Their salaries are: $13.87, $14.02, $15.56, $15.75, and $16.32. What is the average salary for the health record analysts? Round to two decimal places.

Chapter 2   Matching Quiz

Match the definitions with the term.

Definitions:

a. One or more parts of a whole

b. The part of a fraction that is above the line and signifies the number of parts of the denominator taken

c. Any of the set of nonnegative integers

d. A measure used to compare an event over time; a comparison of the number of times an event did happen (numerator) with the number of times an event could have happened (denominator)

e. The relation of one part to another or to the whole with respect to magnitude, quantity, or degree

f. The value obtained by dividing the sum of a set of numbers by the number of values

g. The part of a fraction below the line signifying division that functions as the divisor of the numerator and, in fractions with 1 as the numerator, indicates into how many parts the unit is divided

h. The number resulting from the division of one number by another

i. Numbered or proceeding by tens; based on the number 10; expressed in or utilizing a decimal system, especially with a decimal point

j. The process of approximating a number

Terms:

1. _____ Numerator   6. _____ Whole number
2. _____ Rate   7. _____ Proportion
3. _____ Fraction   8. _____ Decimal
4. _____ Average   9. _____ Rounding
5. _____ Denominator   10. _____ Quotient

Chapter 2   Review

Complete the following exercises.

1. Convert the fraction $\frac{1}{5}$ to a quotient and then a percentage.
2. Round the following percentages to two decimal places.
    a. 16.981%
    b. 13.655%
    c. 0.569%
    d. 98.990%
    e. 98.999%

    Round the following percentages to one decimal place.
    f. 0.698%
    g. 53.123%
    h. 0.075%
    i. 34.337%
    j. 3.876%

3. Convert the following:
    a. Convert $\frac{1}{6}$ to a percentage with two decimal places.
    b. Convert 0.65 to a percentage with two decimal places.
    c. Convert 34% to a fraction. Calculate to its simplest form.
    d. Convert 34% to a decimal.

4. Convert the following fractions to their simplest form:

    a. $\dfrac{3}{9}$

    b. $\dfrac{4}{8}$

    c. $\dfrac{1}{5}$

d. $\dfrac{3}{5}$

e. $\dfrac{124}{248}$

5. Review the following table to verify that the calculations are correct. If any are incorrect, note which ones and provide the correct answers.

Community Hospital Administrator's Semiannual Reference Report Discharges by Day of Week January 1, 20XX to June 30, 20XX		
Day	**Number of Patients**	**Percent of Patients**
Sunday	1,187	19.1%
Monday	755	11.3%
Tuesday	1,085	16.3%
Wednesday	1,031	15.5%
Thursday	1,024	17.0%
Friday	808	12.1%
Saturday	773	11.6%
Totals	**6,663**	**100.0%**

6. A physician on your staff performed 44 cardiac catheterizations last month. 34 of those treated were male. What is the ratio of male patients to female patients who had cardiac catheterizations? What is the proportion? Round to one decimal point.

7. It was reported in your department meeting that over the past year your hospital decreased the number of employees by four percent. Last year there were 389 people employed; how many are employed this year? Round to a whole number.

8. Your manager needs to purchase a computer for the new receptionist in your department. The usual price is $1,100. The local supply company gives the facility a 13 percent reduction on all items they purchase. What price will your manager pay?

9. Your beginning salary as an analyst in the HIM department is $14.50 per hour. You are due to receive a 3.4 percent cost-of-living raise in your next paycheck. Your performance evaluation is coming up in one month, and you believe you should get an additional 5 percent increase based on your excellent performance. What should your hourly wage be after your next paycheck, and what do you anticipate it will be after your performance evaluation?

10. Last year, you purchased equipment in the HIM department for $14,250. You have been told that the equipment you bought has depreciated in value by 20 percent. What is the value of the equipment now?

11. You just scored 40 points out of a possible 50 on your health information test. What percentage of available points did you earn?

12. Last year, the number of hospitals in your state decreased from 320 to 240. What is the percentage of decrease?

13. Review the following table and determine the average birth weights and average age of mother. Calculate to one decimal place.

Community Hospital Births March 1 through March 31, 20XX			
Birth	Birth Weight in Pounds	Mother's No.	Mother's Age
1	5.6	1	18.5
2	6.7	2	19.3
3	5.9	3	15.5
4	6.0	4	34.2
5	3.9	5	25.6
6	9.2	6	29.7
7	10.3	7	24.8
8	11.3	8	26.6
9	6.9	9	17.3
10	7.1	10	26.5
11	5.9	11	24.7
12	5.7	12	23.2
13	5.2	13	21.4
14	6.9	14	22.9
15	10.2	15	31.5
Totals			

For the following questions, refer to the following Quarterly Coding Professional Accuracy Report.

14. Are the calculations of the percentage of records accurately coded for each month and the total for the quarter correct?

15. Coding professional D determined her accuracy rate for the quarter to be 95.9 percent. She would like you to recalculate her accuracy rate because she thinks it is incorrect in the report.

Community Hospital
Quarterly Coding Professional Accuracy Report
January–March 20XX

	January			February			March			Total		
	# Records	# Correct	% Correct	# Records	# Correct	% Correct	# Records	# Correct	% Correct	# Records	# Correct	% Correct
Coding professional A	560	504	90.0%	544	495	91.0%	270	243	90.0%	1,374	1,242	90.4%
Coding professional B	540	503	93.1%	523	491	93.9%	531	494	93.0%	1,594	1,488	93.4%
Coding professional C	500	440	88.0%	445	401	90.1%	493	435	88.2%	1,438	1,276	88.7%
Coding professional D	620	583	94.0%	588	570	96.9%	584	551	94.3%	1,792	1,704	95.1%
Coding professional E	480	408	85.0%	432	392	90.7%	465	397	85.4%	1,377	1,197	86.9%
Totals	**2,700**	**2,438**	**90.3%**	**2,532**	**2,349**	**92.8%**	**2,343**	**2,120**	**90.5%**	**7,575**	**6,907**	**91.2%**

CHAPTER 3

Patient Census

Learning Objectives

At the conclusion of this chapter, you should be able to

- Explain, differentiate, and apply the following terms: inpatient admission, inpatient census, hospitalization, complete master census, daily inpatient census, inpatient service day, total inpatient service days, and admission and discharge on the same day (A&D), leave of absence and leave of absence day, recapitulation
- Distinguish between an interhospital (interfacility) transfer and an intrahospital transfer
- Compute daily census and inpatient service days using the admission and discharge data provided
- Calculate census and inpatient service days with data given for newborns and transfers
- Determine the average daily inpatient census for a patient care unit given inpatient service days for any such unit
- Utilize software to complete spreadsheets

Key Terms

Average daily inpatient census	Daily inpatient census	Leave of absence
Calculation of inpatient service days	Hospitalization	Patient care unit (PCU)
	Inpatient admission	Patient day
Calculation of transfers	Inpatient census	Recapitulation
Census day	Inpatient service day	Total inpatient service days
Complete master census	Intrahospital transfer	

Hospitals keep track of patient census statistics to determine when they have the largest number of patients and when that number drops. They can then tell when the busiest times of the year are in order to increase staffing, whether there are any patient care units being overburdened by large number of patients, and which units have a decrease in patients. Resources allocated to those units may change throughout the year to accommodate the units with more patients. Policies regarding low census may be enforced when needed and staff may be asked to take time off. Hospital administration will also review the census by individual physicians because they are interested knowing if any of the members of their medical staff are not admitting their patients to the facility, and if so, the reasons for that.

Inpatient Census

Hospital management uses census data for various purposes, including planning, budgeting, and staffing. The **inpatient census** indicates the number of patients present in the healthcare facility at a particular point in time. Hospitals include only inpatients in their calculations. A patient's hospitalization refers to the period of time in an individual's life when he or she is a patient in a single hospital without interruption except by possible intervening leaves of absence.

A staff member, usually a member of the nursing staff, on each **patient care unit (PCU)** is designated to count the patients on that unit each day. A PCU is an organizational entity of a healthcare facility organized both physically and functionally to provide care. For example, the intensive care unit (ICU) would be considered a PCU. In some small facilities, PCUs may be designated by location, such as 2-West or 3-North.

The inpatient census-taking time is usually at midnight but may occur at any time as long as the time is consistent for the entire facility; that is, each PCU conducts the census at the same time. Around midnight is actually a good time to take the census because patients are usually in their beds. It would be difficult to account for all patients at 8:00 a.m., for example, because they might be in an exam room, with radiology, in surgery, with their healthcare provider, or just taking a walk in the hospital.

In a manual system, the census taker fills out a form to be sent to a central collection area (usually the nursing office, information systems, admissions, health information department, or any other office designated by the administration). The names of patients admitted, discharged, and transferred to or from a PCU appear on the form. This makes it easier for the central collection area to discover any discrepancies in the data from the PCUs and to know where each patient is located at all times.

In a computerized system, the necessary data are first entered into the computer as admissions, discharges, or transfers and then verified at the designated time by the responsible person on each PCU.

> **Tip:** A PCU is an organizational entity of a healthcare facility such as a medicine unit, surgery unit, or special unit such as the ICU or cardiac care unit (CCU). This should not be confused with medical services, which refer to the activities relating to medical care performed by physicians, nurses, and other healthcare professionals and technical personnel under the direction of a physician.

Figure 3.1 shows a form for a manual daily census summary for a nursing home.

Complete Master Census

In addition to reporting the head count to the central collection area, each PCU reports, in written form or via computer, the number of patients admitted, discharged, and transferred in or out that day. This is commonly referred to as the ADT system in a facility. The central

Figure 3.1.   Daily census summary at Community Manor Nursing Home

To be completed daily at 12:01 a.m. by charge nurse			Community Manor Nursing Home Daily Census Summary	
Hall: ____A ____B ____C ____D			**Date** _____	
Initial admits—New residents			Date	Time
				a.m.–p.m.
				a.m.–p.m.
				a.m.–p.m.
				a.m.–p.m.
Discharged to home or transfer			Date	Time
				a.m.–p.m.
				a.m.–p.m.
				a.m.–p.m.
Transfer to hospital	Location		Date	Time
				a.m.–p.m.
				a.m.–p.m.
				a.m.–p.m.
				a.m.–p.m.
Out on leave—Pass	Date Left	Time	Returned	Time
		a.m.–p.m.		a.m.–p.m.
		a.m.–p.m.		a.m.–p.m.
		a.m.–p.m.		a.m.–p.m.
Deceased			Date	Time of Death
				a.m.–p.m.
				a.m.–p.m.
				a.m.–p.m.
Return from hospital stay			Date	Time
				a.m.–p.m.
				a.m.–p.m.
				a.m.–p.m.
				a.m.–p.m.

Charge nurse: _____

collection area then uses the census from all the units to compile a total census for the facility, sometimes referred to as the **complete master census**. The complete master census shows the names of patients present at a particular point in time and their location. In most facilities this is a computerized process that is linked with the facility's master patient index, billing system, and other electronic health record systems.

> **Tip:** In this book, the term *transfer* in a hospital setting refers to an intrahospital transfer. **Intrahospital transfers** are patients who are moved from one PCU to another within the facility. The transfers in and transfers out on an individual PCU may not be equal because it is possible to transfer more patients in than transfer out and vice versa. However, the total intrahospital transfers in must always equal the intrahospital transfers out.

Exercise 3.1

Answer the following questions.

1. A PCU has a count of 20 patients at 1 a.m. on September 1 and 30 patients at the same time on September 2. Could the counts have been different if the PCU had taken a census at 12:01 a.m. on both days?

2. Would you accept the different PCUs in the hospital taking censuses at different times as long as each unit is consistent within itself?

3. A patient transferred at 5 p.m. to unit A from unit B is counted in unit A's 12:01 a.m. census as one additional patient present. Would that patient still be included in unit B's 12:01 a.m. census?

4. What term is used to describe a patient who is transferred from one PCU to another within the same facility?

5. On July 1, your community hospital has 124 patients who are staying overnight in their facility. In addition, 231 patients have come in to the hospital for various tests and treatments. Which of these patients would be included in the inpatient census count, the 124 patients, the 231 patients, or the 355 patients?

Daily Inpatient Census

The **daily inpatient census** includes the number of inpatients present at the census-taking time each day *and* any inpatients who were both admitted after the previous census-taking time and discharged before the next census-taking time. Thus, a patient admitted to the hospital at 8 a.m. on June 1 and discharged at 10 p.m. that same day would not be present for the midnight head count. Therefore, he or she would not appear on the census report. However, the patient must be accounted for separately in some manner. For example, 20 patients are on a particular PCU. One patient was admitted at 10:00 a.m. and discharged at 7:00 p.m. If there are no other discharges, the daily inpatient census for this day is 21. You add the patient who was admitted and discharged to the 20 patients already on the unit.

Exercise 3.2

Answer the following questions.

1. The census at 12:01 a.m. on June 1 is 110. Three patients were admitted on June 1 at 6:00 a.m. and discharged later that same day. One patient admitted at 6:00 a.m. died at 5:30 p.m. the same afternoon. What is the PCU's daily inpatient census for June 1?

2. Which would be the better form of data to keep permanently, census or daily inpatient census? Why?

3. Community Hospital's census at 12:01 a.m. on September 19 was 327. On that day, 12 patients were admitted and 10 patients were discharged. Calculate the inpatient census for September 19.

4. Community Hospital's CCU census at 12:01 a.m. on December 2 was 14. Four patients were admitted to the CCU on December 2, one patient was discharged to the medicine unit, and one patient died. Calculate the inpatient census for the CCU for December 2.

5. The census in the telemetry unit at Community Hospital on May 1 was 26 patients. Two patients were admitted after stent insertions and three patients were transferred into the unit from the ICU. On the same day, four patients were discharged and one patient was transferred to ICU. One patient was admitted at 7:00 p.m. and was transferred at 9:00 p.m. to another facility. What will the daily inpatient census be for May 1?

Inpatient Service Days

An **inpatient service day** is a unit of measure denoting the services received by one inpatient in one 24-hour period. The 24-hour period is the time between the census-taking hours on two successive days. The usual 24-hour reporting period begins at 12:01 a.m. and ends at midnight. One inpatient service day is counted for each **inpatient admission** when a patient is admitted and discharged on the same day. If this is not done, credit for the services given to that patient is lost.

There are a number of important issues concerning inpatient service days. These include:

- One unit of one service day is not usually divided or reported as a fraction of a day.

- The day of admission is counted as an inpatient service day, but the day of discharge is not.

- The days a patient does not occupy a bed due to leave of absence are excluded because he or she is not present at the census-taking hour. A **leave of absence** day is a day occurring after the admission and prior to the discharge of a hospital inpatient when the patient is not present at the census-taking hour because he or she is on an authorized leave of absence from the healthcare facility. An absence of less than one day is not considered a leave of absence in compiling statistics. A leave of absence is not common in short-term acute care hospitals because lengths of stay are usually short. However, long-term care facilities such as nursing homes, mental health facilities, drug and alcohol abuse and rehabilitation facilities, or facilities for the developmentally disabled may still use them for special reasons such as a special holiday or outing for the patient or a group of patients, a family wedding, a funeral, or if the physician is trying to determine how well a patient would fare outside the facility. Leave of absence days are always written as a physician order. When the patient or the physician believes the advantages of an absence from the facility outweigh the advantages of uninterrupted **hospitalization**, the hospital has the choice of discharging and then readmitting the patient or granting a leave of absence.

Inpatient service day is the correct term to use for what is commonly referred to as a **patient day**, inpatient day, bed occupancy day, or **census day**. The operative word here is service, that is, the number of patients who received service on a particular day. The correct wording reflects the hospital function of providing services to patients each day. If 20 patients are provided services in one 24-hour period, the number of inpatient service days for that calendar day is 20.

Exercise 3.3

Differentiate among census, inpatient census, daily inpatient census, and inpatient service days. Will the figure representing an inpatient service day for any one day be the same as a daily inpatient census or inpatient census?

Total Inpatient Service Days

The term **total inpatient service days** refers to the sum of all the inpatient service days for each of the days during a specified period of time. For example, if the inpatient service days for June 1, 2, and 3 are 100, 105, and 101, the total for the three days is 306. Typically, total inpatient service days are calculated monthly, quarterly, semiannually, or annually.

Exercise 3.4

Given the following inpatient service days for Community Hospital, a 75-bed facility, what is the total number of inpatient service days provided in June?

Date June	Inpatient Service Days	Date June	Inpatient Service Days	Date June	Inpatient Service Days
1	70	11	68	21	68
2	71	12	67	22	71
3	72	13	65	23	70
4	68	14	69	24	73
5	69	15	70	25	70
6	71	16	72	26	69
7	73	17	73	27	67
8	74	18	75	28	65
9	69	19	70	29	69
10	70	20	69	30	72

Exercise 3.5

Complete the following exercises.

1. The time for taking the inpatient census must always be _____.
   a. Variable
   b. Consistent
   c. 12:00 p.m.
   d. 11:59 a.m.

2. Patient day or inpatient day is more correctly termed _____.
   a. Inpatient service day
   b. Daily inpatient census
   c. Total inpatient service day(s)
   d. Census

3. The inpatient census at 12:01 a.m. is 24. Two patients were admitted at 1 p.m. One patient died at 3:15 p.m., and the other patient was discharged at 10:00 p.m. The inpatient service days for that day are _____.
   a. 22
   b. 24
   c. 25
   d. 26

4. The difference between the census and the daily inpatient census is that any patients admitted and discharged the same day are added to _____.
   a. The census to compute the daily inpatient census
   b. The 12:01 a.m. (or other designated time) head count to compute the daily census
   c. Both a and b
   d. Neither a nor b

5. Which of the following should be used when calculating the number of inpatients who received service on a particular day?
   a. The inpatient census
   b. The daily inpatient census
   c. Total inpatient service days
   d. Census

Calculation of Inpatient Service Days

The **calculation of inpatient service days** is the measurement of services received by all inpatients in one 24-hour period (the time between the census-taking hours on two successive days). The usual reporting period begins at 12:01 a.m. and ends at 12:00 a.m. (midnight). Moreover, one inpatient day must be counted for each inpatient admitted and discharged on the same day between two successive census-taking hours.

Example: The definitions of census, inpatient service day, and total inpatient service days provide clues for actual computation. The sample shown in table 3.1 includes all of a hospital's inpatient care units. A summary of all such units helps the administration review the hospital's overall level of activity.

> **Tip:** Sometimes you may be asked by the administration to exclude PCUs such as ICUs and obstetrical units from the inpatient service days. Units such as these are often studied separately because the intensity of service on these units varies greatly from the intensity of services provided on medical and surgical units. Moreover, hospital administration may want information regarding usage on these units in order to determine equipment and staffing needs. Hospitals may use inpatient service days to track trends from month to month or year to date.

Table 3.2 shows a sample of how hospital administration can use inpatient service days data to determine performance.

Table 3.1. Sample inpatient service days display

Sample Inpatient Service Days	
Number of patients in hospital at 12:01 a.m. on November 1	257
Plus the number of patients admitted on November 1	+ 45
Subtotal	302
Minus the number of patients discharged (including deaths) on November 1	− 24
Number of patients in hospital at 11:59 p.m. on November 1 (subtotal)	278
Plus the number of patients both admitted and discharged on November 1	+ 4
Total inpatient service days for November 1	282

Table 3.2. Year-to-date inpatient service days

Community Medical Center September 20XX Year-to-Date Inpatient Service Days			
Service	**Actual**	**Budget**	**Prior Year**
Medicine	13,762	15,000	15,608
Surgery	8,953	13,500	11,634
ICU	3,874	3,500	3,623
Step-down	679	1,500	1,278
Rehabilitation	1,646	2,500	2,136
Obstetrics	1,730	2,200	2,188
Psychiatry	1,002	1,800	872
Newborn	1,689	1,800	2,099
Neonatal ICU	2,875	3,900	2,643
Pediatrics	645	1,000	833
Total	**36,855**	**46,700**	**42,914**

This medical center's analysis of its inpatient service days can be examined to determine how well the facility is doing year to date and to compare its performance with the previous year. This can lead to discussions by administration concerning marketing of their services or examination of whether there are enough practitioners in those services that may not be doing as well as in the previous year.

Before beginning the actual calculation of census data and inpatient service days, it is important to understand the term **calculation of transfers**. The calculation of transfers occurs on the PCU census. Transfers in and out of the unit are shown as subdivisions of patients admitted to and discharged from the unit.

Example: Following are some sample figures listed in a format frequently used by the central collection area.

Note: A/D indicates admitted and discharged the same day; adm, admissions; bir, births; dis, discharges; inpt, inpatients; NB, newborns; A/C, adults and children; serv, service; and trf, transfer.

A head count at 12:01 a.m. on June 1 shows 48 adult and children inpatients and two newborns. Using this starting point, add the number of admissions (2) and transfers in (1) to the number of adult and children inpatients (48) to arrive at a total of 51.

	↓		+		+	↓										
	12:01 a.m. Census		Adm		Trf	Total		Dis	Dis	Trf	**11:59 p.m.** Census			Serv Days	
Day	A/C	NB	A/C	Bir	in	A/C	NB	A/C	NB	out	A/C	NB	A/D	A/C	NB
6/1	**48**	2	**2**	1	**1**	**51**	3	1	2	1	49	1	1	50	1

Add the births (1) to the newborns present at 12:01 a.m. to arrive at a total of three.

		↓		+			↓									
	12:01 a.m. Census		Adm		Trf	Total		Dis	Dis	Trf	**11:59 p.m.** Census			Serv Days	
Day	A/C	NB	A/C	Bir	in	A/C	NB	A/C	NB	out	A/C	NB	A/D	A/C	NB
6/1	48	**2**	2	**1**	1	51	**3**	1	2	1	49	1	1	50	1

Subtract the discharges A/C (1) and the transfers out A/C (1) from the number of adults and children (51) for an 11:59 p.m. census of 49.

						↓		–		–	↓					
	12:01 a.m. Census		Adm		Trf	Total		Dis	Dis	Trf	**11:59 p.m.** Census			Serv Days	
Day	A/C	NB	A/C	Bir	in	A/C	NB	A/C	NB	out	A/C	NB	A/D	A/C	NB
6/1	48	2	2	1	1	**51**	3	**1**	2	**1**	**49**	1	1	50	1

Finally, subtract the newborns that were discharged (2) from the total number of newborns (3) for an 11:59 p.m. census of 1.

						↓			—			↓				
	12:01 a.m. Census		Adm		Trf	Total		Dis	Dis	Trf	**11:59 p.m.** Census			Serv Days	
Day	A/C	NB	A/C	Bir	in	A/C	NB	A/C	NB	out	A/C	NB	A/D	A/C	NB
6/1	48	2	2	1	1	51	**3**	1	**2**	1	49	**1**	1	50	1

The last three columns are discussed later in this chapter.

The following points should resolve any confusion:

- The terms *transfers in* and *transfers out* refer to intrahospital transfers, that is, transfers within the hospital. Transfers in and out of the hospital (called interhospital or interfacility transfers) are included in admissions and discharges. It is common for healthcare providers to use the term *transfer,* as in "The patient was transferred to the nursing home." However, this is really a discharge from the hospital and an admission to the nursing home.

- Transfers in and out of any specific medical care unit may or may not be equal, but they must be equal for the overall hospital **recapitulation.** Every patient transferred into a unit on any given day has to have been transferred out of another unit. Failure of these data to balance may mean that a unit neglected to report transfers correctly. It is essential that someone in the central collection area identify the source of error.

- The data of 49 adults and children and one newborn (the inpatient census at 11:59 p.m. on June 1) must be the same as the actual head count. If they are not the same, a unit may have reported admissions, discharges, or births incorrectly. Again, someone in the central collection area is responsible for finding the error.

- Newborns are considered separately for all computations based on census data. They should be reported separately unless otherwise directed by administration, medical staff, or other persons using the statistical data produced. Births are considered newborn admissions. As mentioned earlier, services provided to newborns differ in intensity from those provided to the rest of the hospital inpatients.

- The census at the close of one day (11:59 p.m.) is the inpatient census at the beginning of the next day and is commonly referred to as the number of patients remaining. This may be a good time to discuss the terminology used in inpatient settings. The hospital may be referred to as the "house," as in "How many patients are in the house?" This refers to the number of patients in the hospital.

Patients Admitted and Discharged on the Same Day

Going back to the last three columns from the previous problem, the number of patients who were admitted and discharged on the same day (A/D) must be added to the 11:59 p.m. census to show that they received services. These are the inpatient service days. As discussed previously, patients who are not present at either of two successive head-counting times still must be accounted for and credited with a day's care. (A patient admitted and discharged on the same day may be referred to as in and out [I&O] or admission/discharge [A&D] or any number of other terms or abbreviations.)

To compute inpatient service days, add the number of patients admitted and discharged on the same day (A/D) to the 11:59 p.m. census data. Note the 50 and 1 in the last two columns for June 1.

Tip: The census for the next day must begin with the 11:59 p.m. census data and not inpatient service days. Calculate under the assumption that the patients admitted and discharged on the same day and the transfers are not newborns.

Recapitulation of Census Data

The process of verifying the data obtained by the process described previously is called the monthly or yearly recapitulation of census data, meaning a concise summary of the data. The total number of patients admitted and born during the month or year is added to the patients-remaining census with which the month or year began. From this sum, the number of discharges (including deaths) during the month or year is subtracted. The resulting data are the number of patients remaining at the end of the month or year. This number should equal the actual head count at 11:59 p.m. the last night of that month or year. Hospital staff often abbreviate this as "recap." Table 3.3 shows a sample monthly census recapitulation.

When you recap (or summarize) monthly (or annual) census data, you are verifying that the columns have been added correctly. This procedure also verifies that no error was made in the original data on one or more lines. This is accomplished by taking the 12:01 a.m. inpatient census at the beginning of the period, adding total admissions and transfers in, and subtracting total discharges and transfers out. The resultant data represent the ending census on the last day of the period (month or year).

Table 3.3. Sample monthly census recapitulation

Community Hospital		
	Adults and Children	**Newborns**
Number of patients in hospital at 12:01 a.m. on October 1	48	2
Add the number of patients admitted in October	+ 100	+ 7
Subtotal	148	9
Subtract the number of patients discharged (including deaths) in October	− 110	− 5
Number of patients in hospital at 11:59 p.m., October 31	38	4

Exercise 3.6

Complete the following exercises.

1. Using the data given in the example on page 39, calculate the census for June 2. Then fill in the blanks in the table below. Did the transfers in and transfers out balance?

	12:01 a.m. Census		Adm		Trf	Total		Dis	Dis	Trf	11:59 p.m. Census			Serv Days	
Day	A/C	NB	A/C	Bir	in	A/C	NB	A/C	NB	out	A/C	NB	A/D	A/C	NB
6/1	48	2	2	1	1	51	3	1	2	1	49	1			
6/2			3	1	2			4	1	2					

2. What data will you use to begin June 3, and why?

3. Fill in the blanks in the table below. What are the inpatient service days for June 2 and 3?

	12:01 a.m. Census		Adm		Trf	Total		Dis	Dis	Trf	11:59 p.m. Census			Serv Days	
Day	A/C	NB	A/C	Bir	in	A/C	NB	A/C	NB	out	A/C	NB	A/D	A/C	NB
6/1	48	2	2	1	1	51	3	1	2	1	49	1	1	50	1
6/2	49	1	3	1	2	54	2	4	1	2	48	1	1		
6/3			1	1	1			3	0	1			0		

4. Would a newborn ever be considered an A/D?

5. At this point, you have inpatient service days for three successive days. The total of these data, excluding newborns, for June 1, 2, and 3 is 145 (50 + 49 + 46). What will you need to know and do to get the hospital total inpatient service days for the entire month of June?

Exercise 3.7

Using the information supplied for June 1, fill in the blanks in the table below.

	12:01 a.m. Census		Adm		Trf	Total		Dis	Dis	Trf	11:59 p.m. Census			Serv Days	
Day	A/C	NB	A/C	Bir	in	A/C	NB	A/C	NB	out	A/C	NB	A/D	A/C	NB
6/1	230	12	20	4	3			19	3	2			1		
6/2			21	4	1			19	4	1			0		
6/3			23	6	0			24	5	0			3		
6/4			25	5	1			23	4	1			1		
6/5			24	4	2			18	3	2			2		

Exercise 3.8

Two hundred and fifty adults and children were in the hospital at 12:01 a.m. on August 1. There were 23 newborns at 12:01 a.m. on August 1. During August, the following data were compiled:

Admissions:	
Adults and children	1,353
Newborns	73
Discharges (including deaths):	
Adults and children	1,348
Newborns	65

1. What would the inpatient census for adults and children be on August 31 at 11:59 p.m.?

2. What would the inpatient census be for newborns on August 31?

3. Can the inpatient service days be computed with the information supplied in the previous question? Explain why or why not.

4. The surgery unit in Community Hospital has reported the following data. Do these data look correct? Explain your answer.

Day	12:01 a.m. Census	Adm	Trf in	Total	Dis	Trf out	11:59 p.m. Census	A/D	Serv Days
8/1	20	4	2	26	2	8	16	1	16

5. On March 1, the telemetry unit at Community Hospital has reported the 15 patients on the unit at 12:01 a.m. During March, the following data were collected:

Admissions	240
Discharges (including deaths)	232

What would the inpatient census be on March 31 at 11:59 p.m. in the telemetry unit?

Exercise 3.9

This exercise consists of two worksheets for calculating a month's inpatient census and inpatient service days. Using the data provided for May 1, complete the first worksheet. If your findings do not match the data for May 31, you have made an error either in your column additions or on one or more of the horizontal lines above the total. You must correct this error to ensure the validity of the monthly totals. If the column additions are correct, continue on to the second worksheet for the recap. This exercise could be placed on an electronic spreadsheet.

Worksheet 1

Day	12:01 a.m. Census A/C	12:01 a.m. Census NB	Adm A/C	Adm NB	Trf in	Total A/C	Total NB	Disch A/C	Disch NB	Trf out	11:59 p.m. Census A/C	11:59 p.m. Census NB	A/D	Serv Days A/C	Serv Days NB
1	165	3	29	0	8	194	3	10	0	7	185	3	0		
2	185	3	24	4	7			12	3	6			1		
3			18	3	3			16	2	2			0		
4			17	2	5			15	2	4			0		

(continued on next page)

Worksheet 1 (*continued*)

Day	12:01 a.m. Census A/C	NB	Adm A/C	NB	Trf in	Total A/C	NB	Disch A/C	NB	Trf out	11:59 p.m. Census A/C	NB	A/D	Serv Days A/C	NB
5			13	0	1			12	1	3			0		
6			20	0	6			19	2	4			0		
7			21	0	14			17	0	12			0		
8			27	1	10			23	3	8			3		
9			23	4	6			22	3	14			2		
10			22	2	8			15	1	10			1		
11			17	3	7			14	4	5			3		
12			19	3	6			17	2	4			0		
13			14	1	4			12	2	2			0		
14			15	4	5			19	3	7			0		
15			20	14	8			13	0	6			1		
16			23	3	6			15	4	2			0		
17			17	1	3			13	3	1			1		
18			15	0	2			21	1	6			2		
19			17	0	7			25	3	2			1		
20			13	2	3			27	4	4			0		
21			12	1	5			21	2	5			3		
22			10	0	1			17	4	1			2		
23			9	2	4			18	1	4			0		
24			23	4	3			12	3	2			2		
25			15	2	4			22	2	3			1		
26			13	3	2			9	1	4			0		
27			21	1	3			29	1	0			2		
28			29	2	5			22	4	4			3		
29			23	4	1			25	3	2			1		
30			15	1	4			21	2	3			0		
31			16	4	2			18	3	2			3		
Totals															

Worksheet 2

Recap of Monthly Data for Adults and Children: May 20XX (Enter numbers from worksheet 1.)		
12:01 a.m. Census A/C		165
Admissions Adult and Children	+	_____
Transfers in	+	_____
Total A/C	=	_____
Discharges Adult and Children	–	_____
Transfers out	–	_____
11:59 p.m. Census A/C on May 31	=	
Recap of Monthly Data for Newborns:		
12:01 a.m. Census NB		
Newborn Admissions	+	_____
Total NB	=	_____
Discharges NB	–	_____
11:59 p.m. Census NB on May 31	=	
Serv Days A/C (total inpatient service days excluding newborns) _____		
Serv Days NB (total newborn service days) _____		
Total inpatient service days _____		

Average Daily Inpatient Census

The **average daily inpatient census** is the average number of inpatients present in the hospital each day for a given period of time. The total inpatient service days for any period (usually a month or a year) represent the inpatient service days for all the calendar days in that period. The formula for calculating average daily inpatient census is:

$$\frac{Total\ inpatient\ service\ days\ for\ a\ period\ (excluding\ newborns)}{Total\ number\ of\ days\ in\ the\ period}$$

When calculating the average daily inpatient census for a month, you need to know how many days there are in each month. Remember the nursery rhyme?

Thirty days hath September, April, June, and November.
All the rest have thirty-one.
Excepting February alone,
Which has twenty-eight days clear,
But twenty-nine each Leap Year.

Example: In the second worksheet in exercise 3.9, the answer was 6,653 inpatient service days for adults and children and 155 inpatient service days for newborns for the month of May. According to the formula, the average daily inpatient census is computed by dividing 6,653 by 31 (number of days in May). The result, rounded to a whole number, is 215.

Tip: Because patient load can fluctuate, the administration is very interested in the hospital's average daily inpatient census. For example, many healthcare facilities in southern states experience a rise in average daily inpatient census during the winter months and a decrease during the summer months due to seasonal visitors. The average daily inpatient census is a measure of use and a reference for anticipated revenues.

As mentioned earlier, adults and children are calculated separately from newborns unless otherwise directed by the hospital's administration. Newborn census data can distort statistics related to resource use. For example, it costs less to maintain a newborn nursery than it does to staff other PCUs. If the average daily inpatient census is consistently low over a specified period, it may be appropriate to close PCUs to reduce expenses. In this example, the average daily newborn census is calculated by dividing 155 by 31. The result is 5.0 or 5.

Tip: Whether to round to a whole number is the individual hospital's decision. What is important is that the hospital act consistently. There is a difference between working with data representing people (because you cannot have a portion of a person) and working with percentages that represent numbers. Many facilities use a whole number when calculating the census and fractions with other healthcare statistics. (Refer to chapter 2 to review rounding.)

Example: A 150-bed hospital reports 3,489 inpatient service days for December. To compute the average daily inpatient census for December, divide 3,489 by 31 (number of days in December). The average daily inpatient census is 113 when rounded to a whole number. This means that, on average, 113 patients were in the facility during each day in December.

Again, this number is important to administration because they will want to know how many patients are being served each month in order to determine staffing and supply needs for practitioners and to monitor the overall financial performance of the facility.

Average Daily Newborn Census

The formula for calculating the average daily newborn census follows the same pattern as the formula for calculating the average daily inpatient census of adults and children.

$$\frac{\textit{Total newborn inpatient service days for a period}}{\textit{Total number of days in the period}}$$

Example: A hospital with 20 bassinets had 552 newborn inpatient service days during April. Divide the total number of newborn inpatient service days (552) by the number of days in the period (30 days in April) to obtain the average daily newborn census (18.4, or 18).

> **Tip:** When administrators and physicians ask for the average daily inpatient census, they may not always indicate to exclude newborns. Clarify the information by asking if newborns should be included or excluded from your computations.

Average Daily Inpatient Census for a Patient Care Unit

The hospital's administration often finds it helpful to know the average use of a specific medical care unit (for example, to know whether additional beds are needed for the ICU). Statistics are the basis for decision making. The formula for calculating the average daily inpatient census for a care unit is:

$$\frac{Total\ inpatient\ service\ days\ for\ the\ unit\ for\ the\ period}{Total\ number\ of\ days\ in\ the\ period}$$

Example: A hospital with a 24-bed CCU reports 740 inpatient service days for July. To compute the average daily inpatient census, divide 740 by 31 (number of days in July). The average daily inpatient census, rounded to a whole number, is 24. This indicates that the CCU is, on average, filled to capacity each day. Administration may want to consider this information closely to determine if additional beds and staffing may be needed. Table 3.4 lists the calculation of census statistics.

> **Tip:** Do not confuse the terms regarding the census and inpatient service days. Inpatient census refers to patients present at the census-taking time. Some healthcare facility staff may just say "census"—they are referring to the inpatient census. The average inpatient census is the mean number of hospital inpatients present in the hospital each day for a given period of time. The inpatient service days include any patients who were admitted and discharged on the same day.

Table 3.4 Calculation of census statistics

Indicator	Numerator	Denominator
Average daily inpatient census	Total number of inpatient service days for a given period	Total number of days for the same period
Average daily inpatient census for NBs	Total number of NB inpatient service days for a given period	Total number of days for the same period
Average daily inpatient census for a PCU	Total number of inpatient service days for a PCU for a given period	Total number of days for the same period

> **Tip:** Some of the exercises in this textbook cover leap years. A leap year is a year in which an extra day is added to the calendar at the end of February, giving February 29 days. Therefore, regular years have 365 days; leap years have 366. Leap years only occur on an even-numbered year, so if the example is an odd year, one not need consider a leap year as a possibility.

Exercise 3.10

Complete the following exercises.

1. Community Hospital has 200 beds and 25 newborn bassinets. The total inpatient service days for May was 5,297 for adults and children and 486 for newborns.
   a. What is the average daily inpatient census for adults and children? Round to a whole number.
   b. Determine the average daily newborn census. Round to a whole number.

2. A 150-bed, 15-bassinet hospital has 4,350 inpatient service days for adults and children and 360 newborn service days during June.
   a. What is the average daily inpatient census, excluding newborns? Round to a whole number.
   b. Determine the average daily newborn census. Round to a whole number.

3. Compute the average daily newborn census for a 125-bed, 10-bassinet hospital with 3,001 inpatient service days for adults and children and 298 inpatient service days for newborns during February (not a leap year). Round your answer to a whole number.

4. If you need to calculate the average daily inpatient census of the surgical unit, where can you obtain the surgical unit's inpatient service days?

5. Community Hospital's burn unit has twelve beds. The inpatient service days for December were 358. What is the average daily inpatient census for the burn unit during December? Round your answer to a whole number.

Chapter 3   Matching Quiz

Match the definition with the term.

Definitions:

a. The period during an individual's life when he or she is a patient in a single hospital without interruption except by possible intervening leaves of absence

b. The mean number of hospital inpatients present in the hospital each day for a given period of time

c. The number of inpatients present at census-taking time each day plus any inpatients who were both admitted and discharged after the census-taking time the previous day

d. The number of inpatients present in a healthcare facility at any given time

e. The authorized absence of an inpatient from a hospital or other facility for a specified period of time occurring after admission and prior to discharge

f. A change in medical care unit, medical staff unit, or responsible physician during hospitalization

g. An organizational entity of a healthcare facility organized both physically and functionally to provide care

h. A unit of measure equivalent to the services received by one inpatient during one 24-hour period

i. A concise summary of data

j. The sum of all inpatient services days for each of the days during a specified period of time

Terms:

1. _____ Inpatient census
2. _____ Leave of absence
3. _____ Recapitulation
4. _____ Daily inpatient census
5. _____ Intrahospital transfer

6. _____ Average daily inpatient census
7. _____ PCU
8. _____ Total inpatient services days
9. _____ Patient day
10. _____ Hospitalization

Chapter 3 Review

1. What is an intrahospital transfer?

2. Differentiate between the terms *inpatient census* and *daily inpatient census*.

3. Is it possible that the transfers into a PCU may not equal the transfers out of the same PCU on the same day?

4. When must transfers in and transfers out be equal?

5. At 11:59 p.m. on February 1, the Community Hospital census was 427. On February 2, 37 patients were admitted, 33 were discharged, and 2 were admitted and discharged that day. In their CCU the census on February 1 was 16. On February 2, six patients were admitted, four were discharged, and one was admitted and later that day died in the CCU. Answer the following questions and round the answers to whole numbers.

   a. Calculate the hospital inpatient census for February 2.

   b. Calculate the hospital daily inpatient census for February 2.

   c. Calculate the CCU inpatient census for February 2.

   d. Calculate the CCU inpatient service days for February 2.

6. In 20XX, a hospital had 175 beds for adults and children from January 1 through June 30. On July 1, the hospital increased its beds to 250 and the number remained at

250 through December 31. During the first six months, 30,875 patient days of service were provided to the hospital's adults and children. During the last six months, 36,982 days of service were provided. Answer the following questions and round the answers to whole numbers. This is a non-leap year.

a. What was the average daily inpatient census for the first six months: 169, 170, 171, or 172?

b. What was the average daily inpatient census for the entire year: 184, 185, 186, or 187?

c. The same hospital provided 12,345 newborn days of service in its 35-bassinet nursery during the year. What was the average daily newborn census: 31, 32, 33, or 34?

d. The same hospital's new surgery unit has 55 beds. During July, the unit provided 1,705 days of service. What was the average daily inpatient census for the surgery unit in July: 52, 53, 54, or 55?

e. Do you think the hospital's administration provided enough beds for the new surgery unit?

7. Using the statistics from the following monthly report from the nursing administration of Community Hospital, an acute care facility, calculate the current month's (November) average daily inpatient census for each nursing unit and the totals. Note that this facility's policy is to round to a whole number.

	Unit	Number of Beds	Inpatient Service Days	Average Daily Inpatient Census
	Community Hospital **Inpatient Statistical Report** **Average Daily Inpatient Census by Nursing Unit** **November 20XX**			
A	Medicine/Surgery	40	1,108	
B	Pediatrics	40	997	
C	Obstetrics	25	733	
D	Rehabilitation	15	400	
E	CCU	20	592	
F	Surgical ICU (SICU)	15	445	
G	Medicine ICU (MICU)	20	585	
Total Adult and Children		175		
I	Newborn Nursery	20	588	
J	Special Care Nursery	10	201	
K	Neonatal ICU (NICU)	10	285	
Total Nursery				

8. Community Hospital reported the following for the month of July, 20XX. Round your answers to whole numbers.

Community Hospital July, 20XX		
	Adults and Children	**Nursery**
Beginning census on July 1	92	6
Admissions	301	54
Discharges and Deaths	286	50
Inpatient Service Days	3,198	300

    a. Calculate the average daily inpatient census for adults and children.

    b. Calculate the average daily inpatient census for the nursery.

    c. What will the census for adults and children be at 11:59 p.m. on July 31?

    d. What will the nursery census be at 11:59 p.m. on July 31?

9. Metropolitan Hospital has a large, busy rehabilitation unit. The 30-bed unit reported the following inpatient service days for the week of April 6. Using the information listed here, what is the average daily inpatient census for the week of April 6 through April 12? Round to three digits after the decimal.

Metropolitan Hospital Rehabilitation Unit Inpatient Service Days April 6–April 12, 20XX	
Day	**Inpatient Service Days**
April 6	29
April 7	28
April 8	29
April 9	26
April 10	27
April 11	28
April 12	29

10. Children's Hospital reported the following statistics for March 20XX. Calculate the average daily inpatient census for each unit and the total. Round each calculation to a whole number.

Children's Hospital Inpatient Service Days March 20XX			
Unit	Number of Beds	Inpatient Service Days	Average Daily Inpatient Census
Pediatrics Surgical	30	833	
Hematology Oncology	20	566	
Neurology/Neurosurgical	30	756	
Renal/Gastroenterology/Endocrinology	20	555	
Respiratory	30	897	
Cardiac Medicine/Surgical	20	589	
Infant Care Unit	10	281	
Pediatric Intensive Care	20	540	
Total	**180**		

11. Community Hospital has 15 bassinets with 286 newborn inpatient service days during October. What is the average daily census for October? Round to a whole number.

12. The planning committee for Metropolitan Hospital is studying the activity of their burn unit which has 15 beds. During the third quarter of the year, (July, August, and September) there were 1,356 inpatient service days. What is the average daily census for this period? How could this information be important to the planning committee at Metropolitan Hospital? Round to a whole number.

13. University Hospital is a 765-bed facility with 250,415 inpatient service days for the past year. What was their average daily census for the period? Round to a whole number.

14. In February 20XX (a leap year) Children's Hospital reported that they had 500 inpatient service days in their neurosurgery unit. What was the average inpatient daily census? Round to a whole number.

15. Of the 500 inpatient service days in the above example, 386 were Dr. Smith's patients. What percentage of inpatient service days did Dr. Smith have in the neurosurgery unit? Round to one decimal place.

CHAPTER 4
Percentage of Occupancy

Learning Objectives

At the conclusion of this chapter, you should be able to

- Identify the beds that are included in a bed count
- Compute the bed occupancy percentage for any period given the data representing bed count and inpatient service days for adults and children and the occupancy percentage for newborn
- Differentiate and apply the direct and indirect bed turnover rate
- Calculate the percentage of occupancy for a period when there has been a change in the number of beds during that period

Key Terms

Bed capacity	Hospital newborn bassinet	Observation patient
Bed count	Inpatient bed count	Occupancy percent
Bed count day	Inpatient bed occupancy	Occupancy ratio
Bed occupancy ratio	rate	Percent of occupancy
Bed turnover rate	Newborn bassinet count	Percentage of occupancy
Certificate of need (CON)	Newborn bassinet count	Swing bed hospital
Hospital inpatient beds	day	Total bed count days

Typically, a healthcare facility is licensed by the state to operate with a specific number of beds. When a new facility wants to open its doors for patient care or when an existing hospital wants to add services or major medical equipment, it may need to apply to the state for a **certificate of need (CON)** to prove that patient care beds or equipment are needed in the area. CON programs are designed to contain healthcare facility costs and prevent the duplication of services and construction. Even though the federal mandate to require a CON has been repealed, 36 states, the District of Columbia, and Puerto Rico have maintained their CON program. States that have kept their CON programs are also responsible for reviewing the needs of outpatient and long-term care facilities and other free-standing facilities (NCSL 2015). Even the fourteen states that do not require a CON have some mechanisms to regulate costs and duplication of services. When granted a CON, the facility is licensed for the specific number of beds requested and is responsible for reporting its bed count.

Percentage of Occupancy

One of the indicators of a facility's financial well-being is the percentage of occupancy. From a facility's perspective, a high percentage of occupancy indicates a positive financial outlook. Conversely, a low percentage of occupancy can mean that the facility may need to work to attract more patients. Percentage of occupancy can also reveal the health of a community. For example, in winter months, a hospital that has a high percentage of occupancy may reflect that there are many cases of influenza or respiratory illnesses in the community.

Inpatient Bed Count

A **bed count**, also called an **inpatient bed count**, is the number of available hospital inpatient beds, both occupied and vacant, on any given day. Bed complement is a third term for bed count that may still be encountered although it is less common. The term **hospital inpatient beds** refers to accommodations for the patient, including supporting services such as food, laundry, and housekeeping for hospital inpatients. It excludes those for the newborn nursery but could include incubators and bassinets in nurseries for premature or sick newborn infants. In a hospital, the bed count includes those beds set up for normal use, whether or not they are occupied. A bed count may be reported for the entire hospital or for any of its units.

Bed capacity is used to denote the number of beds that a facility has been designed and constructed to house, rather than the actual number of beds set up and staffed for use. To avoid confusion, it is preferable to use bed count. Normally, when counting inpatient beds, only those in areas designed for such accommodations and set up, staffed, equipped, and in all respects ready for the care of inpatients are counted. This is an important consideration because regulatory agency surveyors often verify bed count and location against licensed beds and appropriate staffing levels. The bed count may be used in various reports, from those prepared for accrediting agencies to those for regulatory agencies. In a hospital, the number of available beds in the facility or a unit may remain constant for long periods of time. At times, however, the number can change. For example, a significant number of beds may be unavailable for use during a major remodeling or renovation project, but the number will increase after the project is completed. Another example occurs during a disaster, natural or otherwise. Regular beds may be occupied, so additional beds would be set up in alcoves, hallways, offices, or other areas that are not considered patient rooms. These beds do not become a part of the regular bed count, which can result in a percentage of occupancy over 100 percent. Some facilities refer to these as disaster beds. Other types of beds excluded from the bed count are those in treatment areas such as examining rooms, emergency services, physical therapy, labor rooms, and recovery rooms.

Labor Room Beds and Newborn Bassinets

An obstetrics patient may be admitted directly to a labor room bed instead of to a postpartum bed where she may spend the majority of her hospital stay. Labor room beds are not included in the bed count because they are used only temporarily before the patient delivers.

Newborn beds, called bassinets, are computed separately from the bed count. The **newborn bassinet count** is the number of available **hospital newborn bassinets**, both occupied and vacant, on any given day. A hospital newborn bassinet includes accommodations for the newborn plus supporting services such as food, laundry, and housekeeping for hospital newborn inpatients.

Emergency Services Department Beds

Emergency services department (ESD) beds are normally considered outpatient beds. In some instances, however, the hospital provides an observation bed in the ESD. If observation beds meet the qualifications of being set up, equipped, and staffed for inpatient use, they may be counted in the bed count depending on what the particular facility has decided and on state-licensing compliance.

A patient under observation, an **observation patient**, is one who presents with a medical condition that imposes a significant degree of instability and disability and who needs to be monitored, evaluated, and assessed to determine whether he or she should be admitted for inpatient care or discharged for care in another setting. A patient can occupy a special bed set aside for this purpose or a bed in any unit of the hospital (that is, the ESD, a medical unit, or obstetrics). Usually hospital administration decides on the terms to describe and classify outpatients who occupy hospital beds and information systems to track these patients.

Exercise 4.1

1. In the event of a disaster, extra beds may be set up to meet the immediate needs of the situation. Would these beds be part of the bed count? Explain your answer.

2. Compare and contrast the terms bed count, bed complement, and bed capacity.

Bed Count Days

A **bed count day** is a unit of measure denoting the presence of one inpatient bed, whether or not it is occupied, set up, and staffed for use in one 24-hour period. The term **total bed count days** refers to the sum of inpatient bed count days for each of the days during a specified period of time. Bed count days also may be referred to as the maximum number of patient days or potential days because they represent a statistical probability of every bed being occupied every day.

> **Example:** A hospital has an inpatient bed count of 100. During June, the bed count days would be 100 (number of beds) × 30 (the number of days in June) or 3,000. If every hospital bed were filled each day for a certain period (for example, a month), the inpatient bed occupancy rate would be 100 percent for that month. This is because each bed was occupied the maximum number of times it could have been occupied.

We can also use this for newborn bassinets. An inpatient bassinet count day is a unit of measure denoting the presence of one inpatient bassinet (either occupied or vacant) set up and staffed for use in one 24-hour period. The term total bassinet count days refers to the sum of inpatient bassinet count days for each of the days in the period under consideration.

> **Example:** A hospital has a bassinet count of 15. The bed count days in June would be 15 (number of bassinets) × 30 (the number of days in June) or 450.

All the rates in this text can be determined by remembering this general rule: A rate is the number of times something has happened compared with the number of times something could have happened. The equation is

$$Rate = \frac{Part}{Base}$$

or

$$\frac{The\ number\ of\ times\ something\ happened}{The\ number\ of\ times\ it\ could\ have\ happened}$$

The number of times "something happened" is expressed in terms of inpatient service days. The number of times "it could have happened" is expressed in terms of bed count days (bed count multiplied by the number of calendar days). Refer to chapter 2 for the discussion on rates.

> **Tip:** Rates are expressed with a % sign or "per population" factor. For example, 45.6% or 45 per 10,000, depending on the formulas.

Inpatient Bed Occupancy Ratio/Percentage

Occupancy percentages also are referred to as rates or ratios. The **bed occupancy ratio** is the proportion of beds occupied, defined as the ratio of inpatient service days to bed count days during a specified period of time. The inpatient service days are used to represent the actual occupancy (number of times something happened), and the bed count represents the possibility for occupancy (number of times it could have happened). The formula for determining bed occupancy ratio is:

$$\frac{Total\ inpatient\ service\ days\ in\ a\ period \times 100}{Total\ bed\ count\ days\ in\ the\ period\ (Bed\ count \times Number\ of\ days\ in\ the\ period)}$$

Synonymous terms for bed occupancy ratio are **percent of occupancy**, occupancy rate, **occupancy percent**, **inpatient bed occupancy rate**, and **occupancy ratio**. The ratio is usually expressed as a percent and can be computed for any specified day or as a daily average in any period of time.

> **Example:** On September 1, 207 inpatient service days were provided in a 225-bed hospital. Making the appropriate substitutions in the previously stated formula, the bed occupancy ratio for September 1 is calculated as follows:
>
> $$\frac{(207 \times 100)}{225} = \frac{20,700}{225} = 92.0\%$$

The bed occupancy ratio for September 1 is 92 percent. This simply means that on September 1, 92 percent of the beds were occupied.

Tip: You might prefer to compute a decimal fraction and then multiply by 100. Another option is to convert to a percentage by moving the decimal point two places to the right as

$$\frac{207}{225} = 0.92 = 0.92 \times 100 = 92.0\%$$

Another example of bed occupancy ratio for the period of a month by patient care unit is shown in table 4.1.

Example: The total bed occupancy ratio for October is 84.6% percent. Additionally, as the example shows, it is possible to compute the bed occupancy rate for individual patient care units (PCUs).

In another example, a hurricane hit a small coastal town on November 17, 20XX. The local hospital is licensed for 70 beds. All 70 beds were occupied; an additional 10 beds (disaster beds) were set up in the facility and occupied. The calculation for the percentage of occupancy for November 17 would be:

$$\frac{(80 \times 100)}{(70 \times 1)} = \frac{8,000}{70} = 114.3\%$$

Table 4.1. Examples of bed occupancy ratios

Community Hospital October 20XX		
Patient Care Unit/Bed Count	Inpatient Service Days	Percentage of Occupancy (Rounded to One Decimal Point)
Medicine/24 beds	587	$\frac{(587 \times 100)}{(24 \times 31)} = \frac{58,700}{744} = 78.9\%$
Surgery/16 beds	432	$\frac{(432 \times 100)}{(16 \times 31)} = \frac{43,200}{496} = 87.1\%$
Psychiatric/4 beds	124	$\frac{(124 \times 100)}{(4 \times 31)} = \frac{12,400}{124} = 100.0\%$
Obstetrics/6 beds	169	$\frac{(169 \times 100)}{(6 \times 31)} = \frac{16,900}{186} = 90.9\%$
Total/50 beds	1,312	$\frac{(1,312 \times 100)}{(50 \times 31)} = \frac{131,200}{1,550} = 84.6\%$

This is an example of an instance where the percentage of occupancy is greater than 100 percent. This often happens in a disaster. It is important to note that even though 10 additional beds were set up temporarily to handle the increased patient load, only the 70 beds are used in the denominator because they are the normal number of beds available. Remember that disaster beds or other beds set up for temporary use are not counted in the bed count.

Exercise 4.2

Using the information in the following table, calculate the percentage of occupancy for each day of the month and for the entire month. Round to one decimal place.

	Community Hospital April 20XX 80 beds					
Date	Inpatient Service Days	Percentage of Occupancy		Date	Inpatient Service Days	Percentage of Occupancy
1	75			16	56	
2	77			17	71	
3	72			18	78	
4	79			19	57	
5	73			20	52	
6	74			21	53	
7	76			22	50	
8	60			23	55	
9	69			24	58	
10	54			25	68	
11	59			26	64	
12	63			27	80	
13	65			28	70	
14	66			29	62	
15	67			30	61	

Exercise 4.3

Using the information in the following table, calculate the percentage of occupancy for each unit of Children's Hospital as well as the total percentage of occupancy. Round to one decimal place.

Unit	Number of Beds	Inpatient Service Days	Percentage of Occupancy
Children's Hospital June 20XX			
Pediatrics Surgical	30	833	
Hematology Oncology	20	566	
Neurology/Neurosurgical	30	756	
Renal/Gastroenterology/ Endocrinology	20	555	
Respiratory	30	897	
Cardiac Medicine/Surgical	20	589	
Infant Care Unit	10	281	
Pediatric Intensive Care	20	540	
Total			

Change in Bed Count

Occasionally, a hospital changes its bed count during a period of time. This expansion or reduction would be considered a permanent change and is not designed to meet a temporary or emergency situation.

For example, a hospital changes its official bed count from 50 to 75 on May 15 and goes on to provide a total of 1,700 inpatient service days for the entire month. How is the maximum number of bed count days determined for the month of May? Multiply 50 beds by the first 14 days of the month and 75 beds by the remaining 17 days of the month, and then add the products.

$$14 \times 50 = 700$$
$$17 \times 75 = 1,275$$
$$700 + 1,275 = 1,975$$

The maximum number of bed count days for May is 1,975. Now compute the bed occupancy ratio. The calculation is:

$$\frac{(1,700 \times 100)}{1,975} = \frac{170,000}{1,975} = 86.1\%$$

The bed occupancy ratio for May is 86.1 percent.

This procedure provides the most accurate result. Compare the previous computation with what would have happened if 50 beds had been used for the entire month. The calculation is:

$$\frac{(1,700 \times 100)}{(50 \times 31)} = \frac{170,000}{1,550} = 109.7\%$$

If 75 beds had been used for the entire month, the calculation would be:

$$\frac{(1,700 \times 100)}{(75 \times 31)} = \frac{170,000}{2,325} = 73.1\%$$

Obviously, there is a significant difference in the results. This example illustrates how easy it can be to present an inaccurate statistical picture. Because many administrative decisions are made on the basis of statistical presentations, the health information management practitioner has an important responsibility in providing accurate data and validating computerized statistics.

Exercise 4.4

Community Hospital began the year 20XX, a non-leap year, with 102 beds. On March 1, it had expanded the number of beds to 116. From April 1 through June 30, the hospital reported 120 beds. The hospital increased to 124 beds from July 1 through October 31. Finally, the hospital completed its expansion process on November 1 to end the year with 130 beds. Use these data to answer the questions below. Round to one decimal place.

Community Hospital Annual Statistics, 20XX			
Month	Bed Count (A/C)	Inpatient Service Days	Percentage of Occupancy
January	102	2,765	
February	102	2,897	
March	116	2,987	
April	120	3,123	
May	120	3,078	
June	120	3,245	
July	124	3,459	
August	124	3,598	
September	124	3,634	
October	124	3,687	
November	130	3,760	
December	130	3,792	

1. Calculate the percentage of occupancy for each month.

2. Calculate the percentage of occupancy for each quarter (January through March, April through June, July through September, and October through December).

3. Calculate the percentage of occupancy for the year.

Exercise 4.5

Using the statistics in the following report generated for University Hospital, calculate the percentage of occupancy for the month of January. Round to one decimal place.

University Hospital January 20XX			
PCU	**Inpatient Service Days**	**Bed Count**	**Percentage of Occupancy**
Medicine	3,752	130	
Rehabilitation/Neurology	600	35	
Orthopedics/Trauma	485	20	
Medicine/Surgical Oncology	1,803	60	
Pediatrics	2,142	80	
Critical Care:			
Medicine ICU	1,603	55	
Surgical ICU (Adult)	1,584	55	
Transplant	895	30	
Surgical ICU (Pediatrics)	923	40	
Total			

Newborn Bassinet Occupancy Ratio/Percentage

Typically, newborn occupancy ratios are computed separately. If every bassinet were full every day in the period, the hospital would have the maximum potential bassinet occupancy. The formula for determining newborn bassinet occupancy is:

$$\frac{Total\ newborn\ inpatient\ service\ days\ for\ a\ period \times 100}{Total\ newborn\ bassinet\ count \times Number\ of\ days\ in\ the\ period}$$

Table 4.2 lists the calculations of inpatient bed occupancy rates.

Table 4.2. Calculations of inpatient bed occupancy rates

Rate	Numerator	Denominator
Inpatient bed occupancy rate	Total number of inpatient service days for a given period × 100	Total number of inpatient bed count days for the same period
Newborn bassinet occupancy rate	Total number of newborn inpatient service days for a given period × 100	Total number of bassinet bed count days for the same period

Example: During July, a hospital with a bassinet count of 30 provided 874 newborn inpatient service days of care. According to the formula, the newborn bassinet occupancy ratio for July would be:

$$\frac{(874 \times 100)}{(30 \times 31)} = \frac{87,400}{930} = 94.0\%$$

Real-World Example: A rural hospital has a very low percentage of occupancy for the past year as indicated in table 4.3.

Table 4.3. Sample percentage of occupancy report

Hospital Board of Directors Report Percentage of Occupancy Report July 20XX–June 20XX	
Month	**Percentage of Occupancy**
July	16.4
August	22.4
September	20.4
October	21.3
November	17.1
December	28.2
January	31.7
February	28.1
March	24.6
April	16.9
May	20.7
June	22.3

The hospital board of directors of this facility is concerned that if the last year's percentage of occupancy continues much longer, they face the possibility of having to close the facility. The long-term care facility in town, however, is at full capacity and has had to turn patients away. The vice president of finance has asked the board to consider turning some beds in the facility to long-term beds and become a **swing bed hospital**. A swing bed hospital is one in which the hospital participating in Medicare has approval to provide post-hospital skilled care. That is, the hospital can use its beds for either acute care or skilled nursing care as needed. That is exactly what this hospital board decided. Now, many of its beds are being used for skilled nursing care resulting in an improved percentage of occupancy (Sauers 2016a and 2016b).

Exercise 4.6

Use the statistics in the following report generated for Community Hospital to make the following three calculations (non-leap year). Round to one decimal place.

Community Hospital Annual Statistics 20XX		
Newborn bassinets January–March: 10 April–June: 15 July–September: 20 October–December: 30		
Month	**Newborn Inpatient Service Days**	**Percentage of Occupancy**
January	270	
February	256	
March	300	
April	309	
May	315	
June	350	
July	410	
August	451	
September	475	
October	655	
November	730	
December	779	

1. Calculate the percentage of occupancy for each month.

2. Calculate the percentage of occupancy for each quarter (January through March, April through June, July through September, and October through December).

3. Calculate the percentage of occupancy for the year.

Bed Turnover Rate

The **bed turnover rate** refers to the number of times a bed, on average, changes occupants during a given period of time or the average number of admissions per bed per time period. The bed turnover rate is useful because two time periods may have the same percentage of occupancy, but the turnover rates may be different. For example, if a unit such as an obstetrics unit has a high turnover rate, this could be an indication that the unit can accommodate more patients because the patients have a shorter length of stay (LOS). Conversely, a rehabilitation unit might have a low turnover rate because the patients in that unit have a longer LOS. The bed turnover rate is a measure of the frequency of bed use. It demonstrates the net effect of changes in occupancy rate and LOS. See chapter 5 for a discussion of LOS.

Following are two formulas for determining bed turnover rate. The direct formula is:

$$\frac{Number\ of\ discharges\ (including\ deaths)\ for\ a\ period}{Average\ bed\ count\ during\ the\ period}$$

The indirect formula is:

$$\frac{Occupancy\ rate \times Number\ of\ days\ in\ a\ period}{Average\ length\ of\ stay}$$

Although the most accurate formula has not been determined, administrators of short-stay hospitals place a growing emphasis on bed turnover rate as a measure of hospital services used, especially when it is related to occupancy and LOS. When occupancy goes up and LOS goes down, or vice versa, the bed turnover rate can improve recognition of the net effect of these changes.

Turnover rates can be used in comparing one facility with another or in comparing utilization rates for different time periods or for different units of the same facility. For example, the occupancy rate for one hospital can be essentially the same in two time periods, but the turnover rate may be lower because of a longer LOS in one time period. In other words, bed turnover rate can be a measure of intensity of utilization.

Exercise 4.7 demonstrates both formulas and yields basically the same turnover rate for a short-stay hospital.

Exercise 4.7

<table>
<tr><td colspan="1" style="text-align:center">Community Hospital
Annual Statistics, 20XX
Non-leap year
200 beds</td></tr>
<tr><td>Patients discharged (includes deaths): 7,054
Average length of stay: 9 days
Bed occupancy rate: 85 percent</td></tr>
<tr><td>1. Apply the direct formula for the turnover rate. Round to one decimal place.</td></tr>
<tr><td>2. Apply the indirect formula for the turnover rate. Round to one decimal place.</td></tr>
<tr><td>Answers:

Turnover rate (direct formula):</td></tr>
<tr><td>Turnover rate (indirect formula):</td></tr>
</table>

Chapter 4   Matching Quiz

Match the definition with the term:

Definitions:

a. The number of available hospital inpatient beds

b. A unit of measure that denotes the presence of one newborn bassinet, either occupied or vacant, set up and staffed for use in one 24-hour period

c. The sum of inpatient bed count days for each of the days in a period

d. A state-directed program that requires healthcare facilities to submit detailed plans and justifications for the purchase of new equipment, new buildings, or new service offerings that cost in excess of a certain amount

e. A patient who presents with a medical condition with a significant degree of instability and disability and who needs to be monitored, evaluated, and assessed to determine whether he or she should be admitted for inpatient care or discharged for care in another setting

f. The number of available newborn bassinets

g. Percent of occupancy, percentage of occupancy, occupancy ratio

h. A unit of measure denoting the presence of one inpatient bed set up and staffed for one 24-hour period

i. The number of beds that a facility has been designed and constructed to house

j. The average number of times a bed changes occupants during a given period of time

Terms:

1. ____Certificate of need
2. ____Newborn bassinet count day
3. ____Observation patient
4. ____Bed capacity
5. ____ Bed count/Inpatient bed count

6. ____ Bed turnover rate
7. ____ Total bed count days
8. ____ Bed occupancy ratio
9. ____ Newborn bassinet count
10. ____ Bed count day

Chapter 4   Review

Community Hospital compiled the following annual statistics for 20XX (non-leap year): Use this table to answer questions 1, 2, and 3.

Community Hospital Annual Statistics, 20XX		
	Inpatient Service Days	**Bed Count**
January–June	35,872	175
July–December	36,894	200
December 31 only	201	200
Newborn	12,732	40

Select the correct answer to each of the following questions, rounding to one decimal place.

1. The inpatient occupancy rate (without newborns) for 20XX was ____.
   a. 37.4%
   b. 98.4%
   c. 99.2%
   d. 106.3%

2. The newborn bassinet occupancy rate for 20XX was ____.
   a. 84.7%
   b. 85.2%
   c. 86.2%
   d. 87.2%

3. The bed occupancy rate for December 31 was ____.
   a. 87.3%
   b. 99.5%
   c. 100.0%
   d. 100.5%

The following table is a report of the first quarter of 20XX (January–March) from a 400-bed medical center regarding its insurance categories. In this example, deaths are included in discharges. Round all to one decimal place. This is a non-leap year. Use the following table to answer questions 4, 5, and 6.

Community Medical Center Inpatient Service Days and Number of Discharges by Insurance Category January–March 20XX		
Insurance Category	**Inpatient Service Days**	**Number of Discharges**
Third-party Contracts	5,849	598
Medicare	9,427	1,450
Medicaid	13,604	2,011
County Coverage	5,340	802
Private Pay	3,564	315
No Insurance	2,598	480
Total	**40,382**	**5,656**

4. Calculate the occupancy rate for:
   a. Total
   b. Medicare
   c. Private pay

5. Using the direct formula, calculate the bed turnover rate for:
   a. Total
   b. Medicare
   c. Private pay

6. What is the total average daily inpatient census for this period of time?

7. The following table is a report of the annual inpatient service days of Community Hospital for 20XX. The hospital has an inpatient bed count of 250 and a bassinet count of 30. Calculate the percentage of occupancy for each month for adults/children and for newborns. This is a non-leap year. Round to one decimal place.

Community Hospital Annual Statistics, 20XX				
	Inpatient Service Days		**Percentage of Occupancy**	
Month	**Adults/Children**	**Newborn**	**Adults/Children**	**Newborn**
January	7,250	874		
February	6,532	788		
March	7,354	820		

(continued on next page)

Community Hospital Annual Statistics, 20XX				
	Inpatient Service Days		Percentage of Occupancy	
Month	Adults/Children	Newborn	Adults/Children	Newborn
April	7,365	895		
May	7,235	866		
June	7,132	756		
July	7,501	875		
August	7,523	796		
September	7,196	856		
October	7,362	878		
November	7,065	821		
December	7,175	801		
Total				

8. Community Hospital, a 120-bed facility, reported that in March there were 545 discharges (including deaths). Using the direct formula, what was the bed turnover rate for March?

9. Which of the following beds should be counted in the bed count?

   a. A hospital inpatient bed

   b. A labor room bed

   c. An observation bed

   d. An extra bed set up during a disaster

10. On October 1, a hurricane hit a small coastal community that has a community hospital licensed for 50 beds. Hospital staff set up 10 additional beds around the facility and used three labor room beds and two treatment room beds in order to help take care of patients. Which of the following would be the denominator used to determine the percentage of occupancy for October 1?

   a. 50

   b. 60

   c. 63

   d. 65

11. The 15-bed surgical intensive care unit at Memorial Hospital had 400 inpatient service days during March. What is the percentage of occupancy? Round to one decimal place.

12. On February 12, a fire occurred at a local dry cleaning plant, and the inpatient service days for the local hospital (120 beds) was reported to be 130. What is the bed occupancy rate for February 12? Round to one decimal place.

13. What is the bed occupancy rate for the 15-bassinet Children's Hospital NICU during March if the inpatient service days was 400? Round to one decimal place.

14. During January through June, (non-leap year) a 50-bed hospital had 9,001 inpatient service days. What is the percentage of occupancy? Round to one decimal place.

15. During the period July through December the same hospital as above added 25 beds making its total bed count 75. During July through December there were 12,765 inpatient service days. Calculate the percentage of occupancy, rounding to one decimal place, for:

a. July through December

b. January through December

Length of Stay

Learning Objectives

At the conclusion of this chapter, you should be able to

- Explain, differentiate, and apply the following terms: length of stay (LOS), discharge days, and leave of absence day
- Compute the length of stay for one patient, the average length of stay, and the average length of stay (ALOS) for newborns
- Calculate the total length of stay for a group of discharged patients
- Discover the relationship between length of stay and utilization management
- Utilize software to complete spreadsheets

Key Terms

Admission date	Discharge days	Length of stay (LOS)
Average duration of hospitalization	Duration of inpatient hospitalization	Medicare severity diagnosis-related groups (MS-DRGs)
Average length of stay (ALOS)	Inpatient days of stay	Military time
Days of stay	Leave of absence	Total length of stay
Discharge date	Leave of absence day	Utilization management

Length of stay is an indicator of the amount of resources used in a healthcare facility. The longer the length of stay, the more resources used by the patient. Length of stay is also used to compare diagnoses, MS-DRGs, physicians, and other hospitals.

Length of Stay

Length of stay (LOS) is the number of calendar days a patient stays in the hospital, from admission to discharge. The healthcare facility uses LOS data in utilization management.

Utilization management is a program that evaluates the facility's efficiency in providing necessary services in the most cost-effective manner, including LOS, while also evaluating the level of care required. Its goal is to eliminate over- and underutilization of services. Part of the utilization management process involves reviewing LOS for continued medical necessity. For example, is it more appropriate to continue to treat the patient in an acute-care facility or to transfer the patient to a subacute or rehabilitation facility?

LOS data also are used in financial reporting, for example, to compare patients within the same Medicare severity diagnosis-related group (MS-DRG). MS-DRGs are payment groups, designed for the Medicare population, that recognize severity of illness, resource use, and patient complexity. Patient complexity refers to the characteristics that a patient has, including physical, mental, social, and financial issues, that will determine how a physician will care for the patient. Managing complex patients takes more healthcare practitioner time and uses more resources, including lab, x-ray, and medications, than a patient with fewer problems.

Patients who have similar clinical characteristics and similar costs are assigned to an MS-DRG, which is linked to a fixed payment amount. A particular MS-DRG average length of stay (ALOS) can be compared with the overall healthcare facility's MS-DRG ALOS to determine whether there are too many extreme values, also known as outliers. The **average length of stay (ALOS)** is the average number of days that inpatients discharged during the period under consideration stayed in the hospital. This is discussed in more detail later in this chapter. LOS data for patients with the same diagnosis or procedure treated by various physicians are compared to evaluate any extremes. For example, it is important for hospital administration to be aware of physician differences in LOS because these may be indicative of different types of treatment for the same condition by different physicians.

Discharge Days

Chapter 3 introduced the concept of inpatient service days, which are compiled while the patient is hospitalized. This chapter discusses **discharge days**, which are days calculated after the patient has been discharged from the hospital. Discharge days, **days of stay**, **inpatient days of stay**, and **duration of inpatient hospitalization** are other terms used for LOS.

A discharge occurs at the end of the patient's inpatient stay. Discharges include deaths, so the term discharge may refer both to patients who leave the hospital alive and those who have died. Some patients are transferred to other facilities to continue their care. Hospital staff may refer to these patients as transfers but they are counted as discharges.

In general, every day that a patient is in the hospital is counted as a day except the day of discharge. The LOS for one patient is determined by subtracting the **admission date** from the **discharge date** *when the patient is admitted and discharged within the same month*. The day of admission is counted in computing the number of discharge days or LOS, but the day of discharge is not.

For longer stays when the patient's stay extends beyond one or more months, days must be added to calculate the LOS.

Example: For a patient admitted on March 30 and discharged on April 4, subtract March 30 from March 31 and add the 4 days in April ($31 - 30 = 1$ in March + 4 days in April = 5 days). The LOS is one day if the patient is admitted and discharged on the same day. These types of patients are also called admissions and discharges (A&Ds) or in and outs.

Table 5.1 shows how to calculate the LOS for a sampling of discharged patients.

Table 5.1. Example LOS calculation

Date Admitted	Date Discharged	LOS
9/25	9/25	1 day
9/25	9/26	1 day (9/26 − 9/25 = 1 day)
9/25	9/30	5 days (9/30 − 9/25 = 5 days)
9/25	10/4	9 days (5 days in September + 4 days in October = 9 days)
9/25	11/4	40 days (5 days in September + 31 days in October + 4 days in November = 40 days)

Exercise 5.1

Calculate the LOS for the following discharged patients in an acute care facility.

Date Admitted	Date Discharged	LOS
7/9	7/10	
9/12	9/22	
3/10	3/24	
6/17	7/18	
10/20	11/25	

Exercise 5.2

Calculate the LOS for the following discharged patients in this long-term care facility. Keep in mind that 2012 is a leap year.

Date Admitted	Date Discharged	LOS
1/1/2009	11/01/2014	
4/07/2012	12/31/2013	
6/28/2011	1/23/2012	
2/1/2012	3/15/2013	
10/30/2013	7/07/2014	

Calculating Length of Stay in an Outpatient Setting

It is possible to calculate LOS in an outpatient facility or physician's office. For example, a patient arrived at 8:05 a.m. and was taken to the examining room at 8:22 a.m. Because the hour is the same in both cases (8 a.m.), simply subtract the minutes (22 − 05 = 17 minutes). This patient waited 17 minutes before being taken to the examining room.

If a patient arrived at 8:05 a.m. and was taken into the examining room at 9:15 a.m., subtract the minutes first (15 − 05 = 10 minutes) and then subtract the hour (9 − 8 = 1). The patient waited 1 hour and 10 minutes. Note that the second set of minutes, the taken time (15), is greater than the first set of minutes (05), the arrival time.

If the first set of minutes (arrived) is greater than the second set of minutes (taken), additional steps must take place. Subtract one hour from the second hour (taken) and increase the number of minutes on the second time by 60. It sounds a little confusing, but the following should clear up the issue. Let's say a patient arrived at 1:11 p.m. and was taken to the examining room at 3:02 p.m. The "arrival" minutes of 11 are greater than the "taken" minutes of 02.

- Subtract one hour from 3:02, which will equal 2:02
- Now the one hour (60 minutes) you took from the 3:02 needs to be added to the :02
- The "time" is now 2:62. It is now possible to subtract the 1:11 from 2:62
- 2:62 − 1:11 = 1 hour and 51 minutes, which was the patient's wait time

The next two calculations concern the amount of time between two times when one is before 12:59 and one is after 12:59. Consider this first example: A patient arrived at the physician's office at 11:47 a.m. and was taken to the examination room at 1:27 p.m.

First add 12 hours to the time that occurred after 12:59. In this case that would be 1:27 + 12 = 13:27. This changes the time to **military time**. Military time is time measured in hours numbered to 24 (as 0100 or 2300) from one midnight to the next.

- Next, note that the "arrived" minutes (47) are greater than the "taken" minutes (27)
- Subtract one hour from the 13:27. This equals 12:27.
- Add the 60 minutes from that hour to the "taken" minutes. This would be 27 + 60 = 87.
- The "time" is now 12:87.
- Then, subtract 11:47 from 12:87. That is 12 − 11 = 1 and 87 − 47 = 40.
- The patient waited for 1 hour and 40 minutes.

Consider this second example: A patient arrives at the outpatient clinic at 11:21 a.m. and is taken to the examination room at 2:33 p.m.

- In this case, first add 12 hours to the time that occurred after 12:59. This would be 2:33 + 12 = 14:33.
- Note that the "arrived" minutes (21) are less than the "taken" minutes of 33.
- Subtract the minutes 33 − 21 = 12.
- Now, subtract the 11:00 from 14:00 which equals 3.
- The patient waited for 3 hours and 12 minutes.

Exercise 5.3

1. Calculate the time it takes to see patients in this physician's office.

Time Admitted	Time Seen by Physician	Time between Checking In at Reception and Being Seen by Physician
8:00 a.m.	8:17 a.m.	
1:22 p.m.	2:05 p.m.	
10:30 a.m.	11:43 a.m.	
1:30 p.m.	3:00 p.m.	
2:15 p.m.	2:56 p.m.	

2. Metropolitan Hospital, a very large urban hospital, promises patients that there will be no more than a 60-minute wait between the time they arrive (sign in) at the emergency services department until they are triaged. Calculate the wait time between arrival and triage. The hospital selected 10 patients at random to check the times.

   a. Calculate the wait time for each patient.

   b. What is the average wait time?

   c. Is the hospital in compliance with its own guidelines?

Patient	Time of Arrival	Time Patient was Triaged	Wait Time
Patient A	8:00 a.m.	8:23 a.m.	
Patient B	8:23 a.m.	8:56 a.m.	
Patient C	8:56 a.m.	9:20 a.m.	
Patient D	9:45 a.m.	10:46 a.m.	
Patient E	10:20 a.m.	1:45 p.m.	
Patient F	11:20 a.m.	1:50 p.m.	
Patient G	12:15 p.m.	2:40 p.m.	
Patient H	1:05 p.m.	2:56 p.m.	
Patient I	3:27 p.m.	5:05 p.m.	
Patient J	4:05 p.m.	4:56 p.m.	

Total Length of Stay

The **total length of stay** is the sum of the days stayed of any group of inpatients discharged during a specified period of time. Total LOS also may be referred to as total discharge days. Although the total LOS and inpatient service days may approximate each other over a long period of time, they are not interchangeable. The reason for this is that inpatient service days are counted concurrently and discharge days are counted after discharge.

Example: A patient hospitalized for a period beyond an entire year and into a second year (for example, a rehabilitation patient) would be credited with 365 inpatient service days at the end of the first year, but no discharge days. When the patient is discharged from the hospital in the second year, all the discharge days from admission to discharge are counted at that time, increasing the discharge days for the second year by at least 365.

If the patient stays in the hospital for two or more years (as often happens in long-term facilities), all 730+ discharge days are assigned to one year in calculating the duration of inpatient hospitalization. These types of patients increase the number of discharge days for any year, making the total number much larger than inpatient service days for the same period.

Why calculate both inpatient days of service and total LOS? Each is meaningful in its own right. Inpatient service days are useful in the analysis of current utilization of hospital facilities related to the entire hospital, a clinical unit, or a service department. They are used to compute various daily averages and occupancy ratios. The total LOS can be used to analyze LOS for groups of discharged patients with similar characteristics such as age, disease, treatment, clinical service, or day of week admitted.

Exercise 5.4

Using the table below, answer the following questions for this group of 15 patients discharged from Community Hospital on 10/20/20XX.

Community Hospital Discharge List October 20, 20XX				
Pt. Name	**Age**	**Clinical Service**	**Admission Date**	**LOS**
Schulman	71	Surgery	9/18	
Hubbard	40	Medicine	9/12	
Miraboto	35	Obstetrics	10/18	

(continued on next page)

Pt. Name	Age	Clinical Service	Admission Date	LOS
Tatum	23	Obstetrics	10/18	
Rankins	71	Medicine	9/28	
Lampton	90	Medicine	9/4	
Hruska	45	Surgery	10/5	
Adman	17	Obstetrics	10/19	
Savage	37	Medicine	9/1	
Beachton	46	Medicine	10/1	
Sanders	14	Obstetrics	10/17	
Pavalchik	62	Surgery	9/26	
Walters	57	Surgery	9/30	
Harding	51	Medicine	10/1	
Clay	82	Medicine	10/10	
Total				

Community Hospital
Discharge List
October 20, 20XX

Calculate the following:

a. LOS for each individual patient

b. Total LOS for all patients

c. Total LOS for medicine service patients

d. Total LOS for surgery service patients

e. Total LOS for obstetrics service patients

f. Total LOS for patients 25 years of age and younger

g. Total LOS for patients age 26 to 40 years old

h. Total LOS for patients age 41 to 55 years old

i. Total LOS for patients age 56 to 70 years old

j. Total LOS for patients over age 70

k. What percentage of medicine discharges were there? Round to one decimal place.

Average Length of Stay

The average length of stay (ALOS) is the average number of days that inpatients discharged during the period under consideration stayed in the hospital. The formula for calculating ALOS is:

$$\frac{Total\ length\ of\ stay\ (discharge\ days)}{Total\ discharges\ (including\ deaths)}$$

In general, inpatient LOS is decreasing in US hospitals. Several trends in healthcare have contributed to this reduction in ALOS, including improved medical technology, changes in medical practice, an increase in outpatient visits, financial pressures on healthcare facilities, and changes in types of care provided, including managed care, home care, and skilled nursing units in hospitals (Kalra et al. 2010). Synonymous terms for ALOS include **average duration of hospitalization** and average stay.

The formula above does not include the LOS for newborns. Most hospitals calculate the ALOS for newborns separately because newborns ordinarily stay the same length of time as their mothers. In addition, when compared with many other classifications of patients, normal newborn stays are relatively short. In contrast, newborn stays in the newborn intensive care unit tend to be quite long, sometimes months at a time. Therefore, inclusion of both mothers and newborns would distort the total ALOS.

A critical care access hospital monitors the ALOS very closely because the Centers for Medicare and Medicaid Services CMS requires an annual ALOS of 96 hours. Each month, the health information manager reports the hospital's monthly and cumulative ALOS to the board of directors.

Exercise 5.5

Complete the following exercises.

1. In April, Community Hospital reported 923 discharge days for adults and children and 107 discharge days for newborns. During the month, 192 adults and children and 37 newborns were discharged. Calculate the ALOS for adults and children for the month of April. Round to one decimal place.

2. Using the table in exercise 5.4, compute the ALOS for the following groups of patients:
   a. All patients
   b. Medicine service patients
   c. Surgery service patients
   d. Obstetrics service patients
   e. Patients 25 years of age and younger
   f. Patients age 26 to 40 years old
   g. Patients age 41 to 55 years old
   h. Patients age 56 to 70 years old
   i. Patients over age 70

3. Using the semiannual report below from University Medical Center, calculate the ALOS for each service. Round to one decimal place.

University Medical Center January–June, 20XX			
Clinical Units	Discharges	Discharge Days	ALOS
Medicine	12,280	61,400	
Surgery	10,320	51,762	
Neurology	12,464	68,320	
Oncology	6,228	61,280	
Orthopedics	4,906	20,624	
Rehabilitation	1,926	48,250	
Urology	678	2,698	
Psychiatry	936	22,400	
Ophthalmology	385	804	
Obstetrics/Gynecology	3,528	8,820	
Pediatrics	3,148	18,388	
Total			

Average Newborn Length of Stay

As stated earlier, newborn LOS is usually calculated separately. The formula for calculating average newborn LOS is:

$$\frac{Total\ newborn\ discharge\ days}{Total\ newborn\ discharges\ (including\ deaths)}$$

The hospital stay for a newborn is generally just long enough to identify any early healthcare concerns and to determine that the family is able to care for the infant. Table 5.2 lists the calculations for LOS statistics.

Table 5.2 Calculations for LOS statistics

Indicator	Numerator	Denominator
ALOS	Total LOS (discharge days) for a given period	Total number of discharges, including deaths, for the same period
ALOS for NBs	Total LOS (discharge days) for all NB discharges and deaths for a given period	Total number of NB discharges, including deaths, for the same period

Exercise 5.6

Using the table below, calculate the ALOS for newborns in each month and then compute the annual ALOS. Round to one decimal place.

University Hospital Annual Newborn Discharge Statistics 20XX			
Month	**Newborn Discharges**	**Discharge Days**	**Newborn ALOS**
January	103	278	
February	128	427	
March	107	247	
April	148	302	
May	152	327	
June	143	396	
July	162	422	
August	163	433	
September	183	568	
October	179	485	
November	164	459	
December	159	407	
Total			

Leave of Absence Days

Another data element that is significant in some hospitals is the number of leave of absence days. A **leave of absence** is a physician-authorized absence of an inpatient from a hospital or other facility for a specified period of time occurring after admission and prior to discharge. This means that the physician writes an order that the patient can leave the facility and return at a later date. The healthcare facility will hold the bed until the patient returns or it is determined that the patient is absent without leave.

A **leave of absence day** is determined when the patient is not present at the census-taking hour. A leave of absence involves an overnight pass, or, more frequently given in longer-stay facilities, a weekend pass; thus, the patient would not be present when the census is taken.

Leave of absence data are important for administrative purposes as well as for the analysis of the services provided and care patterns. Leave of absence days are usually excluded or tabulated separately when computing bed occupancy, calculating inpatient service days, or preparing an inpatient census. Another issue with leave of absence days is that insurance companies generally do not pay for days outside the hospital. Thus, if the days are being used in conjunction with financial data, they may need to be separated from the actual days in the hospital. However, they are included when considering discharge days and computing ALOS. Leave of absence days do not occur very often in acute care facilities; however, hospitals that generally have longer lengths of stay, such as rehabilitation, mental health, or chronic care hospitals, will use the leave of absence as a way for the patient to adjust to time away from the facility, so it is ordinarily considered part of the patient's treatment. If the leave of absence is not considered part of the patient treatment, the physician may elect to discharge and then readmit the patient rather than grant a leave of absence.

Exercise 5.7

Using the statistics in the tables below, determine the following calculations for Community Hospital.

1. Compute the LOS for each of the patients in the table below. (Remember that 2012 was a leap year.) If no year is specified, assume it is not a leap year and both dates are in the same year.

Admitted	Discharged	LOS
1/10	1/31	
7/8	7/30	
1/1/2012	2/1/2015	
11/20	11/20	
6/19/2011	1/4/2012	

2. What is the total LOS for this group of patients?

Using the information in the table below, answer questions 3 through 7. Round to one decimal place.

Community Hospital Annual Statistics, 20XX		
	Number of Discharges	Discharge Days
Total Adults and Children	15,672	67,392
Total Newborns	1,502	3,453
The following services are included in the above totals:		
Medicine	9,455	40,780
Surgery	4,650	22,957
Obstetrics	1,567	3,655

3. Compute the ALOS for adult and children patients.

4. Compute the ALOS for newborn patients.

5. Compute the ALOS for medicine patients.

6. Compute the ALOS for surgery patients.

7. Compute the ALOS for obstetrics patients.

Answers:
Adults and Children ALOS:
Newborns ALOS:
Medicine ALOS:
Surgery ALOS:
Obstetrics ALOS:

8. Calculate the ALOS for the following Medicare patients. Round to one decimal place.

Community Hospital **Medicare Discharge Statistics** **July 20XX**			
Unit	**Medicare Discharges**	**Medicare Discharge Days**	**ALOS**
Medicine	478	3,411	
Surgery	253	2,566	
Rehabilitation	261	4,507	
Skilled Nursing	394	11,132	

Exercise 5.8

Last month, Community Hospital compiled the discharge statistics shown in the following table. Notice that the last three days are missing. Prepare a spreadsheet on a software program and enter the information from the chart. Then use the discharge lists for July 29, 30, and 31 to enter the missing data into the appropriate columns for medicine, surgery, obstetrics, and newborn discharged patients and their corresponding discharge days.

Finally, compute the ALOS for medicine service, surgery service, obstetrics service, and newborn service and then compute the ALOS for adults and children (medicine, surgery, and obstetrics).

Community Hospital Discharge List July 29, 20XX				
Patient Name	Age	Service	Admission Date	LOS
Andres, Michael	47	Medicine	7/21	8
Barty, Stephen	34	Surgery	7/21	8
Christenson, Andrea	17	OB	7/27	2
Christenson, Baby Boy	NB	NB	7/27	2
Denison, William	15	Surgery	7/19	10
Henry, Christopher	67	Surgery	7/17	12
Jackson, Michelle	39	OB	7/25	4
Katon, Marie	41	OB	7/25	4
Williamson, Baby Boy	NB	NB	7/24	5

Community Hospital Discharge List July 30, 20XX				
Patient Name	Age	Service	Admission Date	LOS
Adams, Paul	34	Medicine	7/23	7
Butler, Thomas	65	Medicine	7/24	6
Carson, Johnnie	67	Surgery	7/24	6
Daniels, George	45	Medicine	7/22	8
Finley, Joyce	24	OB	7/28	2

(continued on next page)

Community Hospital Discharge List July 30, 20XX				
Patient Name	Age	Service	Admission Date	LOS
Finley, Baby Girl	NB	NB	7/28	2
George, Michael	32	Surgery	7/21	9
Jacquinta, Marlene	29	OB	7/27	3
Jacquinta, Baby Boy	NB	NB	7/27	3
Katosh, Joseph	82	Medicine	7/25	5
Kettison, Jack	78	Medicine	7/18	12
Kettison, Mary	76	Surgery	7/24	6
Laytham, Clint	50	Surgery	7/25	5
Matson, Dorianne	76	Medicine	7/23	7
Nettleson, Andy	43	Surgery	7/24	6
Pierce, Otto	92	Medicine	7/19	11
Ransom, Jackson	54	Medicine	7/28	2
Springer, Mary	32	Surgery	7/27	3
Tatum, Neal	76	Surgery	7/28	2
Wallace, Mattie	19	OB	7/28	2
Zininsky, Maureen	32	OB	7/28	2

Community Hospital Discharge List July 31, 20XX				
Patient Name	Age	Service	Admission Date	LOS
Allan, Randy	52	Medicine	7/23	8
Banta, Janet	76	Medicine	7/25	6
Cox, David	56	Surgery	7/27	4
Dunning, Stephen	15	Surgery	7/26	5
Epp, Melvin	65	Medicine	7/26	5

(continued on next page)

Community Hospital Discharge List July 31, 20XX				
Patient Name	Age	Service	Admission Date	LOS
Farmer, Jaimie	19	OB	7/29	2
Finley, Baby Girl	NB	NB	7/28	3
Finney, G. W.	54	Surgery	7/23	8
Fry, Benedict	83	Surgery	7/24	7
Girard, Katherine	73	Medicine	7/25	6
Halford, Harold	65	Surgery	7/26	5
Kilpatrick, Susan	19	OB	7/25	6
Kilpatrick, Baby Boy	NB	NB	7/26	5
Martindale, Amanda	18	OB	7/28	3
Martindale, Baby Boy	NB	NB	7/28	3
Martindale, Baby Boy	NB	NB	7/28	3
Nachtigall, Brian	22	Medicine	7/23	8
Niazi, Baby Boy	NB	NB	7/25	6
Poepperling, Wanda	56	Medicine	7/25	6
Trotman, Baby Girl	NB	NB	7/23	8

Community Hospital Student Name July 20XX											
	Medicine		Surgery		Obstetrics		Subtotal		Newborn		Total	
Date	No. Pts.	Dis Days	No. Pts.	Dis Days	No. Pts.	Dis Days	No. Pts.	Dis Days	No. Pts.	Dis Days	No. Pts.	Dis Days
1-July	8	40	2	25	5	16			6	23		
2-July	6	36	8	80	3	10			3	10		
3-July	4	21	4	23	1	4			1	4		
4-July	11	47	3	42	4	10			4	10		
5-July	15	77	5	23	3	7			2	5		
6-July	6	52	7	56	2	5			3	7		

(*continued on next page*)

	Medicine		Surgery		Obstetrics		Subtotal		Newborn		Total	
Date	No. Pts.	Dis Days	No. Pts.	Dis Days	No. Pts.	Dis Days	No. Pts.	Dis Days	No. Pts.	Dis Days	No. Pts.	Dis Days
7-July	5	71	9	123	6	13			5	10		
8-July	8	63	1	4	3	9			2	13		
9-July	9	72	4	26	2	6			3	9		
10-July	7	34	9	112	3	8			3	8		
11-July	2	9	3	27	1	2			1	2		
12-July	5	28	4	16	2	5			1	3		
13-July	4	29	6	119	2	7			2	7		
14-July	9	26	8	95	2	6			2	6		
15-July	7	45	4	81	4	8			5	11		
16-July	6	37	2	15	3	8			3	8		
17-July	4	52	9	37	3	10			2	10		
18-July	3	55	6	30	3	9			3	10		
19-July	4	8	4	16	4	10			4	10		
20-July	8	63	3	37	2	6			3	9		
21-July	3	29	5	23	1	3			0	0		
22-July	5	35	8	78	4	9			4	9		
23-July	5	34	4	32	2	4			3	8		
24-July	8	53	1	5	3	6			2	6		
25-July	7	26	2	62	2	2			2	4		
26-July	2	23	3	42	4	12			3	7		
27-July	3	23	4	53	1	5			4	11		
28-July	5	25	2	10	3	10			2	8		
29-July												
30-July												
31-July												
Total												

Community Hospital
Student Name
July 20XX

Chapter 5   Matching Quiz

Match the definitions with the terms.

Definitions

   a. Time measured in hours numbered to 24 (such as 0100 or 2300) from one midnight to the next

   b. The total number of patient days for an inpatient episode, calculated by subtracting the date of admission from the date of discharge

   c. The authorized absence of an inpatient from a hospital or other facility for a specified period of time occurring after admission and prior to discharge

   d. The year, month, and day that an inpatient was formally released from the hospital and room, board, and continuous nursing services were terminated

   e. The year, month, and day of inpatient admission, beginning with a hospital's formal acceptance of a patient who is to receive healthcare services while receiving room, board, and continuous nursing services

   f. The mean length of stay for hospital inpatients discharged during a given period of time

   g. A program that evaluates the healthcare facility's efficiency in providing necessary care to patients in the most effective manner

   h. The sum of the days of stay of any group of inpatients discharged during a specific period of time; also called discharge days

   i. A day occurring after the admission and prior to the discharge of a hospital inpatient when the patient is not present at the census-taking hour because he or she is on leave of absence from the healthcare facility

   j. Payment groups designed for the Medicare population that recognize severity of illness, resource use and patient complexity

Terms:

1. ____MS-DRG	**6.** ____Leave of absence
2. ____Utilization management	**7.** ____Admission date
3. ____Length of stay	**8.** ____Discharge date
4. ____Total length of stay	**9.** ____Average length of stay
5. ____Military time	**10.** ____Leave of absence day

Chapter 5   Review

   1. The number of discharge days for a patient admitted January 23 to February 15 is _____.

     a. 21 days

     b. 22 days

     c. 23 days

     d. 24 days

2. Determine the length of stay for the following patients:

Patient	Admitted	Discharged (same year as admission)	LOS
A	6/25	6/25	
B	6/25	7/4	
C	6/25	8/1	
D	6/25	9/2	

Use the information in the table below for questions 3, 4, and 5.

3. Determine the length of stay for the following individual patients who were all discharged on July 12 of the same year as the admission year:

Patient	Admitted	LOS
A	7/4	
B	7/5	
C	6/20	
D	3/12	
E	4/17	
F	3/1	
G	6/23	
H	6/25	
I	4/7	
J	5/6	

4. The total length of stay for the patients is _____.
   a. 523
   b. 577
   c. 602
   d. 645

5. The average length of stay for these patients is _____.
   a. 52.3 days
   b. 57.7 days
   c. 60.2 days
   d. 64.5 days

6. When a patient is authorized to be absent from the health care facility and plans to return at a later date, this is referred to as (a) _____.

   a. Absent without leave

   b. Leave of absence

   c. Discharge day

   d. Total leave

7. What is the wait time for a patient who arrives at a physician's office at 8:20 a.m. and is seen by the physician at 9:30 a.m.

   a. 68 minutes

   b. 70 minutes

   c. 1 hour, 5 minutes

   d. 50 minutes

8. For a long-term-care patient admitted in July of one year and discharged in March of the next year, the discharged days are counted in the first year. True or false?

   a. True

   b. False

Use the following Information to answer questions 9 through 12.

Patient arrives at the hospital's surgery center	5:30 a.m.
Patient called back to the prep area	6:12 a.m.
Patient prep completed	7:58 a.m.
Patient taken to surgical suite	8:20 a.m.
Surgery started	8:35 a.m.
Surgery ended	9:50 a.m.
Patient taken to recovery room	10:03 a.m.
Patient taken to hospital room	11:45 a.m.

9. What is the patient's wait time from the time of arrival to the surgery center and begin taken to the surgery prep area?

   a. 42 minutes

   b. 43 minutes

   c. 45 minutes

   d. 60 minutes

10. How long was the surgical prep time?

    a. 100 minutes

    b. 103 minutes

    c. 106 minutes

    d. 120 minutes

11. How long was the surgery?
    a. 60 minutes
    b. 65 minutes
    c. 70 minutes
    d. 75 minutes

12. What was the total time from the time of the patient arriving at the hospital to the time the patient arrived in the hospital room?
    a. 5 hours, 15 minutes
    b. 6 hours, 15 minutes
    c. 300 minutes
    d. 400 minutes

Use the table below to answer questions 13, 14, and 15. Round to one decimal place.

Service	Discharges	Discharge Days
Medicine	6,658	37,284
Surgery	7,820	48,481
Obstetrics	2,389	4,790
Newborn	2,214	4,456

13. What is the average length of stay for the medicine service?
    a. 15.6 percent
    b. 5.6 days
    c. 6.9 days
    d. 17.8 days

14. What is the average length of stay for the newborn service?
    a. 2.0 percent
    b. 2.0 days
    c. 2.1 days
    d. 4.9 days

15. What is the average length of stay for all services?
    a. 2.0 days
    b. 4.7 days
    c. 4.9 days
    d. 5.0 days

CHAPTER 6

Death (Mortality) Rates

Learning Objectives

At the conclusion of this chapter, you should be able to

- Calculate the following death rates: hospital, gross, net, postoperative, anesthesia, postoperative, maternal, newborn, fetal, cancer, crude, and case fatality
- Compare the differences in the four types of anesthesia used
- Distinguish between a direct obstetrical death and indirect obstetrical death

Key Terms

Anesthesia death rate
Cancer mortality rate
Cancer registrar
Cancer registry
Case fatality rate
Centers for Medicare and
   Medicaid Services
Complication
Crude death rate
Dead on arrival
Death rate
Disposition
Early fetal death
Fetal death
Fetal death rate

Gross death rate
Hospital death rate
Hospital live birth
Infant death
Institutional death rate
Intermediate fetal death
Late fetal death
Maternal death
Maternal death rate
Mortality
Mortality rate
Neonatal death
Neonatal period
Net death rate
Newborn

Newborn death
Newborn death rate
Newborn mortality rate
Perinatal death
Postneonatal death
Postoperative death rate
Postpartum
Prepartum
Stillbirth
Surgical death rate
Surgical operation
Surgical procedure
World Health Organization
   (WHO)

Death rates have always been important information for health agencies and hospitals in evaluating the quality of medical care. It may also be useful to examine death rates based on certain characteristics, such as socioeconomic status, geography or location, age, and cause of death. Death rate information is used by a variety of industries in addition to healthcare. For example, the automobile industry uses death rate information to determine the likelihood of drivers and passengers dying in some car models compared with others. Handgun advocates look at death rates to determine the likelihood of someone dying a violent death while using a firearm. Organizations such as the American Heart Association, the American Cancer Association, and other groups are interested in looking at death rates to help bring attention to their causes and to raise money for research. Researchers use death rates to show causes of death in certain populations. All this information can help improve the quality of medical care given to patients.

An article in the *Journal of the American Medical Association* calling for more emphasis on a new medical specialty—intensive care specialists, or intensivists—showed that having such intensive care experts could reduce death rates. The study showed that having high numbers of intensivists was associated with lower hospital mortality and lower intensive care unit (ICU) mortality (Pronovost et al. 2002). The patients cared for by intensivists had reduced ICU and hospital death rates and lengths of stay. Health information management (HIM) practitioners— and anyone else who relies on statistical information—must remember that numbers count, not only in reports and records, but also in the human equation.

Death rate data also are important in helping public health agencies plan for health services. For example, the **Centers for Medicare and Medicaid Services (CMS)** publishes information on death rates among Medicare patients, specific ethnic groups, and patients in particular diagnosis categories, to name a few. The CMS is the division of the Department of Health and Human Services that is responsible for developing healthcare policy in the United States and for administering the Medicare program and the federal portion of the Medicaid program. CMS also publishes Hospital Compare at Medicare.gov that gives healthcare providers information about hospitals in their area, including death rates, which can be indicators of the quality of care given to patients. HIM practitioners must understand basic death rates and be ready to calculate or verify other data pertaining to mortality.

Guidelines for Calculating Death Rates

When calculating death rates, the following guidelines should be considered:

- Because death rates are ordinarily small, the calculation is usually carried out to three decimal places and rounded down to two places.
- Death is a type of discharge or **disposition**. Any data representing total discharges include deaths for that period. Thus, deaths are always assumed to be included in the total discharges in the denominator unless otherwise specified.
- If deaths of **newborn** inpatients are included in the numerator, all discharges of newborn inpatients must be included in the denominator. Ordinarily, newborns are included in the gross death rate unless a facility chooses to calculate their death rate separately.
- Patients who are **dead on arrival** (DOA) are not included in the gross death rate because DOAs are not admitted to the hospital.
- Patients who die in the emergency services department are not included in the gross death rate because they were not admitted to the hospital.
- Patients who die in the hospital while outpatients are not included in the gross death rate.

- **Fetal death** is the death of a product of human conception before its complete expulsion or extraction from the mother, regardless of the duration of the pregnancy; also called stillborn. Fetal deaths are not included in the hospital death rate but are often calculated separately. It is a good idea to put a zero in front of the decimal (for example, 0.23%) to show the casual observer that the rate is less than 1 percent.

Gross (Hospital) Death Rate

The **gross death rate** is defined as the number of inpatient deaths for a given period of time divided by the total number of live discharges and deaths for the same time period. A synonymous term for hospital death rate is **hospital death rate**.

When computing hospital death rates, the concept of number of occurrences versus number of times something could have occurred still applies. That is, every patient discharged from the hospital could possibly have died. Of course, this does not happen, but it is still a statistical possibility. Therefore, the formula for calculating the hospital death rate (gross death rate) is the number of patient deaths divided by the number of patient discharged alive and deaths, as shown:

$$\frac{Number\ of\ inpatient\ deaths\ (including\ NB)\ in\ a\ period\ \times 100}{Number\ of\ discharges\ (including\ A\&C\ and\ NB\ deaths)\ in\ the\ same\ period}$$

Example: If a hospital had seven deaths and 520 discharges for a month, the gross death rate would be

$$\frac{(7 \times 100)}{520} = 1.35\%$$

This concept can be explored more specifically by means of the formula referred to as the **case fatality rate**:

$$\frac{Number\ of\ people\ who\ die\ of\ a\ disease\ in\ a\ specified\ period\ \times 100}{Number\ of\ people\ who\ have\ the\ disease}$$

The case fatality rate is the total number of deaths due to a specific illness during a given time period divided by the total number of cases during the same period.

Using the example of patients with acute myocardial infarction, every patient discharged with the diagnosis of acute myocardial infarction has the potential to die. Thus, the formula is

$$\frac{Number\ of\ patients\ with\ acute\ myocardial\ infarction\ who\ died \times 100}{Number\ of\ patients\ discharged\ with\ a\ diagnosis\ of\ acute\ myocardial\ infarction}$$

If a hospital had 40 acute myocardial infarction discharges last year and eight deaths, the death rate would be

$$\frac{(8 \times 100)}{40} = 20.00\%$$

If 50 kidney transplant patients were discharged in the past year and two died, the calculation would be:

$$\frac{(2 \times 100)}{50} = 4.00\%$$

Example: The case fatality rate can be used to examine the death rates by physician. If Dr. Howard discharged 600 patients in the past year and 27 died, the formula would be:

$$\frac{(27 \times 100)}{600} = 4.50\%$$

Exercise 6.1

1. Using the data below, calculate the gross death rate at Community Hospital for May. Deaths are not included in the discharges. Round to two decimal places.

Community Hospital December 20XX Data	
Total adult and children live discharges	645
Total adult and children deaths	4
Total newborn live discharges	87
Total newborn deaths	1
Answer:	

2. The HIM professional reported to the quality improvement committee at Community Hospital that there were 58 patients with influenza discharged from the hospital in January. Of those, three died. What is the case fatality rate for influenza for January? Round to two decimal places.

3. Last year, University Hospital had 15 liver and pancreas transplants. Three patients died. What is the case fatality rate for this surgery at University Hospital? Round to two decimal places.

Exercise 6.2

The table below is a sample report for a hospital showing the discharges and deaths for the last quarter of the year. Notice that this report lists the patient discharges and deaths by physicians on the medical staff. Calculate the death rate for each physician and the total for this quarter. Deaths are not included in the discharges. Round to two decimal places.

Community Hospital October–December 20XX Discharges and Deaths—By Primary Care Physician			
Physician Number	**No. of Live Discharges**	**No. of Deaths**	**Gross Death Rate**
Dr. 097	12	3	
Dr. 123	204	4	
Dr. 256	12	1	
Dr. 372	92	4	
Dr. 431	124	6	
Dr. 537	79	2	
Dr. 638	107	4	
Dr. 725	85	3	
Dr. 800	100	1	
Dr. 901	158	8	
Total			

Tip: You may notice when computing your rates that sometimes your answer may be a whole number, such as 6 percent, or there may be a zero in the hundredths place as in 6.1 percent. When asked to compute to two decimal places, always add the zeros. Your answers would read 6.00 percent and 6.10 percent.

Net Death Rate

Various reporting or accrediting agencies sometimes request the **net death rate**, also referred to as the **institutional death rate**. Usually, adult, child, and newborn statistics are kept separately. However, when calculating the net death rate, newborn deaths are included in the inpatient deaths with the adult/children deaths. Historically, hospital inpatient deaths were classified as either those that occurred less than 48 hours after admission and those deaths that occurred 48 hours or more after admission.

The net death rate came into use because it was felt that healthcare providers should not be held accountable for a death that occurred less than 48 hours after admission because they would not have had enough time to directly affect the patient's condition; only emergency treatment could be provided during this period of time. However, with the technology available today, many authorities believe this concept is no longer valid. Regardless of this consideration, the net death rate excludes deaths under 48 hours and is less than the gross death rate.

The formula for calculating the net death rate is

$$\frac{Total\ number\ of\ inpatient\ deaths\ (including\ NB)\ minus\ deaths < 48\ hours\ for\ a\ given\ period \times 100}{Total\ number\ of\ discharges\ (including\ NB\ deaths)\ minus\ deaths < 48\ hours\ from\ the\ same\ period}$$

Example: Last month, Community Hospital had 255 discharges, including nine deaths. Three of the deaths were patients who were in the hospital less than 48 hours. The net death rate would be calculated as follows:

$$\frac{[(9-3)\times100]}{(255-3)} = \frac{600}{252} = 2.38\%$$

Exercise 6.3

Using the data in the table below, calculate the net death rate at Community Hospital for April. Discharges do not include deaths. Round to two decimal places.

Community Hospital April 20XX Deaths	
Total adult and children live discharges	409
Total adult and children deaths	7
Deaths < 48 hours	2
Deaths ≥ 48 hours	5
Total newborn live discharges	68
Total newborn deaths	2
Deaths < 48 hours	1
Deaths ≥ 48 hours	1
Answer:	

Exercise 6.4

Using the information in the table below, calculate the net death rate for each service and the total net death rate at Community Hospital for December. In this exercise deaths are included in the discharges. Round to two decimal places.

| | | Community Hospital December 20XX Deaths | | |
Service	No. of Discharges (includes Deaths)	Total Deaths	Deaths < 48 hours	Net Death Rate
Medicine	372	7	3	
Surgery	301	4	3	
Psychiatric	107	4	2	
Rehabilitation	74	6	3	
Total				

Postoperative Death Rate

The **postoperative death rate**, also called the **surgical death rate**, refers to the number of deaths occurring after an operation has been performed. Standard instructions for computing the postoperative death rate involve the ratio of deaths within 10 days after surgery to the total number of patients operated on during that period.

A **surgical operation** is defined as one or more surgical procedures performed at one time for one patient via a common approach or for a common purpose. A **surgical procedure** is any single, separate, systematic process upon or within the body that can be complete in itself; is normally performed by a physician, dentist, or other licensed practitioner; can be performed either with or without instruments; and is performed to restore disunited or deficient parts, remove diseased or injured tissues, extract foreign matter, assist in obstetrical delivery, or aid in diagnosis.

The formula for calculating the postoperative death rate is

$$\frac{Total\ number\ of\ deaths\ (within\ 10\ days\ after\ surgery) \times 100}{Total\ number\ of\ patients\ who\ were\ operated\ on\ for\ the\ period}$$

Some healthcare practitioners question the usefulness of this calculation in evaluating the effectiveness of a healthcare facility's medical care. Thus, rather than compute a total postoperative death rate, some hospitals evaluate the relationship of deaths following specific operations (for example, abdominal aortic aneurysm repair or coronary artery bypass grafts).

Tip: The standard formula for a rate applies here as well. All individuals who have surgery have the potential to die. The only difference here is that convention places a time limit of 10 days. After 10 days, concerns other than the surgery may cause the death of a patient. The denominator includes the patients operated on and not the number of operations because one patient may have several operations during a hospital stay.

Exercise 6.5

Using the information in the table below, calculate the postoperative death rate for each surgeon at Community Hospital during the semi-annual period of July through December. Round to two decimal places.

	Community Hospital July–December 20XX Number of Surgery Patients and Deaths, by Surgeon		
Physician Number	No. of Surgery Patients	No. of Deaths within 10 Days after Surgery	Postoperative Death Rate
Dr. 102	298	6	
Dr. 237	247	4	
Dr. 391	110	2	
Dr. 518	144	2	
Dr. 637	206	8	
Dr. 802	82	3	
Dr. 900	120	3	
Total			

Exercise 6.6

Using the information in the table that follows, calculate the postoperative death rate at Community Hospital during July. Round to two decimal places.

Community Hospital July 20XX Deaths Surgery Service	
Discharges (Does not include deaths)	483
Deaths	9
Within 10 days after surgery	5
More than 10 days after surgery	4
Number of operations	495
Number of patients operated on	480
Answer:	

Exercise 6.7

Using the information in the table below, calculate the postoperative death rate at Community Hospital for each MS-DRG listed for January through June and the total for this semiannual period. Round to two decimal places.

MS-DRG	MS-DRG Title	No. of Surgery Patients	No. of Deaths within 10 Days after Surgery	Postoperative Death Rate
	Community Hospital **January–June 20XX** **Selected MS-DRGs—Postoperative Deaths** **Number of Surgery Patients and Deaths** **Surgery Service**			
139	Salivary gland procedures	12	1	
217	Cardiac valve & oth maj cardiothoracic proc w card cath w CC	427	5	
239	Amputation for circ sys disorders exc upper limb & toe w MCC	8	2	
327	Stomach, esophageal & duodenal proc w CC	84	3	
338	Appendectomy w complicated principal diag w MCC	6	1	
405	Pancreas, liver & shunt procedures w MCC	62	4	
469	Major joint replacement or reattachment of lower extremity w MCC	212	3	
625	Thyroid, parathyroid & thyroglossal procedures w MCC	207	1	
652	Kidney transplant	27	4	
736	Uterine & adnexa proc for ovarian or adnexal malignancy w MCC	143	4	
Total				

Anesthesia Death Rate

The definition of **anesthesia death rate** is the ratio of deaths caused by anesthetic agents to the number of anesthetics administered during a specified period of time. Because anesthesia deaths occur so infrequently, some hospitals might choose, instead, to evaluate the relationship between a death and a specific type of anesthetic for a special study.

There are three major types of anesthesia: general, regional, and local. When general anesthesia is administered, the patient is unconscious and has no sensations. General anesthesia is given intravenously or inhaled. When regional anesthesia is given, the patient may be awake or may be sedated. Regional anesthetics remove the ability to feel any pain or sensations in a specific region of the body. A peripheral nerve block is a type of regional anesthetic that blocks pain and sensations around a specific nerve or group of nerves. These are often used on the hands, arms, feet, legs, or face. Spinal and epidural anesthesia are types of regional anesthesia and are used near the spinal cord and the spinal nerves and block pain and sensation in an entire region of the body, such as the abdomen, hips, or legs. Local anesthesia numbs a small area of the body. This involves an injection of an anesthetic, in this case, a numbing agent, placed directly into the area to block pain. During the procedure the patient may also receive medication to help him or her relax (WebMD 2014).

The formula for calculating the anesthesia death rate is:

$$\frac{Total\ deaths\ caused\ by\ anesthetic\ agents \times 100}{Total\ number\ of\ anesthetics\ administered}$$

Example: If anesthetics were given 2,000 times to surgical patients and one patient death was attributed to anesthesia during the past year, the anesthesia death rate would be computed as follows:

$$\frac{(1 \times 100)}{2,000} = \frac{100}{2,000} = 0.05\%$$

Tip: The fact that anesthesia deaths occur infrequently is reason to always check the placement of the decimal point in calculations of anesthesia death rates.

Exercise 6.8

Using the information in the table below, calculate the anesthesia death rate for University Hospital for January through June. Round to two decimal places.

University Hospital July–December 20XX Surgery Service	
Discharges (Does not include deaths)	2,642
Deaths:	59
Within 10 days	12
After 10 days	42
Number of operations	2,645
Number of patients operated on	2,636
Number of anesthetics administered	2,636
Number of deaths due to anesthetic agents	3
Answer:	

Exercise 6.9

Using the information in the table below, compute individually the number of deaths due to the administration of general, regional, and local anesthesia. Round to two decimal places.

University Hospital January–June 20XX Surgery Service	
Discharges (Does not include deaths)	2,642
Deaths	54
Within 10 days	12
After 10 days	42
Number of operations	2,645
Number of patients operated on	2,636

(continued on next page)

University Hospital January–June 20XX Surgery Service	
Number of anesthetics administered	2,636
General anesthesia	1,072
Regional anesthesia	1,017
Local anesthesia	547
Number of deaths due to anesthetic agents	7
General anesthesia	4
Regional anesthesia	2
Local anesthesia	1
Answers: General anesthesia:	
Regional anesthesia:	
Local anesthesia:	

Maternal Death Rate

A **maternal death** is defined as the death of any woman from any cause related to or aggravated by pregnancy or its management (regardless of duration or site of pregnancy, but not from accidental or incidental causes). An example of an accidental death would be a motor vehicle accident or a fall down a flight of stairs. An example of an incidental death would be a suicide or homicide.

Many healthcare facilities also differentiate between direct obstetrical deaths and indirect obstetrical deaths. A *direct obstetrical death* is a death directly related to the pregnancy, for example, a patient who died after a C-section because of a nick to the uterine artery that resulted in hemorrhage. An *indirect obstetrical death* is not directly due to obstetrical causes, even though the physiologic effects of the pregnancy are partially responsible for the death. An example of an indirect obstetrical death is diabetes. A pregnant woman can have **complications** of the diabetes that are aggravated by the pregnancy, but the cause of death is the diabetes and not the pregnancy. When computing the **maternal death rate**, hospitals usually classify only direct obstetrical deaths as maternal deaths and include only those deaths that occur during hospitalization. Nonmaternal deaths (deaths resulting from accidental or incidental causes not related to pregnancy or its management) are not included. A woman who dies after an abortion is considered a maternal death, as is an obstetrical patient who dies in the **prepartum** period (that is, the time period occurring before childbirth—some facilities refer to these as *antepartum* deaths) of a cause due to pregnancy. If the healthcare facility's service classification system includes a breakdown of obstetrical discharges into delivered, aborted, not delivered, and **postpartum** (the time after childbirth), all these should be included in the total obstetrical discharges in the denominator of the formula (and in the numerator if the mother dies).

The formula for calculating the maternal death rate is:

$$\frac{\textit{Number of direct maternal deaths for a period} \times 100}{\textit{Number of obstetrical discharges (including deaths) for the period}}$$

Example: At University Hospital, a mother died immediately after delivery. The hospital's annual obstetrics/gynecology discharges are classified as: delivered, 4,782; aborted, 97; not delivered (prepartum), 186; and postpartum, 46.

Please note in this example that some patients are divided into prepartum (not delivered) and postpartum cases. A patient who comes into the hospital in labor but does not deliver and is discharged home is considered a prepartum patient; a patient who comes into the hospital after delivery with an infection of the C-section incision site is considered a postpartum patient. A postpartum patient may be admitted to the hospital following her delivery for a variety of reasons such as hemorrhage or infection. When reporting this in obstetrical statistics, many hospitals will classify this as an "undelivered patient, postpartum" to distinguish these obstetrical patients from delivered patients.

The calculation of the hospital maternal mortality rate is:

$$\frac{(1 \times 100)}{(4,782 + 97 + 186 + 46)} = \frac{100}{5,111} = 0.02\%$$

Tip: The maternal death rate calculation is usually rounded to two places.

Computing Population Statistics for Maternal Mortality Rate

As noted in chapter 1, researchers frequently use vital statistics information for public health and policy studies. Researchers use a number other than 100 in the numerator because they are not interested in determining percentages but, rather, the number of times something occurs in the population. For example, researchers may use 100,000 to determine how often something occurred per 100,000 people, 10,000 to determine how often it occurred per 10,000 people, and so on.

The following vital statistics formula for maternal mortality rate may be used in the United States:

$$\frac{\textit{Number of deaths attributed to maternal conditions during a period} \times 100,000}{\textit{Number of births during the period}}$$

Example: During the year, a community hospital reported 1,307 **hospital live births** and two deaths after abortions. The vital statistics maternal mortality rate would be calculated as follows:

$$\frac{(2 \times 100,000)}{1,307} = \frac{200,000}{1,307} = 153.02 \text{ per } 100,000 \text{ births}$$

$$\frac{(2 \times 10,000)}{1,307} = \frac{20,000}{1,307} = 15.30 \text{ per } 10,000 \text{ births}$$

$$\frac{(2 \times 1,000)}{1,307} = \frac{2,000}{1,307} = 1.53 \text{ per } 1,000 \text{ births}$$

Exercise 6.10

Using the information in the table below, calculate Community Hospital's maternal death rate for May. These are all direct maternal deaths. Round to two decimal places.

Community Hospital May 20XX Obstetrical Unit	
Discharges (Does not include deaths)	
Delivered	227
Aborted	4
Undelivered, prepartum	32
Undelivered, postpartum	17
Deaths	
Delivered	1
Aborted	2
Undelivered, prepartum	1
Undelivered, postpartum	2
Answer:	

Exercise 6.11

Last month, The Women's Hospital reported 123 obstetrical discharges and five deaths. (The deaths are included in the discharges.) The causes of the five deaths were

- Injuries due to spousal abuse
- Injuries due to an automobile accident
- Suicide
- Hemorrhage after C-section due to severed uterine artery
- Pre-eclampsia

Calculate the direct maternal death rate for this hospital. Round to two decimal places.

Exercise 6.12

Using the annual statistics in the table below, calculate the maternal death rate and the abortion death rate for University Hospital. These are all direct maternal deaths. Deaths are included in the discharges. Round to two decimal places.

University Hospital Annual Statistics 20XX Obstetrical Service	
Discharges and Deaths	
Delivered	1,032
Aborted	57
Undelivered, prepartum	92
Undelivered, postpartum	85
Deaths:	
Delivered	3
Aborted	2
Undelivered, prepartum	1
Undelivered, postpartum	1
Answers:	
Maternal death rate:	
Abortion death rate:	

Another statistic that is used in the description of maternal deaths is one by the **World Health Organization (WHO)**. The WHO is an organization formed by the United Nations in 1948 and is the direct and coordinating authority on international health within the United Nations system. The WHO describes a maternal death as the death of a woman while pregnant or within 42 days of termination of pregnancy from any cause related to or aggravated by the pregnancy. It includes all pregnancies no matter the length of the pregnancy or the location (uterine or ectopic) of the pregnancy, except those deaths from accidental or incidental causes.

The formula for the WHO maternal mortality rate is as follows:

$$\frac{\textit{Number of maternal deaths} \times 100,000}{\textit{Number of live births}}$$

Exercise 6.13

In 2010 there were 3,999,386 live births in the United States (Martin et al. 2012). According to the Centers for Disease Control and Prevention there were 825 documented maternal deaths (CDC 2016) in the United States. What is the maternal mortality rate per 100,000 population? Calculate to the nearest whole number.

Newborn Death Rate

Statistical tabulations for vital events related to pregnancy and newborns can provide valuable information on reproductive health. They also can provide data on national and international trends.

Types of infant deaths and their definitions are discussed in table 6.1.

Table 6.1.   Definitions describing infant deaths

Type of Death	Definition
Newborn death	Death of a liveborn infant born in the hospital who later dies during the same admission
Neonatal death	Death of a liveborn infant within the **neonatal period** of 27 days, 23 hours, and 59 minutes from the moment of birth
Postneonatal death	Death of a liveborn infant from 28 days of birth to the end of the first year of life (through 364 days, 23 hours, 59 minutes from the moment of birth)
Infant death	Death of a liveborn infant at any time from the moment of birth to the end of the first year of life (through 364 days, 23 hours, 59 minutes from the moment of birth)
Perinatal death	An all-inclusive term referring to both stillborn infants and neonatal deaths

The formula for calculating the **newborn death rate** (also called the **newborn mortality rate**) is:

$$\frac{Total\ number\ of\ newborn\ deaths\ for\ a\ period \times 100}{Total\ number\ of\ newborn\ discharges\ (including\ deaths)\ for\ the\ period}$$

Tip: When computing newborn mortality rates, the answer should be rounded to two places. This is important because newborn death rates are usually very small. When healthcare facilities report discharges, they typically include deaths in the discharge figures because a death is a type of a discharge.

Example: If University Hospital had 2,567 newborn discharges and two newborn deaths in one year, its newborn mortality rate would be calculated as:

$$\frac{(2 \times 100)}{2,567} = \frac{200}{2,567} = 0.08\%$$

Computing Population Statistics for Neonatal and Infant Mortality Rates

Researchers frequently use birth certificate data for public health and policy studies. Similar vital statistics formulas are used in the United States. Following are two examples of vital statistics formulas.

Neonatal mortality rate formula:

$$\frac{Number\ of\ neonatal\ deaths\ during\ a\ period \times 1,000}{Number\ of\ live\ births\ during\ the\ period}$$

Infant mortality rate formula:

$$\frac{Number\ of\ infant\ deaths\ (neonatal\ and\ postneonatal)\ during\ a\ period \times 1,000}{Number\ of\ live\ births\ during\ the\ period}$$

Example: If a hospital had 4,270 births, three newborn deaths, and 4,269 newborn discharges, the vital statistics neonatal mortality rate would be calculated as follows:

$$\frac{(3 \times 1,000)}{4,270} = \frac{3,000}{4,270} = 0.70\ per\ 1,000$$

Exercise 6.14

1. Using the information in the table below, calculate Community Hospital's annual newborn death rate. In this exercise, the deaths are included in the discharges. Round to two decimal places.

Community Hospital Annual Statistics 20XX Newborn Service	
Births	487
Newborn deaths	3
Newborn discharges and deaths	486
Answer:	

2. Using the information in the table below, calculate the newborn death rate for April at Community Hospital. In this exercise, the deaths are included in the discharges. Round to two decimal places.

Community Hospital Newborn Unit April 20XX	
Births	52
Discharges and deaths	52
Deaths	2
Answer:	

3. In 2013, there were 15,867 neonatal deaths in the United States while there were 3,932,181 live births during the same year (CDC 2013). What is the neonatal mortality rate per 10,000 population? Round to a whole number.

Fetal Death Rate

A hospital fetal death is defined as a death prior to the complete expulsion or extraction from the mother (in a hospital facility) of a product of human conception (fetus and placenta) regardless of the duration of pregnancy. The death is indicated by the fact that after such expulsion or extraction, the fetus does not breathe or show any other evidence of life (for example, beating of the heart, pulsation of the umbilical cord, or definite movement of voluntary muscles). Typically, hospitals are required to report fetal deaths to a state agency. However, the reporting method varies according to individual state laws, statutes, and regulations.

Because fetal deaths are not considered patient deaths, they are not included in any other calculation of deaths but, instead, are calculated separately. Determination of whether to include fetal death data in a specific hospital's statistics requires an investigation of the facility's needs by hospital administration, medical staff, and reporting agencies. Fetal deaths are classified as listed in table 6.2.

Both intermediate and late fetal deaths constitute what is commonly termed a **stillbirth**. The formula for calculating the **fetal death rate** is:

$$\frac{\textit{Total number of intermediate and/or late fetal deaths for a period} \times 100}{\textit{Total number of live births} + \textit{Intermediate and late fetal deaths for the period}}$$

Example: During November, a hospital had 207 live births, one early fetal death, two intermediate fetal deaths, and three late fetal deaths. To determine the fetal death rate for the hospital, the total number of intermediate and late fetal deaths (5) is multiplied by 100 and divided by the total number of live births and the intermediate and late fetal deaths (207 + 5). The calculation is as follows:

$$\frac{(5 \times 100)}{(207 + 5)} = \frac{500}{212} = 2.36\%$$

Tip: Keep in mind that the denominator in the fetal death rate formula does not include discharges. If you remember the formula for rates discussed in chapter 2, that is, the number of times something actually happened in relation to the number of times it could have happened, it becomes clear that every birth could be a fetal death. And, be sure to include the intermediate and late fetal deaths in the denominator. This is an exception to the general rule of using discharges in the denominator for death statistics.

Table 6.3 lists the calculations of hospital-based mortality rates.

Table 6.2. Classifications of fetal death

Classification	Length of Gestation	Weight
Early fetal death	Less than 20 weeks gestation	500 grams or less
Intermediate fetal death	20 weeks completed gestation, but less than 28 weeks	501 to 1,000 grams
Late fetal death	28 weeks completed gestation	Over 1,000 grams

Table 6.3. Calculation of hospital-based mortality rates

Rate	Numerator	Denominator
Gross death rate (Hospital death rate)	Total number of inpatient deaths, including NBs, for a given period × 100	Total number of discharges, including A&C and NB deaths, for the same period
Net death rate (Institutional death rate)	Total number of inpatient deaths, including NBs, minus deaths < 48 hours for a given period × 100	Total number of discharges, including A&C and NB deaths, minus deaths < 48 hours for the same period
Postoperative death rate	Total number of deaths within 10 days after surgery for a given period × 100	Total number of patients operated on for the same period
Anesthesia death rate	Total number of deaths caused by anesthesia agents for a given period × 100	Total number of anesthetics administered for the same period
Maternal death rate	Total number of direct maternal deaths for a given period × 100	Total number of maternal (obstetrical) discharges, including deaths, for the same period
Newborn death rate	Total number NB deaths for a given period × 100	Total number of NB discharges, including deaths, for the same period
Fetal death rate	Total number of intermediate and late fetal deaths for a given period × 100	Total number of live births plus total number of intermediate and late fetal deaths for the same period

Tip: Remember that newborn births are the same as newborn admissions.

Exercise 6.15

Community Hospital reported the following statistics for the month of February. Calculate the fetal death rate. Round to two decimal places.

Community Hospital February 20XX Newborn Service	
Live births	37
Newborn discharges and deaths	36
Fetal deaths:	
Early	1
Intermediate	4
Late	3
Answer:	

Exercise 6.16

Using the information in the table below, calculate the newborn mortality rate and fetal death rate at Community Hospital for the year. In this exercise, deaths are included in the discharges. Round to two decimal places.

Community Hospital January–December 20XX Newborn Service	
Live births	307
Newborn discharges and deaths	306
Newborn deaths	3

(*continued on next page*)

Community Hospital January–December 20XX Newborn Service	
Fetal deaths:	
Early	5
Intermediate	4
Late	2
Answers:	
Newborn death rate:	
Fetal death rate:	

Cancer Mortality Rate

A **mortality rate** measures the risk of death for the cause under study in a defined population during a given time period. The cancer mortality rate is the proportion of patients who die from cancer. The National Center for Health Statistics collects data on all cancer deaths occurring in the United States and classifies them by sex, age, race, and cancer site so that mortality for a given time period can be determined for the entire country or selected areas (Shambaugh et al. 1994).

The formula for calculating the **cancer mortality rate** for a population is

$$\frac{Number\ of\ cancer\ deaths\ during\ a\ period \times 100,000}{Total\ number\ in\ population\ at\ risk}$$

Example: In 2013, 584,881 people died from cancer in the United States. The estimated 2013 census for the US population was 316,094,000 (US Census Bureau 2013). The formula for calculating the cancer mortality rate per 100,000 people in 2013 would be:

$$\frac{Number\ of\ cancer\ deaths\ in\ 2013}{Population\ at\ risk}$$

Using the statistics provided here, the calculation is

$$\frac{584,881 \times 100,000}{314,094,000} = \frac{58,488,100,000}{314,094,000} = 185.0 \text{ deaths from cancer per 100,000 population}$$

This is a **crude death rate** because it encompasses deaths in a given population for a given period of time frame divided by the estimated population for the same period of time. In other words, it is based on the entire US population. One can calculate specific rates for the risk of a particular cancer occurring in a population or its subgroups, such as a particular age group or sex.

Knowledge of healthcare statistics is an essential tool for cancer registrars. A **cancer registrar** is an individual who is responsible for maintaining a complete summary of the history, diagnosis, treatment, and disease status for every cancer patient seen in the healthcare facility. Hospital cancer registries were developed as organized programs in hospitals to collect information about cancer patients. Their primary goal is to help improve treatment of cancer through various methods, including comparing different types of therapies used to treat cancer. The American College of Surgeons Commission on Cancer offers the opportunity for hospitals and treatment centers to become accredited. Accurate cancer data is vital to the fight against cancer, and cancer registrars are critical to capturing that data. Hospital and other cancer registry data are reported to population-based (central or regional) registries.

When you are calculating the cancer death rate in your own facility, use the formula for a rate—that is the number of deaths from a specific diagnosis of cancer divided by the number of discharges of that same diagnosis of cancer.

For example, Community Hospital had five cases of prostate cancer patients who died last year. There were a total of 189 prostate cancer patients discharged in the same time period. The rate of prostate cancer deaths was 2.65%.

$$\frac{(5 \times 100)}{189} = \frac{500}{189} = 2.65\%$$

Exercise 6.17

Using the information given in the table below from Community Hospital's Cancer Registry, calculate the death rates for each type of cancer and the total for this annual period. Deaths are included in the discharges. Round to two decimal places.

Community Hospital Cancer Registry Annual Report Selected Cancers Reported 20XX			
Type of Cancer	No. of Discharges and Deaths	No. of Deaths	Cancer Death Rate
Breast	311	15	
Prostate	208	17	
Digestive System	102	13	
Lung and bronchus	162	12	

(continued on next page)

Community Hospital Cancer Registry Annual Report Selected Cancers Reported 20XX			
Type of Cancer	No. of Discharges and Deaths	No. of Deaths	Cancer Death Rate
Urinary System	98	13	
Female Reproductive	48	3	
Melanoma of the skin	21	14	
All other sites	215	52	
Total			

Exercise 6.18

Using the statistics in the table below from a multihospital system, calculate the cancer death rate for each hospital listed and for the entire healthcare system. In this exercise, the deaths are included in the discharges. Round to two decimal places.

Community Healthcare System Annual Statistics 20XX			
Hospital	No. of Cancer Discharges and Deaths	No. of Cancer Deaths	Cancer Death Rate
Urban Hospital	15,634	207	
Rural Hospital	6,203	154	
Suburban Hospital	2,073	58	
Total			

Exercise 6.19

Using the information in the table below, calculate the death rates for University Hospital's Cancer Registry for each of the cancers reported and the total for this annual period. In this exercise, the deaths are included in the discharges. Round to two decimal places.

Type of Cancer	No. of Discharges and Deaths	No. of Deaths	Death Rate
University Hospital **Cancer Registry Annual Report** **Selected Cancers Reported** **20XX**			
Oral Cavity and Pharynx	24	1	
Digestive System	198	5	
Respiratory System	242	16	
Bone and Joint	218	4	
Skin (excludes Basal Cell)	34	1	
Breast	190	12	
Female Genital System	47	8	
Male Genital System	228	25	
Urinary System	77	7	
Brain and Other Nervous System	42	19	
Endocrine System	28	1	
Lymphoma	47	6	
Myeloma	25	2	
Leukemia	15	4	
Total			

Chapter 6   Matching Quiz

Match the definition with the terms.

Definitions

a. The number of inpatient deaths that occurred during a given time period divided by the total number of inpatient discharges, including deaths, for the same time period

b. The ratio of deaths within 10 days after surgery to the total number of operations performed during a specified period of time

c. The death of a product of human conception that is fewer than 20 weeks of gestation and 500 grams or less in weight before its complete expulsion or extraction from the mother

d. An all-inclusive term that refers to both stillbirths and neonatal deaths

e. An inpatient who was born in a hospital at the beginning of the current inpatient hospitalization

f. Occurring after childbirth

g. A medical condition that arises during an inpatient hospitalization

h. A term referring to the incidence of death in a specific population

i. The number of newborns who died divided by the total number of newborns, both alive and dead

j. The total number of inpatient deaths minus the number of deaths that occurred less than 48 hours after admission for a given time period divided by the total number of inpatient discharges minus the number of deaths that occurred less than 48 hours after admission for the same time period

Terms:

1. _____ Complication		**6.** _____ Gross death rate
2. _____ Postpartum		**7.** _____ Newborn
3. _____ Newborn death rate		**8.** _____ Postoperative death rate
4. _____ Perinatal death		**9.** _____ Mortality
5. _____ Net death rate		**10.** _____ Early fetal death

Chapter 6   Review

Using the data reported below for the past year, perform the calculations requested below for questions 1 through 10. Round these to two decimal places.

Community Hospital Mortality Report Annual Statistics				
Discharges (includes deaths)		Deaths	
Total adults and children	13,954	Total adults and children	48
Total newborns	1,965	Total newborns	1
The following are included in the discharges:		The following are included in the deaths:	
OB delivered	1,971	Within 10 days postop	3
OB aborted	120	< 48 hours after admission	14

(continued on next page)

Community Hospital Mortality Report Annual Statistics			
OB undelivered, prepartum	27	≥ 48 hours after admission	34
OB undelivered, postpartum	23	Anesthetic death	1
The following are included in the discharges:		Obstetrical deaths:	
Medicine Service Discharges	7,678	Undelivered, prepartum	1
Surgery Service Discharges	4,165	Aborted	1
Patients discharged with a primary diagnosis of cancer	565	Medicine Service Deaths	41
		Surgery Service Deaths	5
		Cancer Deaths	53
		Fetal deaths:	
		Early	5
		Intermediate	4
		Late	3
Admissions			
Total adults and children	14,023	Total patients operated on	4,165
Total live births	1,964	Total anesthetics administered	4,165

1. What is the gross death rate?
   a. 0.030%
   b. 0.31%
   c. 3.10%
   d. 3.11%

2. What is the net death rate?
   a. 0.22%
   b. 2.20%
   c. 0.022%
   d. 22.00%

3. What is the postoperative death rate?
    a. 0.007%
    b. 0.07%
    c. 7.70%
    d. 77.02%

4. What is the anesthesia death rate?
    a. 0.002%
    b. 0.24%
    c. 0.02%
    d. 2.24%

5. What is the maternal death rate?
    a. 0.009%
    b. 0.93%
    c. 0.09%
    d. 9.34%

6. What is the newborn death rate?
    a. 0.05%
    b. 0.50%
    c. 5.08%
    d. 5.10%

7. What is the fetal death rate?
    a. 0.03%
    b. 0.04%
    c. 0.36%
    d. 3.55%

8. What is the death rate for the medicine service?
    a. 0.05%
    b. 0.53%
    c. 5.33%
    d. 5.34%

9. What is the death rate for the surgery service?
    a. 0.12%
    b. 1.20%
    c. 12.00%
    d. 12.04%

10. What is the cancer death rate?
    a. 0.01%
    b. 0.09%
    c. 9.30%
    d. 9.38%

11. Which of the following deaths is also called the institutional death rate?
  a. Crude death rate
  b. Gross death rate
  c. Net death rate
  d. Postoperative death rate

12. Your hospital's cancer registry reported 287 deaths to cancer patients with 3,821 discharges of patients with a primary diagnosis of cancer. What is the cancer death rate?
  a. 0.75%
  b. 7.50%
  c. 7.51%
  d. 75.11%

Use the information in the table below to answer questions 13 through 15. In these exercises, the deaths are included in the discharges; this includes deaths occurring in less than 48 hours and postoperative deaths.

Community Hospital Annual Statistics 20XX				
Service	Discharges	Deaths	<48 hours	Postop
Medicine	1,478	92	8	0
Surgery	1,385	25	10	2
Obstetrics	751	1	0	0
Newborn	753	1	1	0
Psychiatric	486	2	0	0
Rehabilitation	362	22	1	0
Total				
Additional Information				
Anesthetics administered			1,386	
Anesthetic deaths			1	
Patients operated on			1,385	
Total livebirths			753	
Fetal deaths:				
Early			5	
Intermediate			5	
Late			1	

13. What is the gross death rate for the Rehabilitation Service?
    a. 0.67%
    b. 0.68%
    c. 6.07%
    d. 6.08%

14. What is the total hospital net death rate?
    a. 0.24%
    b. 2.36%
    c. 2.37%
    d. 2.74%

15. What is the postoperative death rate?
    a. 0.14%
    b. 1.44%
    c. 14.10%
    d. 14.44%

Hospital Autopsies and Autopsy Rates

Learning Objectives

At the conclusion of this chapter, you should be able to

- Identify alternate terms for autopsy
- Recognize a coroner's case and determine when it would be included in a hospital's autopsy rate
- Calculate the following autopsy rates: gross, net, adjusted hospital, newborn, and fetal
- Utilize software to complete spreadsheets

Key Terms

Adjusted hospital autopsy
  rate
Autopsy
Autopsy rate
Available for hospital
  autopsy
Coroner
Coroner's case

Emergency services
  department
Fetal autopsy rate
Gross autopsy rate
Home healthcare
Hospice
Hospital autopsy
Hospital autopsy rate

Hospital inpatient autopsy
Medical examiner
Morgue
Necropsy
Net autopsy rate
Newborn autopsy rate
Postmortem examination

An **autopsy** is the examination of a dead body to determine the cause of death. Autopsies can confirm or disprove a diagnosis or cause of death. The practice of autopsies has contributed to medical science by correlating changes in organs and tissues with the patient's symptoms. They also support the quality of care provided. Lawsuits are less frequent in cases when the patient was autopsied because the care given can usually be substantiated by the results of the autopsy. An autopsy can be performed on the entire body or a particular body organ.

    Another name for autopsy is **necropsy** or **postmortem** (after death) **examination**. Autopsies are generally performed by either a hospital pathologist or a physician on the medical staff who has been delegated this responsibility. They are usually performed in the hospital **morgue**, but in the case of small hospitals that do not have a morgue, the body may be removed to an off-site lab or a funeral home for the autopsy. Autopsies are classified as *clinical* or *forensic*. A clinical autopsy is one in which permission is granted by the next of kin while a forensic autopsy, on the other hand, is one in which a legal representative has ordered an autopsy to be performed.

Autopsy Rates

The rate of autopsy has declined substantially over the years. It is estimated that before 1972 the autopsy rate was 40 to 60 percent, but by 2003 the rate had decreased to 8.1 percent. Autopsies generally increase when the physician is unable to determine the cause of death, in cases of heart disease and cancer, or when there are external causes of the death. Autopsies are also more generally performed on patients under the age of 25. Disease conditions are usually the cause of death in older patients and they are not ordinarily autopsied (National center for Health Statistics 2011).

Gross Autopsy Rate

The **autopsy rate** is the proportion of deaths that are followed by the performance of an autopsy. A **gross autopsy rate** is the ratio of all inpatient autopsies to all inpatient deaths during any given period of time. Outpatients are considered in other autopsy formulas. The rate is customarily reported as a percentage. Again, the concept of a rate applies here: the number of times something actually happened compared with the number of times it could have happened. Statistically speaking, every patient who dies could be autopsied. Typically, newborn autopsies are included in the gross autopsy rate but may be calculated separately as determined by the hospital's administration or medical staff committee.

The formula for calculating the gross autopsy rate is

$$\frac{Total\ autopsies\ on\ inpatient\ deaths\ for\ a\ period \times 100}{Total\ inpatient\ deaths\ for\ the\ period}$$

Example: During January, University Hospital discharged 1,027 patients. The hospital had 32 deaths (including newborns) and performed 11 autopsies. Using the formula given above, the gross autopsy rate is determined to be 34.38 percent, as follows:

$$\frac{(11 \times 100)}{32} = \frac{1,100}{32} = 34.38\%$$

Tip: Although death rates are usually small, autopsy rates can be fairly large.

Exercise 7.1

1. True or false? In a one-month period, a 300-bed hospital with 20 bassinets reported 18 inpatient deaths. The medical staff performed 6 autopsies. The gross autopsy rate is 32.50 percent.

2. In January, Community Hospital had 185 discharges, 9 deaths, and 2 autopsies. What is the gross autopsy rate? Round to two decimal places.

3. During the last semiannual period, University Hospital had 6,234 discharges, 18 deaths, and 15 autopsies. What is their gross autopsy rate? Round to two decimal places.

Exercise 7.2

Using the information in the following table, calculate the gross death rate, the net death rate, and the gross autopsy rate for Community Hospital for the time period. Round to two decimal places.

Community Hospital Hospital Statistics July–December 20XX	
Total inpatient discharges (including deaths)	724
Total inpatient deaths	19
(<48 hours—included in total inpatient deaths)	(3)
Total autopsies	6
Answers:	
Gross death rate:	
Net death rate:	
Gross autopsy rate:	

Net Autopsy Rate

The **net autopsy rate** is the ratio during any given period of time of all inpatient autopsies to all inpatient deaths, minus any unautopsied coroners' cases. The formula for net autopsy rate differs slightly from the formula for gross autopsy rate in that it excludes bodies that have been removed by the coroner. Because the body has been removed from the hospital it is not considered in this rate.

Certain types of deaths are reportable to the coroner of a particular jurisdiction. A **coroner** is the official (elected or appointed, physician or nonphysician) who is responsible for determining the cause, time, and manner of death in unattended, violent, or unexplained deaths, or in cases in which a law may have been broken. Coroners may also have other duties depending on their state.

In some areas of the country, the coroner has been replaced with a **medical examiner**. The medical examiner is usually an appointed official who is a physician, commonly holding a specialty in pathology or forensic medicine. Large metropolitan areas usually have a forensic pathologist who acts as the coroner and performs the postmortem examination. In smaller areas, the coroner may be a physician practicing in the community who is not trained as a pathologist. It may also be a mortician or sheriff who is also serving as the coroner. A body released to a coroner or medical examiner is not available for autopsy by the hospital pathologist.

The formula for calculating the net autopsy rate is

$$\frac{\textit{Total autopsies on inpatient deaths for a period} \times 100}{\textit{Total inpatient deaths} - \textit{Unautopsied coroners' or medical examiners' cases}}$$

Example: During April, Community Hospital had 14 patient deaths and performed 3 autopsies. One body was released to the county coroner for autopsy. Therefore, one case is subtracted from the denominator because it was not autopsied by the hospital. Dividing the number of inpatient autopsies performed (3) by the total number of bodies available for autopsy (14 − 1 = 13) produces a net autopsy rate of 23.08 percent, as shown in the equation here.

$$\frac{(3 \times 100)}{(14 - 1)} = \frac{300}{13} = 23.08\%$$

Tip: If the coroner or medical examiner requests the hospital pathologist perform the autopsy, it is included in the rate and not subtracted out because the case would not be unavailable for autopsy.

Exercise 7.3

Over the past year, University Hospital had 18,251 discharges (includes deaths), 267 inpatient deaths, and 170 autopsies. The bodies of 20 patients were released to the medical examiner for autopsy. Calculate the gross death, gross autopsy, and net autopsy rates for University Hospital. Round to two decimal places.

Answers:
Gross death rate:
Gross autopsy rate:
Net autopsy rate:

Tip: The net autopsy rate will be higher than the gross autopsy rate because the denominator includes unautopsied coroners' or medical examiners' cases. Because there is a lower number of autopsies in the denominator, the rate will be higher.

Exercise 7.4

Using the information in the table below, calculate the gross death, gross autopsy, and net autopsy rates for University Hospital. In this exercise, the deaths are included in the discharges. Round to two decimal places.

Community Hospital Quarterly Statistics April–June 20XX	
Discharges and Deaths:	
Adults and children	1,080
Newborn	270
Deaths:	
Adults and children	33
Newborn	2
Inpatient autopsies	12
Coroner's cases (unavailable for autopsy)	3

(continued on next page)

Community Hospital Quarterly Statistics April–June 20XX
Answers: Gross death rate:
Gross autopsy rate:
Net autopsy rate:

Exercise 7.5

Create an electronic spreadsheet by entering the information from the following worksheet. Once the information is entered, complete the spreadsheet by entering the formulas to complete the columns and calculate the gross death, gross autopsy, and net autopsy rates for each month and the year for University Hospital. In this exercise, the deaths are included in the discharges. Round to two decimal places.

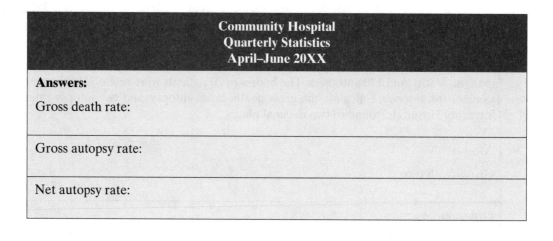

University Hospital Annual Statistics 20XX							
Month	Discharges	Inpatient Deaths	Autopsies	Coroner's Cases	Gross Death Rate	Gross Autopsy Rate	Net Autopsy Rate
January	598	5	2	1			
February	587	6	2	2			
March	607	7	5	1			
April	624	5	1	0			
May	620	6	2	1			
June	599	7	3	2			
July	609	9	5	2			
August	575	5	2	0			
September	611	7	3	1			
October	578	8	4	1			
November	622	6	2	0			
December	572	7	2	2			
Total							

Hospital Autopsies

A **hospital inpatient autopsy** is the postmortem examination that is ordinarily performed in a hospital facility on the body of an inpatient who died during hospitalization. In contrast, a **hospital autopsy** is the postmortem examination of the body of a person who has *at some time* been a hospital patient. Former inpatients may include emergency patients, outpatients, and home care patients.

When determining what autopsies to include in the **hospital autopsy rate**, the following guidelines apply:

- Hospital autopsies are usually performed by the healthcare facility pathologist. However, small hospitals do not always have a pathologist on staff, so responsibility for performing autopsies may be delegated to another physician.

- Normally, hospital autopsies are performed in hospitals. However, a small hospital or a specialty hospital (for example, obstetrical or psychiatric) may not have many deaths and thus may not be equipped with the necessary facilities to perform autopsies. In such cases, the autopsies are performed in another designated place.

- As a general rule, hospital autopsies are performed on inpatients who have died. However, because of the educational value of autopsies, former inpatients who were not in the hospital at the time of death may be considered for hospital autopsies. These individuals may include **emergency services department (ESD)** patients, outpatients, and **home health care** or **hospice** deaths. This is the only case where outpatients are included with inpatient statistics.

    ○ ESD patients are those who are admitted to the emergency services department of a hospital for the diagnosis and treatment of a condition that requires immediate medical, dental, or allied health services in order to sustain life or to prevent critical consequences.

    ○ Outpatients are those who receive ambulatory care services in a hospital-based clinic or department.

    ○ Home health care patients are those who receive care within their own home provided by a home health agency.

    ○ Hospice patients are those who are receiving an interdisciplinary program of palliative care and supportive services that addresses the physical, spiritual, social, and economic needs of terminally ill patients and their families.

- Fetal autopsies are not included in the hospital autopsy rate because a fetus is not considered a patient.

- The essential components for a hospital autopsy are the following:

    ○ The autopsy must be performed by a staff pathologist or a designated physician.

    ○ There must be a consent from the patient's next of kin or legal representative to perform an autopsy, which is filed in the patient's health record. The consent may be for a full body autopsy or a partial autopsy.

    ○ The autopsy report must be filed in the patient's health record.

    ○ The tissue specimens must be filed in the hospital laboratory along with the autopsy report.

Examples of hospital autopsy cases include:

- A patient dies in the hospital and is autopsied by the hospital's pathologist in the local morgue.
- A patient dies in the hospital, and one of the hospital's physicians is designated to perform the autopsy in the absence of the staff pathologist.
- A former patient is pronounced dead on arrival in the hospital's ESD, and the staff pathologist performs the autopsy.

Adjusted Hospital Autopsy Rate

The **adjusted hospital autopsy rate** is the proportion of hospital autopsies performed following the deaths of patients whose bodies are available for autopsy. Although many hospitals calculate the net autopsy rate for various surveys and external reports, the adjusted hospital autopsy rate is a more accurate indication of the hospital's resources for physician education because it includes all autopsies.

The formula for calculating the adjusted hospital autopsy rate is

$$\frac{Total\ hospital\ autopsies \times 100}{Total\ number\ of\ deaths\ of\ hospital\ patients\ whose\ bodies\ are\ available\ for\ autopsy}$$

Patients whose bodies are **available for hospital autopsy** are deceased patients who have, at some point, been a hospital patient. These patients include

- Inpatients (unless the bodies are removed from the hospital by legal authorities such as the coroner or medical examiner). However, if the hospital pathologist or designated physician performs an autopsy while acting as an agent of the coroner or medical examiner, the autopsy is included in the numerator and the death in the denominator of the adjusted hospital autopsy rate formula.
- Other patients, including hospital home care patients, outpatients, and previous hospital patients who have died elsewhere and whose bodies have been made available for the performance of a hospital autopsy.

Example: Community Hospital had 260 discharges in June; seven were deaths. The hospital pathologist performed three of the autopsies. During this period, two home care patients and one outpatient died and were brought to the hospital for autopsy. To determine the adjusted hospital autopsy rate, add all the hospital autopsies performed to determine the numerator (3 inpatients + 2 home care patients + 1 outpatient). The denominator contains all the patients whose bodies were available for autopsy. This includes the seven inpatients, two home care patients, and one outpatient who died in June (7 + 2 + 1).

$$\frac{[(3+2+1) \times 100]}{(7+2+1)} = \frac{600}{10} = 60.00\%$$

Tip: In the previous formulas, outpatients, ESD patients, and home health care patients were not included with the inpatients. When calculating the adjusted hospital autopsy rate, the outpatients, ESD patients, and home care patients would be included if their bodies were autopsied by the hospital pathologist.

Exercise 7.6

During the last quarter, Community Hospital had 22 inpatient deaths, 7 of whom were autopsied. Two of the 22 deaths were coroner's cases, but one was autopsied by the hospital pathologist (included in the seven). In addition, the following bodies were brought to the hospital for autopsy: two former patients who died in the ER, one former inpatient who died in a skilled nursing facility, two former inpatients who died at home, and one patient who died during a round of outpatient chemotherapy. What is the adjusted hospital autopsy rate? Round to two decimal places.

Exercise 7.7

Which of the following represents a hospital autopsy? Select as many as apply:

a. A former inpatient died at home a month after discharge from the hospital, and his body was brought to the hospital for autopsy.

b. The coroner authorized the hospital pathologist to perform an autopsy on a patient who died in the ESD after a car accident.

c. A patient who had been receiving radiation therapy on an outpatient basis at the hospital died at home; her body was brought to the hospital for autopsy.

d. A victim of gunshot wounds who died in the ESD was autopsied by the medical examiner.

e. A cardiac patient died in the ESD, and the hospital pathologist performed the autopsy.

f. The hospital pathologist designated a physician to cover for her while she was away. The physician performed an autopsy on a deceased hospital inpatient.

g. A late fetal death (stillbirth) was autopsied by the hospital pathologist.

Exercise 7.8

Using the information in the following table, calculate the gross death, gross autopsy, net autopsy, and adjusted hospital autopsy rates for University Hospital. In this exercise, the deaths are included in the discharges. Round to two decimal places.

University Hospital Annual Statistics 20XX	
Discharges and Deaths:	
Adults and children	14,892
Newborn	5,223
Deaths:	
Adults and children	362
Newborn	4
Deaths in the ESD and OPD*	12
Autopsies:	
Inpatient	97
ESD/OPD	12
Coroner's cases (unavailable for autopsy)	6
Answers:	
Gross death rate:	
Gross autopsy rate:	
Net autopsy rate:	
Adjusted hospital autopsy rate:	
*ESD = Emergency Services department; OPD = Outpatient department	

Exercise 7.9

Using the information in the following table, calculate the adjusted hospital autopsy rate. Round to two decimal places.

Community Hospital September 20XX Statistics	
Deaths	
Inpatient deaths	12
ESD deaths	2
Home health death	1
Autopsies	
Inpatient autopsies	3
ESD autopsy	2
Home health autopsy	1
Coroner's case (unavailable for autopsy)	2
Answer:	
Adjusted hospital autopsy rate:	

Exercise 7.10

During the first quarter of 20XX, Community Hospital had 24 inpatient deaths, six of whom were autopsied. Of the 24 deaths, two were coroner's cases—one of whom was autopsied by the hospital pathologist (included in the six autopsies) and one removed to be autopsied by the coroner. Additionally, these were also autopsied: one patient who died in the hospital's skilled nursing facility two days after discharge from the hospital, a patient who died in the ESD after a motor vehicle accident, one outpatient who died in the physical therapy department after a fall, and a former patient who died at home while under the care of the hospital's hospice department. Calculate the adjusted hospital rate for Community Hospital for this quarter. Round to two decimal places.

Adjusted hospital rate: _____

Newborn Autopsy Rate

The **newborn autopsy rate** is the proportion of hospital autopsies performed following the deaths of newborns.

The formula for calculating the newborn autopsy rate is

$$\frac{Newborn\ autopsies\ for\ a\ period \times 100}{Total\ newborn\ deaths\ for\ the\ period}$$

Example: Community Hospital had 33 births during the month of June with two newborn deaths. One of the newborns died shortly after birth and was autopsied. Applying the preceding formula, the correct newborn autopsy rate is 50.00 percent.

$$\frac{(1 \times 100)}{2} = \frac{100}{2} = 50.00\%$$

Exercise 7.11

Using the information in the table below, calculate the newborn death rate and the newborn autopsy rate for Community Hospital. In this exercise, the deaths are included in the discharges. Round to two decimal places.

Community Hospital Newborn Statistics January–June 20XX	
Births	210
Discharges and Deaths	208
Deaths	4
Autopsies	3
Answers:	
Newborn death rate:	
Newborn autopsy rate:	

Exercise 7.12

In November 20XX, the newborn unit at Community Hospital reported three stillbirths and two newborn deaths. An autopsy was performed on one of the newborns and two stillbirths. Calculate the newborn autopsy rate for November. Round to two decimal places.

Rate to calculate	Answer
Newborn autopsy rate	

Exercise 7.13

University Hospital reported the following semiannual statistics for January–June 20XX: 966 newborn discharges, five of these were newborn deaths. There were two newborn autopsies. One newborn was born in a taxi on the way to the hospital, was admitted, and later died. It was autopsied. One newborn was born at home and brought to the hospital and admitted. It also died and was autopsied. Calculate University Hospital's newborn death rate and newborn autopsy rate. In this exercise, the deaths are included in the discharges. Round to two decimal places.

Rates to calculate	Answers
Newborn death rate	
Newborn autopsy rate	

Tip: Remember that a newborn is an inpatient who was born in a hospital at the beginning of the current inpatient hospitalizations. A newborn born outside the hospital and then admitted is considered a pediatric admission.

Fetal Autopsy Rate

The **fetal autopsy rate** is the proportion of hospital autopsies performed following the deaths of intermediate and late fetal deaths.

The formula for the fetal autopsy rate is:

$$\frac{\textit{Autopsies performed on intermediate and late fetal deaths for a period} \times 100}{\textit{Total intermediate and late fetal deaths for the same period}}$$

Example: University Hospital newborn service reported 10 fetal deaths last quarter: two early, six intermediate, and two late. Of these, the two late fetal deaths and one intermediate fetal death were autopsied. Applying the formula above, the fetal autopsy rate for this hospital is 37.50 percent.

$$\frac{[(2 \ \textit{late fetal death autopsies} + 1 \ \textit{intermediate fetal death}) \times 100]}{(6 + 2)} = \frac{300}{8} = 37.50\%$$

Table 7.1 lists the calculations for autopsy rates.

Table 7.1.   Calculation of autopsy rates

Rate	Numerator	Denominator
Gross autopsy rate	Total number of autopsies on inpatient deaths for a given period × 100	Total number of inpatient death for the same period
Net autopsy rate	Total number of autopsies on inpatient deaths for a given period × 100	Total number of inpatient deaths minus unautopsied coroner or medical examiner cases for the same period
Adjusted hospital autopsy rate	Total number of hospital autopsies for a given period × 100	Total number of deaths of hospital patients whose bodies are available for autopsy
NB autopsy rate	Total number of autopsies on NB deaths for a given period × 100	Total number of NB deaths for the same period
Fetal autopsy rate	Total number of autopsies on intermediate and late fetal deaths for a given period × 100	Total number of intermediate and late fetal deaths for the same period

Exercise 7.14

Using the information in the following table, calculate the newborn death, fetal death, newborn autopsy, and fetal autopsy rates for the Newborn Service at University Hospital. In this exercise, the newborn deaths are included in the newborn discharges. Round to two decimal places.

University Hospital Newborn Service Statistics July–December 20XX	
Births	687
Discharges and Deaths	686
Newborn deaths	3
Newborn autopsies	2
Fetal deaths:	
Early	4
Intermediate	7
Late	3
Fetal death autopsies:	
Early	10
Intermediate	1
Late	2
Answers:	
Newborn death rate:	
Fetal death rate:	
Newborn autopsy rate:	
Fetal autopsy rate:	

Exercise 7.15

Community Healthcare System reported the statistics in the table below for its four facilities during its past semiannual period. Calculate the newborn death, fetal death, newborn autopsy, and fetal autopsy rates for each facility and for the system as a whole. In this exercise, the deaths are included in the discharges. Round to two decimal places.

Community Healthcare System Newborn Statistics January–June 20XX				
	Urban Hospital	Suburban Hospital	Rural Hospital	Specialty Hospital
Live births	252	247	176	201
Newborn discharges and deaths	250	245	173	200
Newborn deaths	2	2	2	12
Fetal deaths:				
Early	3	1	1	7
Intermediate	4	4	2	8
Late	3	1	1	3
Autopsies:				
Newborn	1	1	1	8
Fetal (late and intermediate)	2	1	2	8
Answers:				
Urban Hospital				
Newborn death rate:				
Fetal death rate:				
Newborn autopsy rate:				
Fetal autopsy rate:				

(*continued on next page*)

Community Healthcare System Newborn Statistics January–June 20XX
Suburban Hospital Newborn death rate:
Fetal death rate:
Newborn autopsy rate:
Fetal autopsy rate:
Rural Hospital Newborn death rate:
Fetal death rate:
Newborn autopsy rate:
Fetal autopsy rate:
Specialty Hospital Newborn death rate:
Fetal death rate:
Newborn autopsy rate:
Fetal autopsy rate:

(*continued on next page*)

Community Healthcare System Newborn Statistics January–June 20XX	
System as a Whole	
Newborn death rate:	
Fetal death rate:	
Newborn autopsy rate:	
Fetal autopsy rate:	

Chapter 7 Matching Quiz

Match the definition with the terms.

Definitions:

a. The place where the bodies of persons who have died are kept until identified and claimed by relatives or released for burial

b. The postmortem examination of the organs and tissues of a body to determine the cause of death or pathological conditions

c. A public officer whose principal duty is to enquire via an inquest into the cause of any deaths that there is reason to suppose is not due to natural causes

d. The total number of autopsies performed by a hospital pathologist for a given time period divided by the number of deaths of hospital patients (inpatients and outpatients) whose bodies were available for autopsy for the same time period

e. The number of autopsies performed on newborns who died during a given period of time divided by the total number of newborns who died during the same period

f. A situation in which the required conditions have been met to allow an autopsy to be performed on a hospital patient who has died

g. A postmortem examination performed on the body of a patient who died during an inpatient hospitalization by a hospital pathologist or a physician of the medical staff who has been designated the responsibility

h. The number of inpatient autopsies conducted during a given time period divided by the total number of deaths of inpatient deaths for the same time period

i. The proportion of hospital autopsies performed following the deaths of patients whose bodies are available for autopsy

j. The total number of autopsies on an inpatient deaths for a given period divided by the total inpatient deaths minus the unautopsied coroners' or medical examiners' cases

Terms:

1. _____ Autopsy

2. _____ Hospital autopsy rate

3. _____ Morgue

4. _____ Newborn autopsy rate

5. _____ Medical examiner

6. _____ Hospital inpatient autopsy

7. _____ Adjusted hospital autopsy rate

8. _____ Gross autopsy rate

9. _____ Net autopsy rate

10. _____ Available for hospital autopsy

Chapter 7   Review

Calculate all rates to two decimal places.

Community Hospital reported the statistics in the following table. Using this information, calculate the rates requested and select the correct calculation for questions 1 through 5.

Community Hospital Annual Statistics 20XX	
Inpatient discharges and deaths:	
Adults and children	8,234
Newborn	820
Inpatient deaths (included in discharges):	
Adults and children	54
Newborn	3
Fetal deaths:	
Early	4
Intermediate	5
Late	3

(*continued on next page*)

Community Hospital Annual Statistics 20XX	
Inpatient autopsies:	
Adults and children	12
Newborn	2
Coroner's cases:	
Unavailable for autopsy	4
Autopsy by hospital pathologist (included in inpatient autopsies)	1
Fetal death autopsies:	
Intermediate and late	4
Former hospital patient brought in for autopsy	2

1. What is the gross autopsy rate?
   a. 24.00%
   b. 24.56%
   c. 0.24%
   d. 2.45%

2. What is the net autopsy rate?
   a. 0.26%
   b. 2.64%
   c. 26.41%
   d. 26.42 %

3. What is the adjusted hospital autopsy rate?
   a. 29.09%
   b. 2.90%
   c. 29.09%
   d. 0.29%

4. What is the newborn autopsy rate?
   a. 0.66%
   b. 0.67%
   c. 6.67%
   d. 66.67%

5. What is the fetal autopsy rate?
   a. 0.50%
   b. 5.00%
   c. 50.00%
   d. 0.050%

Using the information reported by University Hospital for September 20XX in the following table, calculate the rates for questions 6 through 12. Round to two decimal places.

University Hospital September 20XX Statistics	
Discharges and Deaths:	
Total adults and children	1,432
Newborn	123
Total live births	120
Deaths (included in discharges):	
Adults and children	87
Newborn	3
Autopsies:	
Adults and children	23
Newborn	2
Hospital autopsied outpatients	7
Coroner's cases (unavailable for autopsy)	3
Fetal deaths:	
Early	0
Intermediate	5
Late	2
Fetal death autopsies:	
Intermediate and late	4

6. What is the gross death rate?
   a. 0.05%
   b. 0.57%
   c. 5.79%
   d. 57.87%

7. What is the gross autopsy rate?
   a. 0.27%
   b. 27.77%
   c. 27.78%
   d. 2.78%

8. What is the net autopsy rate?
   a. 0.28%
   b. 2.87%
   c. 2.88%
   d. 28.74%

9. What is the adjusted hospital autopsy rate?
   a. 34.04%
   b. 0.34%
   c. 3.40%
   d. 3.04%

10. What is the newborn autopsy rate?
   a. 0.66%
   b. 0.67%
   c. 6.67%
   d. 66.67%

11. What is the fetal death rate?
   a. 0.55%
   b. 5.51%
   c. 55.10%
   d. 0.06%

12. What is the fetal autopsy rate?
   a. 0.05%
   b. 0.57%
   c. 5.71%
   d. 57.14%

13. What is the principal difference between net autopsy rate and adjusted hospital autopsy rate?
   a. The net autopsy rate considers only inpatient deaths.
   b. Hospital autopsy rates include only those deaths in which the bodies are available for autopsy.
   c. Fetal deaths are not counted in hospital autopsy rates.
   d. Legal cases sometimes are excluded from deaths when computing net autopsy rate.

14. In which of the following rates are outpatients who were autopsied counted in an autopsy rate?
   a. Gross autopsy rate
   b. Net autopsy rate
   c. Adjusted hospital autopsy rate
   d. Newborn autopsy rate

15. Hospital autopsies include which of the following?

    a. Inpatients only

    b. Inpatients and outpatients who die in the hospital

    c. Inpatients, outpatients, and home care patients

    d. Inpatients and any other patient who has at some time been a hospital patient

Morbidity and Other Miscellaneous Rates

Learning Objectives

At the conclusion of this chapter, you should be able to

- Make calculations based on morbidity, infection, postoperative infection, complication, consultation, readmission
- Explain the difference between a surgical operation and surgical procedure
- Identify what constitutes a clean surgery case

Key Terms

Cesarean section	Consultation	Morbidity
Cesarean section rate	Consultation rate	Nosocomial infection
Chronic	Delivery	Nosocomial or hospital-
Clean surgical case	Hospital-acquired infection	acquired infection rate
Complication	(HAI)	Postoperative infection rate
Complication rate	Iatrogenic	Surgical operation
Concomitant	Infection rate	Surgical procedure

Health statistics and data are important to facilities because they measure a variety of indicators for a community. Data collected can provide comparisons with other facilities, they can provide information for improved quality of care. Data can help administrators see where additional services are needed and help them plan for the future.

Morbidity Rates

The term **morbidity** refers to the state of being diseased or the number of sick persons or cases of disease in relation to a specific population. Morbidity may be infectious or have other causes. For example, the presence of **concomitant** (taking place at the same time) or **chronic** (of long duration) conditions may constitute comorbidity. Moreover, morbidity may be preexisting (arising prior to admission to the hospital) or **iatrogenic** (occurring because of the patient's treatment).

Infection Rate

Preventing morbidity due to infection is an important clinical and quality management function. Frequently, the healthcare facility establishes a committee whose primary function is to evaluate infections and determine their causes so that recurrence can be avoided. Typically called the Infection Control Committee, or Infection Prevention Committee, it is composed of representatives from medical staff, nursing, pharmacy, laboratory, housekeeping, and health information management (HIM). Charged with the duty of infection prevention, committee members establish procedures for the management and reporting of infections. Effective management of infections acquired in the hospital (**nosocomial infections**), more commonly referred to as **hospital-acquired infections**, sometimes requires finding cases beyond the infections listed by physicians in the medical record. The HIM practitioner can help identify such cases in the course of performing qualitative analysis and coding.

In 1970, the Centers for Disease Control and Prevention (CDC) developed a voluntary reporting system, the National Nosocomial Infections Surveillance (NNIS) System, to monitor the incidence of nosocomial infections, which are also referred to as healthcare-associated infections (HAIs). In 2008, the CDC's Division of Healthcare Quality Promotion developed the National Healthcare Safety Network (NHSN) which includes the previous work of the NNIS. "The NHSN is a secure, internet-based surveillance system that integrates former CDC surveillance systems, including the National Nosocomial Infections Surveillance System (NNIS), National Surveillance System for Healthcare Workers (NaSH), and the Dialysis Surveillance Network (DSN). It is the nation's most widely used healthcare-associated infection tracking system. NHSN allows healthcare facilities to track blood safety errors and important healthcare process measures such as healthcare personnel influenza status" (CDC 2016b).

As defined in chapter 2, the term *rate* refers to the number of times something happened compared with the number of times it could have happened (Rate = Part/Base or R = P/B). Each healthcare facility's medical staff must determine the criteria for inclusion of a patient in both the numerator (infection) and denominator (patients at risk of infection).

Most healthcare facilities differentiate between nosocomial or hospital-acquired infections and exacerbation and recurrence of previous infections. For example, if an obstetrical patient develops a urinary tract infection, a physician must determine whether it was hospital-acquired or due to a recurrence of a previous urinary tract infection. Most Infection Prevention Departments are more interested in determining whether nosocomial infections are attributable to specific patient care units, specific operations, patients with specified diseases, the organized medical staff units, or individual physicians or hospital employees.

The **nosocomial** or **hospital-acquired infection rate** is the number of hospital-acquired infections in the hospital for a given time period divided by the total number of inpatient discharges (including deaths) for the same time period.

The formula for calculating the nosocomial infection rate is

$$\frac{Total\ number\ of\ nosocomial\ infections\ for\ a\ period \times 100}{Total\ number\ of\ discharges, including\ deaths,\ for\ the\ same\ period}$$

Example: In February, Community Hospital had 289 discharges and deaths. Twelve of these patients had hospital-acquired infections. The nosocomial infection rate is 4.15%.

$$\frac{(12 \times 100)}{289} = \frac{1,200}{289} = 4.15\%$$

Infection rates may be calculated separately for specific infections, such as surgical wound infections, puerperal infections (infections that occur immediately after childbirth), and infections of the respiratory tract, urinary tract, bloodstream, and so on.

The formula for calculating the infection rate is:

$$\frac{Total\ number\ of\ infections \times 100}{Total\ number\ of\ discharges\ (including\ deaths)\ for\ the\ period}$$

Example: In May, Community Hospital had 360 discharges, four of whom developed a ventilator-associated pneumonia (VAP) while in the hospital. The infection rate is calculated by placing the number of infections (4) $\times$ 100 in the numerator and dividing by the 360 (discharges) in the denominator.

$$\frac{(4 \times 100)}{360} = \frac{400}{360} = 1.11\%$$

Exercise 8.1

Using the information in the table below, calculate the rates requested for Community Hospital. In this exercise, deaths are included in the discharges. Round to two decimal places.

Community Hospital Annual Statistics 20XX	
Discharges and Deaths	
Adults and children	2,190
Newborn	127

(continued on next page)

Community Hospital Annual Statistics 20XX	
Deaths:	
Adults and children	13
Newborn	1
Nosocomial or Hospital-acquired Infections:	
Adults and children	18
Newborn	2
Answers:	
Hospital-acquired infection rate for adults and children:	
Hospital-acquired infection rate for newborns:	
Total hospital-acquired infection rate for the hospital:	
Gross death rate for this annual period:	

Exercise 8.2

Using the information given in the table below, calculate the rates requested. In this exercise, the deaths are included in the discharges. Round to two decimal places.

Service	University Hospital Semiannual Statistics July–December 20XX		
	No. of Discharges (includes Deaths)	No. of Deaths	No. of Nosocomial Infections
Medicine	2,469	201	52
Surgery	2,890	144	56
Obstetrics	785	2	6
Psychiatry	786	1	4
Rehabilitation	847	18	27
Pediatrics	945	3	3
Newborn	791	1	1
Total			

Answers:

Gross death rate for each service:

Total gross death rate:

Hospital-acquired infection rate for each service:

Total hospital-acquired infection rate for the semiannual period:

Postoperative Infection Rate

Another specific type of infection of great concern to hospitals is the **postoperative infection rate**. This is because a postoperative infection can contribute to the increased morbidity, mortality, and cost of care. Postoperative infections occur, as the name suggests, after surgery. The CDC estimates that surgical site infections account for 31 percent of all hospital-acquired infections (CDC 2016c). Even though hospitals take care to avoid an infection after surgery, one still can occur.

Two terms need to be considered here:

- A *surgical procedure* is defined as any single, separate, systematic process upon or within the body that can be complete in itself; normally is performed by a physician, dentist, or other licensed practitioner; can be performed with or without instruments; and is performed to restore disunited or deficient parts, remove diseased or injured tissues, extract foreign matter, assist in obstetrical delivery, or aid in diagnosis.

- A *surgical operation* is defined as one or more surgical procedures performed at one time for one patient via a common approach or for a common purpose.
  - An example of a surgical operation including more than one surgical procedure is an abdominoperitoneal resection, which involves resection of both the abdomen and the peritoneum.
  - An example of two surgical operations and two surgical procedures is a tonsillectomy followed by a circumcision. Even though the procedures were performed at one time for one patient, the approach to each procedure is different and the two procedures are not performed for a common purpose.

The postoperative infection rate is the ratio of all infections in clean surgical cases to the number of surgical operations performed. A general definition of a **clean surgical case** is one in which no infection existed prior to surgery.

The formula for calculating the postoperative infection rate is:

$$\frac{Total\ number\ of\ infections\ in\ clean\ surgical\ cases\ for\ a\ period \times 100}{Total\ number\ of\ surgical\ operations\ for\ the\ period}$$

Example: During May, a hospital reported that 578 surgical operations were performed. The infection prevention committee reported three postoperative infections in a clean surgical case. According to the formula, the postoperative infection rate for May is 0.52 percent.

$$\frac{(3 \times 100)}{578} = \frac{300}{578} = 0.52\%$$

A postoperative infection may be difficult to determine because it is not always evident whether the patient entered the hospital with an infection or acquired one because of the surgical techniques used. Therefore, the medical staff should provide guidance to the HIM practitioner and the infection prevention department on what constitutes a clean surgical case and which infections should be considered postoperative infections.

Many infection prevention departments use the classifications developed by the NNIS system (now a part of the NHSN). These are developed according to the likelihood and degree of wound contamination at the time of the operation. Wounds are classified as clean, clean-contaminated, contaminated, and dirty or infected wounds.

A clean wound is one in which no inflammation is encountered and the respiratory, alimentary, genital, or uninfected urinary tracts are not entered. Many infection prevention departments report the number of postoperative infections relative to the type of surgery that was performed. For example, if a patient has no infection prior to a coronary artery bypass graft but develops one after surgery, then the infection prevention department would report this as a postoperative infection in a clean case.

A clean-contaminated case is one in which the respiratory, alimentary, genital, or urinary tract is entered. Specifically, operations involving the biliary tract, appendix, vagina, and oropharynx are included in this category. For instance, a patient who develops an infection after an abdominal hysterectomy would be reported as an infection in a clean-contaminated case.

A contaminated wound includes an open, fresh, accidental wound; an operation with a break in sterile technique or gross spillage from the gastrointestinal tract; and incisions in which acute, nonpurulent inflammation is encountered.

A dirty wound is one that involves old traumatic wounds or devitalized tissue, an existing clinical infection or perforated viscera. Organisms were present before the procedure (CDC 2016c).

If you are assisting the infection prevention department with their statistics, be sure to determine how they are classifying your facility's postoperative infections.

Exercise 8.3

Using the information in the table below, calculate the postoperative infection and postoperative death rates for University Hospital during this semiannual period. Round to two decimal places.

University Hospital Surgery Service July–December 20XX	
Number of surgical operations	2,176
Number of patients operated on	2,170
Number of postoperative infections	14
Number of postoperative deaths	8

Answers:

Postoperative infection rate:

Postoperative death rate:

Exercise 8.4

Using the information in the table below, calculate the rates requested. Round to two decimal places.

		Deaths		Infections		No. of Patients Operated On	No. of Surgical Operations
Month	Live Disch	Postop	Other	Postop	Nosocomial		
Jan	540	2	10	2	4	478	479
Feb	660	3	12	3	5	642	648
Mar	680	3	8	1	4	660	663
Apr	669	2	12	4	3	650	653
May	701	5	15	4	2	690	690
Jun	693	3	11	5	3	685	685
Total							

Community Hospital
Semiannual Report
January–June, 20XX

Answers:

1. The month with the lowest postoperative infection rate:

2. The postoperative infection rate for the semiannual period:

3. The month with the highest postoperative death rate:

4. The postoperative death rate for the semiannual period:

5. The gross death rate for the surgical service during the semiannual period:

Exercise 8.5

Using the information below, calculate (the rates requested. In this exercise, the deaths are included in the discharges. Round to two decimal places.

Community Hospital Infection Prevention Committee Report on Infections January–March, 20XX 389 discharges		
Type of Infection	No. of Infections	Infection Rate
Central line-associated bloodstream infections	8	
Catheter-associated urinary tract infections	12	
Ventilator-associated pneumonia	4	
Surgical-site infections	6	
Cardiovascular system infections	2	
Gastrointestinal tract infections	3	
Skin and soft-tissue infections	1	
Ears, nose, and throat infections	9	
Central nervous system infections	7	
Systemic infections	5	

Complication Rate

In addition to infections, healthcare facilities are concerned with any other type of complication that results from or occurs during the course of care. A **complication** is a medical condition that arises during an inpatient hospitalization. According to the Centers for Medicare and Medicaid Services, a complication is a condition that occurs during the patient's hospital stay that extends the length of stay by at least one day in 75 percent of cases.

Complications may be related to the quality of care received by patients. The purpose of collecting a **complication rate** is to determine if changes in the treatment or practice in the facility can prevent them from occurring again.

Examples of complications include blood transfusion reactions, injuries sustained during cardiopulmonary resuscitation, reactions to medications given, vaccination reactions, and patient falls out of bed, just to name a few. Infections, of course, can be complications, but they are generally calculated separately. Any of these examples would change the way the patient was treated from the original reason for hospitalization.

Many facilities calculate these rates at usual intervals: monthly, quarterly, semiannually, or annually.

The general formula for calculating the complication rate is

$$\frac{Total\ number\ of\ complications\ for\ a\ period \times 100}{Total\ number\ of\ discharges\ (including\ deaths)\ in\ the\ same\ period}$$

Example: From July through December, Community Hospital had 32 complications and 2,394 discharges. The complication rate is

$$\frac{(32 \times 100)}{2,394} = \frac{3,200}{2,394} = 1.34\%$$

More often than not, facilities will calculate specific types of complications.

Example: In July, Community Hospital had 18 patients on the Medicine unit who had a blood transfusion. Of those, two developed an adverse reaction to the transfusion. The blood transfusion reaction rate is calculated by placing the number of blood transfusion reactions (2) $\times$ 100 in the numerator and dividing it by the number of blood transfusions.

$$\frac{(2 \times 100)}{18} = \frac{200}{18} = 11.11\%$$

Exercise 8.6

Using the information in the table below for University Hospital, calculate the complication rate for each service and the total for this quarterly period. Round to two decimal places.

Service	University Hospital Statistics January–March 20XX		
	Discharges and Deaths	Complications	Complication Rate
Medicine	2,742	197	
Surgery	2,075	208	
Obstetrics	492	7	
Newborn	490	3	
Total			

Exercise 8.7

Using the information below, calculate the complication rates by physician and the total for this semiannual period for Community Hospital. Round to two decimal places.

	Community Hospital Complication Rate by Physician January–June 20XX		
Physician No.	No. Discharges and Deaths	No. Complications	Complication Rate
102	298	2	
237	247	4	
391	110	3	
518	144	2	
637	206	3	
802	82	1	
900	100	3	
Total			

Cesarean Section Rate

Most hospitals determine the percentage of deliveries that are performed by cesarean section (commonly called C-section) as compared with spontaneous or vaginal deliveries. A **cesarean section** is a surgical operation for delivering a child by cutting through the wall of the mother's abdomen. Hospitals determine the **cesarean section rate**, which is the ratio of all cesarean sections to the total number of deliveries, including cesarean sections, during a specified period of time. Much attention has been given to high C-section rates by specific physicians, hospitals, and areas of the country because of concerns about adverse effects to the mother and child. It may be necessary to report C-section rates to accrediting agencies or the American Medical Association for such reasons as residency programs.

A **delivery** is defined as the process of delivering a live-born infant or dead fetus (and placenta) by manual, instrumental, or surgical means.

> **Tip:** A pregnant mother who delivers has one delivery but may have multiple births. For example, a woman who delivers a live-born infant is counted as one delivery and one live birth whereas a woman who delivers live-born twins is counted as one delivery and two live births. A woman who delivers a stillbirth is counted as one delivery and one intermediate or late fetal death. This is also considered to be one delivery and one birth since a stillbirth is considered to be a birth but not a live birth.

Tip: Sometimes a woman is admitted to the hospital for a condition of her pregnancy but does not deliver her infant during that hospitalization. For example, a woman may be admitted in apparent labor, which turns out to be false labor. In this case, the patient may be classified as an obstetrics patient, not delivered.

The formula for calculating the cesarean section rate is

$$\frac{Total\ number\ of\ C\text{-}sections\ performed\ in\ a\ period \times 100}{Total\ number\ of\ deliveries\ in\ the\ period\ (including\ C\text{-}sections)}$$

Tip: The C-section rate is not based on the number of patients discharged but, rather, on the number of deliveries. A rate compares the number of actual occurrences with the total possible; obviously, only deliveries can be C-sections. Usually the data on deliveries and the number of C-sections for the period are obtained from delivery room personnel.

Example: Four C-sections were performed in a month during which there were 350 deliveries. The C-section rate is calculated by multiplying the number of C-sections (4) by 100 and then dividing that number by the total number of deliveries (350). The C-section rate is 1.14 percent.

$$\frac{(4 \times 100)}{350} = \frac{400}{350} = 1.14\%$$

Exercise 8.8

Using the information in the table below, calculate the C-section rate and the vaginal delivery rate at University Hospital for the semiannual period. Round to two decimal places.

University Hospital Obstetrics Service Semiannual Statistics July–December 20XX	
Admissions	672
Discharges and Deaths:	
Delivered	504
Not delivered	147

(continued on next page)

University Hospital Obstetrics Service Semiannual Statistics July–December 20XX	
Aborted	21
Vaginal deliveries	403
C-sections	101
Answers: C-section rate:	
Vaginal delivery rate:	

Exercise 8.9

Using the information in the table below, calculate the C-section rate, the newborn death rate, and the fetal death rate at University Hospital for the month of July. Round to two decimal places.

University Hospital Newborn Service July 20XX	
Discharges (includes deaths)	130
Births:	
Single live births	125
Multiple live births	1 set of twins 1 set of triplets
Deliveries:	
Vaginal	110
C-section	20

(*continued on next page*)

University Hospital Newborn Service July 20XX	
Deaths:	
Newborn	1
Fetal:	
Early	4
Intermediate	2
Late	2
Answers: C-section rate:	
Newborn death rate:	
Fetal death rate:	

Consultation Rates

A **consultation** is the response by one healthcare professional to another healthcare professional's request to provide recommendations or opinions regarding the care of a particular patient or resident. A patient's attending physician may occasionally request that a consultant (another physician or healthcare practitioner) examine a patient and give an opinion as to his or her condition. Ordinarily the consultant is called in to help identify and treat a patient whose diagnosis is outside the expertise of the attending physician. Consultants are usually specialists in their particular field of medicine. The consultant has the opportunity to visit with the patient and review the medical record and then prepare a consultation report that includes the findings of the examination and recommendations for treating the patient. The consultation report is made a part of the patient's medical record.

The formula for calculating the **consultation rate** is

$$\frac{Total\ number\ of\ patients\ receiving\ a\ consultation \times 100}{Total\ number\ of\ patients\ discharged}$$

Example: During the month of May, Community Hospital's medicine unit had 103 discharges, 14 of whom were seen by a consultant. The consultation rate is 13.59 percent.

$$\frac{(14 \times 100)}{103} = \frac{1,400}{103} = 13.59\%$$

Tip: Close examination of this formula reveals that the definition of a rate applies here. That is, every patient discharged could theoretically have had a consultation.

Exercise 8.10

Using the information in the table below, calculate the consultation rate at Community Hospital for each service and the total for the semiannual period. Round to two decimal places.

Community Hospital Semiannual Statistics July–December 20XX			
Service	Discharges and Deaths	No. of Patients Receiving Consultations	Consultation Rate
Medicine	3,240	962	
Surgery	3,745	827	
Obstetrics	690	35	
Psychiatric	155	10	
Rehabilitation	132	15	
Pediatrics	387	49	
Newborn	685	4	
Total			

Exercise 8.11

Using the information in the table below, calculate the rates requested below for Community Hospital. In this exercise, the deaths are included in the discharges. Round to two decimal places.

Month	Disch Including Deaths	Deaths	Consults	Consultation Rate	Gross Death Rate
January	602	18	119		
February	675	12	107		
March	598	11	92		
April	555	14	74		
May	630	10	105		
June	592	6	96		
July	581	9	85		
August	593	7	72		
September	621	5	89		
October	610	12	56		
November	601	10	95		
December	581	14	82		
Total					

Community Hospital
Surgery Service
Annual Statistics 20XX

1. Consultation rate for each month:

2. Consultation rate for the year for the surgery service:

3. Gross death rate for each month:

4. Gross death rate for the year for the surgery service:

Exercise 8.12

Using the information in the table below, calculate the consultation rates by physician for Community Hospital. Round to two decimal places.

Physician No.	No. of Discharges and Deaths	No. of Consultations	Consultation Rate
	Community Hospital **Consultation Rate by Physician** **January–June, 20XX**		
102	298	12	
237	247	3	
391	110	7	
518	144	8	
637	206	5	
802	82	12	
900	100	10	
Total			

Other Rates

The HIM practitioner may compute and report other rates according to individual healthcare facility needs. External agencies may also ask that additional data and rates be reported. To pursue all the possibilities in this book is impractical. The best rule of thumb is to use the "other rates" formula. You may become so intrigued with this formula that you will volunteer to produce new and useful rates, which is, incidentally, part of the HIM professional's responsibility. The formula for calculating other rates is

$$\frac{\textit{Number of times something happened} \times 100}{\textit{Number of times something could have happened}}$$

Tip: Statistics should not be kept just because they have always been kept. After you assure yourself, the administration, and the medical staff that a particular statistic no longer serves a useful purpose, stop keeping it. Do not be afraid to be creative and imaginative about providing new ideas for statistical computations that will serve a useful purpose, even if only on a temporary, special-study basis.

Table 8.1 lists the calculations for morbidity and other rates.

Table 8.1 Calculations for Morbidity and other rates

Rate	Numerator	Denominator
Infection rate	Total number of infections for a period × 100	Total number of discharges (including deaths) for the same period
Postoperative infection rate	Total number of infections in clean surgical cases for a period × 100	Number of surgical operations for the same period
Complication rate	Total number of complications for a period × 100	Total number of discharges (including deaths) for the same period
C-section rate	Total number of C-sections for a period × 100	Total number of deliveries (including C-sections) in the same period
Consultation rate	Total number of patients receiving consultations for a period × 100	Total number of discharges (including deaths) for the same period
Readmission rate	Number of patients readmitted within 30 days of the previous discharge × 100	Total patients discharged (excluding deaths)

Exercise 8.13

Using the information in the table below, calculate the readmission rates for each month and the semiannual period for University Hospital using the following formula. Round to two decimal places.

$$\frac{\textit{Number of patients readmitted within 30 days of the previous discharge} \times 100}{\textit{Total patients discharged (excluding deaths)}}$$

University Hospital Surgery Service Semiannual Statistics July–December 20XX			
Month	No. of Patients Discharged Alive	No. of Patients Readmitted within 30 Days of the Previous Discharge	Readmission Rate
July	673	38	
August	765	43	
September	789	49	
October	750	32	
November	769	36	
December	778	45	
Total			

Exercise 8.14

Using the information in the table below, calculate the readmission rates requested for Community Hospital. Round to two decimal places.

MS-DRG	Title	No. Live Disch	No. Readmissions within 30 days of Previous Discharge	Readmission Rate
	Community Hospital **Semiannual Statistics, 20XX** **Readmission by Selected MS-DRGs**			
190	COPD with MCC	12	2	
191	COPD with CC	14	5	
192	COPD without CC/MCC	42	11	
193	Simple pneumonia & pleurisy with MCC	8	1	
194	Simple pneumonia & pleurisy with CC	15	4	
195	Simple pneumonia & pleurisy without CC/MCC	97	8	
280	Acute myocardial infarction discharged alive, with MCC	10	3	
281	Acute myocardial infarction discharged alive, with CC	8	2	
282	Acute myocardial infarction discharged alive, without CC/MCC	180	10	
291	Heart failure & shock with MCC	3	1	
292	Heart failure & shock with CC	6	1	
293	Heart failure & shock without CC/MCC	63	2	
469	Major joint replacement or reattachment, lower extremity with MCC	15	2	
470	Major joint replacement or reattachment, lower extremity without MCC	49	4	

Exercise 8.15

Using the information in the table below, calculate the rate of readmitted patients by physician at Community Hospital for each month and for this quarter. Round to two decimal places.

| | | Community Hospital Semiannual Statistics 20XX Readmissions by Physicians | | |
Physician	No. of Live Discharges	No. of Readmissions within 30 days of Previous Discharge	Readmission Rate
102	298	8	
237	247	4	
391	110	3	
518	144	2	
637	206	12	
802	82	6	
900	100	5	
Total			

Exercise 8.16

Using the information in the table below for University Hospital, calculate the rate of accounts turned over to collection for each month and for the period. Use the formula for a rate to make these calculations. Round answers to two decimal places.

| | | University Hospital Semiannual Statistics January–June 20XX | |
Month	No. of Discharges and Deaths	No. of Accounts Turned Over to a Collection Agency	Rate of Accounts Turned Over to a Collection Agency
January	413	36	
February	437	41	

(continued on next page)

University Hospital Semiannual Statistics January–June 20XX		
March	453	43	
April	429	26	
May	463	35	
June	423	20	
Total			

Exercise 8.17

Using the information in the table below, calculate the rates requested for the medicine service at Community Hospital. Round to two decimal places.

Community Hospital Medicine Service Selected Annual Statistics, 20XX	
Total Hospital Discharges: 9,845	
Medicine Service	**Number**
Discharges and deaths	5,967
Complications	236
Hospital-acquired infections	89
Deaths (included in discharges)	71
Payer information:	
Medicare	1,016
Medicaid	923
Third-party insurance	3,237
Self-pay	791
Selected patients:	
Primary diagnosis:	
Asthma	370
Cancer	875
Diabetes and its complications	736

(continued on next page)

Community Hospital Medicine Service Selected Annual Statistics, 20XX	
HIV/AIDS	92
Hypertension	701
Myocardial infarction	561

Answers:

1. Percentage of total hospital patients in the medicine service:

2. Complication rate in the medicine service:

3. Hospital-acquired infection rate in the medicine service:

4. Gross death rate in the medicine service:

5. Percentage of patients in the medicine service with:

    a. Medicare:

    b. Medicaid:

    c. Third-party insurance:

    d. Self-pay:

6. Percentage of patients with:

    a. Asthma:

    b. Cancer:

    c. Diabetes and its complications:

    d. HIV/AIDS:

    e. Hypertension:

    f. Myocardial infarction:

Chapter 8   Matching Quiz

Match the definition with the terms.

Definitions:

   a. The ratio of all infections to the number of discharges, including deaths
   b. Of long duration
   c. A medical condition that arises during an inpatient hospitalization
   d. Accessory; taking place at the same time
   e. The process of delivering a liveborn infant or dead fetus by manual, instrumental, or surgical means
   f. An infection acquired by a patient while receiving care or services in a healthcare organization; also called a hospital-acquired infection
   g. The state of being diseased
   h. Induced inadvertently by a physician or surgeon or by medical treatment or diagnostic procedure
   i. One or more surgical procedures performed at one time for one patient via a common approach of for a common purpose
   j. A surgical case in which no infection existed prior to surgery

Terms:

   1. _____ Morbidity
   2. _____ Infection rate
   3. _____ Delivery
   4. _____ Complication
   5. _____ Clean surgical case

   6. _____ Concomitant
   7. _____ Chronic
   8. _____ Surgical operation
   9. _____ Iatrogenic
   10. _____ Nosocomial infection

Chapter 8   Review

Use the following information to answer questions 1 through 3.

Discharges and Deaths	
Adults and children	8,191
Newborn	809
Surgical procedures	2,376
Surgical operations	2,371
Patients receiving consultations	2,789
Hospital-acquired infections	27
Postoperative infections (included in total HAIs)	6

1. The hospital-acquired infection rate (including newborns) is _____.
   a. 0.03%
   b. 0.30%
   c. 3.00%
   d. 30.00%

2. The consultation rate (including newborns) is _____.
   a. 0.03%
   b. 0.30%
   c. 3.09%
   d. 30.99%

3. What is the postoperative infection rate?
   a. 0.25%
   b. 0.025%
   c. 2.53%
   d. 25.30%

4. A hospital reported the following statistics for the past year: births, 1,702; deliveries, 1,708; C-sections, 360; and obstetrical discharges, 1,827. The C-section rate for that year is _____.
   a. 0.21%
   b. 2.10%
   c. 21.08%
   d. 20.77%

Use the information below to answer questions 5 through 7.

Women's Hospital September, 20XX	
Deliveries	284 Two sets of twins
Births	286
Obstetrical Discharges	287
First-time C-sections	5
Repeat C-sections	4

5. What is the C-section rate for September?
   a. 0.03%
   b. 0.31%
   c. 3.17%
   d. 31.69%

6. What is the percentage of multiple births?
   a. 0.14%
   b. 14.00%
   c. 13.98%
   d. 1.40%

7. What is the percentage of patients with multiple births?
   a. 0.07%
   b. 0.70%
   c. 7.04%
   d. 70.42%

8. A third-party review company reported the statistics in the table below. Calculate the rate of admissions approved for each month and for the quarter. Round to two decimal places.

	July	August	September
Number of admission claims reviewed	875	892	925
Number of claims approved for admission to the hospital	851	888	920

Answers:

July:

August:

September:

Quarter:

Using the information below, answer questions 9 through 12.

| Community Hospital Selected Semiannual Statistics, 20XX | | | | | | |
Month	No. of Patients Discharged Alive	No. of Deaths	No. of Patients Readmission within 30 days	No. of Hospital-acquired Infections	No. of Consultations	No. of Complications
Jan	187	5	7	9	12	3
Feb	207	6	10	7	10	8
Mar	315	8	8	5	15	5
Apr	327	6	6	4	9	7
May	288	5	5	6	11	6
Jun	292	4	9	8	14	4
Total						

9. The readmission rate for the entire semiannual period is _____.
   a. 0.27%
   b. 27.84%
   c. 0.02%
   d. 2.78%

10. What is the hospital-acquired infection rate for the entire semiannual period?
   a. 2.36%
   b. 23.63%
   c. 0.23%
   d. 0.02%

11. The consultation rate for the entire semiannual period is _____.
   a. 0.43%
   b. 0.04%
   c. 4.30%
   d. 43.03%

12. The complication rate for the entire semiannual period is _____.
   a. 0.20%
   b. 0.02%
   c. 20.00%
   d. 2.00%

Using the information below answer questions 13 through 15. In these questions, the discharges include the deaths.

Month	No. of Surgical Operations	No. of Post-op Infections	No. of Deliveries	No. of C-sections	No. of Discharges and Deaths	No. of Deaths
		Community Hospital **Selected Semiannual Statistics, 20XX**				
Jul	127	3	142	4	238	8
Aug	132	2	137	8	264	7
Sept	147	4	130	3	288	8
Oct	140	6	138	9	292	9
Nov	137	3	140	5	246	7
Dec	110	2	152	6	220	3
Total						

13. What is the postoperative infection rate for this semiannual period?
    a. 0.25%
    b. 2.52%
    c. 0.02%
    d. 25.22%

14. What is the C-section rate for this semiannual period?
    a. 4.17%
    b. 40.17%
    c. 0.41%
    d. 0.04%

15. What is the gross death rate for this semiannual period?
    a. 0.27%
    b. 0.02%
    c. 27.13%
    d. 2.71%

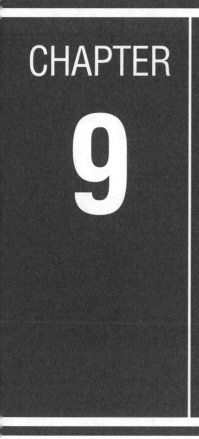

CHAPTER 9

Statistics Computed within the Health Information Management Department

Learning Objectives

At the conclusion of this chapter, you should be able to

- Explain, differentiate, and apply the following terms; full-time equivalent employee, budget, case-mix, fiscal year, variance and variance analysis, payback period, return on investment
- Determine the uses that statistics play in the health information management (HIM) department in terms of unit labor cost, productivity, staffing levels, budgets, and physician profiling
- Differentiate between the operational and capital budgets
- Verify computerized statistical reports and spreadsheets for accuracy
- Calculate common statistics used in the management of an HIM department

Key Terms

Budget	Fiscal year	Release of information (ROI)
Capital budget	Full-time equivalent employee	Return on investment
Case-mix	Operational budget	Spreadsheet
Case-mix index	Payback period	Unit labor cost
Electronic health record	Productivity	Variance
Electronic signature	Profiling	Variance analysis

Statistics computed for use within the health information management (HIM) department usually relate to labor costs, productivity, and staffing and often are used in determining whether the department may be able to hire a new employee, set benchmarks for productivity, determine absentee rates, and so on. The following sections provide examples of common, everyday computations made by HIM staff members.

Health Information Statistics

Health information professionals can improve processes and procedures by keeping track of common statistics such as employee compensation, unit labor costs, staffing and productivity, department budgets and verifying statistical reports generated by the HIM department and others. The HIM professional is at the center of all of this data and can use the data to help make informed decisions.

Employee Compensation and Unit Labor Costs

One example of where health information managers must make effective decisions is in regard to employee compensation and **unit labor cost**.

The annual compensation for an individual employee is calculated by multiplying the number of hours worked per year (2,080 for a full-time employee) by the hourly wage and then multiplying that number by the benefits received. Then add the amount of the benefits to the base salary. A sample calculation follows:

(2,080 hours $\times$ \$15 per hour) $\times$ 30% benefits = \$31,200 $\times$ .30 = \$9,360 + \$31,200 = \$40,560

Tip: A quicker way to compute this is to multiply by 1.3 (if 30% benefits).

2,080 hours $\times$ \$15 per hour $\times$ 1.3 (30% benefits) = \$40,560

To determine the annual productivity, multiply the amount of work completed (for example, lines transcribed, number of records coded, and the like) per day by the number of workdays in the year (5 workdays per week $\times$ 52 weeks per year = 260 workdays). Note that this calculation includes any vacation time or sick leave that an employee may take.

The unit labor cost is determined by dividing the total annual compensation by total annual productivity. For example, coding workload in an HIM Department is commonly measured in number of records coded. To determine the unit coding labor cost, divide the total coding professional annual compensation by the total annual productivity as shown below.

$$\frac{Total\,(sum)\,coding\,professional\,annual\,compensation}{Total\,(sum)\,coding\,professional\,annual\,productivity}$$

Example: Two full-time beginning coding professionals in the HIM department code 20 records per day each. One employee earns \$15.00 per hour and is paid an annual salary of \$31,200; the other employee earns \$15.65 per hour and is paid an annual salary of \$32,552.

To determine the annual productivity, multiply the number of records coded the two employees (20 per day per coding professional or 40 per day) by the number of workdays in the year (5 workdays per week $\times$ 52 weeks per year = 260 workdays).

2(260 workdays $\times$ 20 records) = 10,400 records coded per year

To determine the unit cost, add the two salaries ($31,200 + $32,552 = $63,752) and divide by the total number of records coded by the two employees in one year (10,400). The unit cost is $6.13 per record.

$$\frac{\$63,752}{10,400} = \$6.13$$

Example: This formula can be applied to other employees in the department. For example, if one analyst is compensated at $14.50 per hour and analyzes six records per hour. The employee's annual compensation is $30,160.

To determine the employee's annual productivity, multiply six records per hour by 7.5 hours per day to get 45 records per day. Then multiply 45 by 5 days in the workweek and 52 weeks in the year to get 11,700 records coded per year. The unit cost is $2.58 per record.

$$\frac{\$30,160}{11,700} = \$2.58$$

Tip: Some employers consider 7.5 hours a productive work day, thinking in terms of an 8-hour day minus breaks the employee may take.

Tip: Notice that the unit cost did not consider times that the employee is not working (for example, sick time or vacation time). The unit cost to code one record is still valid because someone has to perform the work even when the employee who normally performs that task is absent.

Exercise 9.1

Complete the exercises below.

1. Accurate Transcription Company hires Transcriptionist A, a full-time employee earning $15.00 per hour and an annual salary of $31,200. She transcribes 1,200 lines per day for a total of 312,000 lines per year. What is the unit medical transcription labor cost for Transcriptionist A (or how much does a line cost when transcribed by Transcriptionist A)?

2. The same transcription company hires Transcriptionist B, a full-time employee earning $14.00 per hour and an annual salary of $29,120. He transcribes 900 lines per day for a total of 234,000 lines per year. What is the unit medical transcription labor cost for Transcriptionist B?

3. University Hospital has eight full-time transcriptionists. Five of them produce 1,000 lines each per day. Of these five, one earns $14.00 per hour, three earn $14.80 per hour, and one earns $16.00 per hour.

   Two other transcriptionists in the department produce 1,100 lines per day. Of these two, one earns $14.25 per hour and the other earns $17.00 per hour. Finally, the eighth transcriptionist produces 1,200 lines per day and earns $14.00 per hour.

   a. What is the difference in cost per line between the employee who produces 1,000 lines per day and makes $14.00 per hour and the employee who produces 1,200 lines per day and makes $14.00 per hour?

   b. What general observations can you make about the unit labor cost and the two employees just mentioned?

   c. What is the difference in cost per line between the employee who produces 1,000 lines per day and makes $16.00 per hour and the employee who produces 1,100 lines per day and makes $14.25 per hour?

   d. What is the total unit cost for medical transcription?

4. The HIM department at Community Hospital has three full-time coding professionals. One is considered the lead coding professional and his salary is $20.35 per hour. One coding professional is a new graduate who makes $15.50 per hour, and the third coding professional is an experienced employee who earns $18.90 per hour. The lead coding professional codes four records per hour; the new coding professional codes three records per hour, and the experienced coding professional codes six records per hour.

   a. Using a 7.5-hour productive day, what is the unit cost per coding professional?

   b. What is the total unit cost for all three coding professionals?

5. University Hospital employs ten full-time coding professionals. Using the information below, determine the individual salary per year, the unit cost of coding for each employee, and the total unit cost for the coding department. Use 7.5 hours per day as a productive work day. Round salary to whole numbers.

Coding Professional	Salary	Records coded per hour	Salary per year	Unit Cost
A	$15.00	4	$31,200	
B	$15.45	5	$32,136	
C	$15.10	4	$31,408	
D	$16.79	6	$34,923	
E	$18.22	6	$37,898	
F	$22.65	6	$47,112	

(continued on next page)

Coding Professional	Salary	Records coded per hour	Salary per year	Unit Cost
G	$16.03	6	$33,342	
H	$16.85	6	$35,048	
I	$21.76	8	$45,261	
J	$17.34	6	$36,067	
Total			**$364,395**	

To justify costs for **release of information (ROI)**—the process of disclosing patient information from the medical record to another party—in the health information department, one HIM professional needed to calculate cost breakdowns.

Unit Costs for Release of Information

The Health Insurance Portability and Accountability Act (HIPAA), commonly referred to as the Privacy Rule, allows a facility to charge a reasonable, cost-based fee for any requests for records made by patients after the first request. Time studies would need to be performed in order to validate the cost. Some activities involved could be:

- Keeping track of the time it takes to review the request and log it into your computer system
- Finding the patient information in the master patient index
- Determining the location of the medical record, either paper or electronic
- Determining whether other departments have portions of the medical record and have possibly made a disclosure
- Retrieving the record if it is a paper record or locating the record online and printing any scanned documents
- Reviewing any previous disclosures made
- Preparing a list of the disclosures
- Preparing an invoice for the patient
- Updating the release of the information log

The HIM department also may consider nonlabor expenses such as those listed in table 9.1. However, the facility's chief financial officer is usually consulted to determine whether other nonlabor costs can be applied.

Another aspect that will need consideration is that some health information departments are copying records onto a CD or thumb drive and giving them directly to a patient. This will affect the cost of the release of information as it does not take as much time to copy the parts of the record onto a CD or thumb drive as it would to produce a paper copy. Also, when health information exchanges become fully operational, it may be possible to move the information from one organization to another. The health information director will need to calculate the time needed to transfer the information rather than copy the information.

Table 9.1. Average record requests per month

<table>
<tr><td colspan="2" align="center">**Community Hospital**
Health Information Department
Release of Information Costs
Average Requests per Month = 410</td></tr>
<tr><td>**Item**</td><td align="center">**Cost per Request**</td></tr>
<tr><td>Postage: $510 per month</td><td>$\dfrac{\$510}{410} = \$1.24$</td></tr>
<tr><td>Service contract (includes copier): $250 per month</td><td>$\dfrac{\$250}{410} = \$0.61$</td></tr>
<tr><td>Equipment (includes copies): $125 per month</td><td>$\dfrac{\$125}{410} = \$0.30$</td></tr>
<tr><td>Supplies (includes toner, printer cartridges, paper): $90 per month</td><td>$\dfrac{\$90}{410} = \$0.22$</td></tr>
<tr><td>Wages: $14.00 per hour = monthly salary of $2,427 ($14.00 × 2,080 hours = $29,120 annual salary, $\dfrac{\$29,120}{12 \text{ months}} = 2,426.66 = \$2,427$ per month)</td><td>$\dfrac{\$2,427}{410} = \$5.92$</td></tr>
<tr><td>**Total**</td><td>**$8.30**</td></tr>
</table>

Exercise 9.2

Using the information in the table below, calculate the cost breakdown per item and the monthly cost for the ROI services at Community Hospital. Round wages to whole numbers.

<table>
<tr><td colspan="2" align="center">**Community Hospital**
Health Information Department
Release of Information Costs
Average Requests per Month = 540</td></tr>
<tr><td>**Item**</td><td align="center">**Cost per Month**</td></tr>
<tr><td>Postage</td><td align="center">$675</td></tr>
<tr><td>Service contract (includes copier)</td><td align="center">$250</td></tr>
<tr><td>Equipment (includes copies)</td><td align="center">$125</td></tr>
<tr><td>Supplies (includes toner, printer cartridges, paper)</td><td align="center">$95</td></tr>
<tr><td>Wages</td><td align="center">$12.00 per hour</td></tr>
<tr><td>**Monthly cost**</td><td align="center">$</td></tr>
</table>

Exercise 9.3

Using the information provided in the table below, complete the following exercises. Round wages to whole numbers.

Community Hospital Health Information Department Release of Information Costs Average Requests per Month = 550	
Item	**Cost per Month**
Postage	$790
Service contract (includes copier)	$265
Equipment (includes copies)	$150
Supplies (includes toner, printer cartridges, paper)	$95
Wages	$13.00 per hour

1. Calculate the cost breakdown for each item.

2. What is the monthly cost for the ROI services?

3. On average, the ROI section brings in $1,800 per month. What is the difference between cost and income?

4. An ROI contract company has approached the director of HIM with a proposal to take over the ROI function for free and they would then charge the third parties for the copies. What are the advantages and disadvantages of this proposal?

5. The HIM department at Community Hospital had 100,000 active records. During January through June 20XX, they received 6,382 requests for records.

   a. What is the request rate for this six-month period? Round to two decimal places.

   b. Of the 6,382 requests, 3,375 were located within the 25-minute time frame which was set as one of the department's quality indicators. What is the rate of compliance in answering these requests for records? Round to two decimal places.

Other Labor Unit Costs

The HIM department also processes patient record (chart) requests, which consumes a great deal of staff time. Responsibilities in maintaining records include

- *Scanning of records*: Some facilities choose to scan the paper record to make it available online. These facilities may have an electronic document management system to help manage all their documents for a patient. This technology allows users to scan documents, move documents from the transcription system to the electronic health record (EHR), enter information online, handle the **electronic signature** of records, which is an electronic signature is any representation of a signature in digital form, including an image of a handwritten signature; text-editable deficiencies, which are those that a physician or other healthcare practitioner can enter through the computer or mobile device in order to make changes to a particular document; index documents as they are entered into the computer system; access information from a variety of locations; and more. The main calculations for this department are productivity and quality. These are regularly computed and used for staffing issues and benchmarking. New technologies will continue to evolve, and managers in health information departments will continue to determine the costs and benefits of these new systems.

- *Provider–patient e-mail*: As patients become more comfortable with e-mailing their physicians through patient portals and as healthcare insurers begin to reimburse physicians for their time used to e-mail patients, this will become an everyday issue for healthcare organizations. E-mail and text messages are considered healthcare business records and thus are subject to the same rules and regulations as any other health record. Facilities will usually make all email messages sent or received part of the patient's medical record. E-mail can be used to schedule appointments, refill prescriptions, transfer department results, or request that information be sent to other providers. Organizations may decide to keep track of the time spent responding to e-mails, gathering information before the e-mail is answered, and deciding what can be answered via e-mail (Pendergrass 2016).

- *Loose papers*: Often these are copies of medical records sent from other healthcare facilities or prenatal records coming from obstetricians that must be included in the EHR. The number of pieces of paper received in the HIM department for filing is a significant factor in determining staffing levels. Loose papers may be measured in inches or by individual pieces, which is a more accurate measure. Because of the time involved in tracking this information, departments may choose to sample this activity for a one-week period several times a year.

- *Performance improvement activities*: HIM managers will often keep track of the activity in the department to determine that they are meeting their performance improvement targets. For example, the coding supervisor may monitor the number of days it takes the coding professionals to code a discharged record. There may be a standard of three days to receive the record after discharge. This is often referred to as the bill "being dropped." Or, they may be responsible for resubmitting claims that have been denied.
  - After the record is coded, the claim will be sent electronically to the third-party payer or to a clearinghouse, which is a go-between contract company between the healthcare provider and the payer. The payer processes the claim and determines the validity of the payment and then reimburses the facility at a prenegotiated rate. If a claim fails the payer's edits and checks, the facility will be notified of the denial in the form of an Explanation of Benefits (EOB) or Electronic Remittance Advice. Failed claims must be reconciled with the original claims, corrections made, and the claims resubmitted (Voth 2016).
  - Qualitative review of the medical record is also a task that the HIM professional performs. This can include reviewing medical reports for quality and adequacy of the documentation to ensure it follows policies of the facility, accreditation agency requirements, and government regulations. Common reports that are reviewed are the discharge summary, history and physical examination, and operative report. HIM professionals may also audit specific types of records for documentation, for example, patients who enter with a myocardial infarction may have certain tests required on admission, and these would be checked to determine that they were completed. Unapproved abbreviations may also be reported as part of HIM department quality checks.

Exercise 9.4

Complete the following exercises.

1. The HIM department at Community Hospital completed a time study, and the data are listed in the table below. Complete the table by determining the number of hours worked in each activity.

Community Hospital Health Information Department Time Allocation Report September 20XX		
Service/Division	**Number of Hours**	**Hours Worked**
Inpatient records:		
Medicine	450 h/w × 4 weeks	
Surgery	460 h/w × 4 weeks	
Pediatrics	12 h/w × 4 weeks	
Psychiatry	10 h/w × 4 weeks	
Obstetrics	60 h/w × 4 weeks	
Newborn	48 h/w × 4 weeks	
Subtotal inpatient records		
ED records:		
Supervisory	5 h/w × 4 weeks	
Correspondence	7 h/w × 4 weeks	
Clerical/Processing	28 h/w × 4 weeks	
Subtotal ED records		
General clinic:		
Supervisory	5 h/w × 4 weeks	
Transcription	0.10 h/record × 370 records	
Clerical/Processing	6 h/w × 4 weeks	
Subtotal general clinic		
Outpatient/Ambulatory surgery		

(*continued on next page*)

Community Hospital Health Information Department Time Allocation Report September 20XX		
Service/Division	**Number of Hours**	**Hours Worked**
Clerical/Primary:	16 h/w × 4 weeks	
Filing	3 h/w × 4 weeks	
Admissions	3 h/w × 4 weeks	
Combining records	1 h/w × 4 weeks	
Tumor registry	1 h/w × 4 weeks	
Correspondence	3 h/w × 4 weeks	
Record completion	12 h/w × 4 weeks	
Supervisory	10 h/w × 4 weeks	
Transcription	0.10 h/record × 720 records	
Coding	0.15 h/record × 1,000 records	
Subtotal outpatient/ Ambulatory surgery		
Total hours worked		

2. What percentage of the total hours is spent in each category of inpatient records, and what percentage is spent in inpatient, emergency department, general clinical, and outpatient/ambulatory surgery records? Round to two decimal places.

Service/Area	% of Time Worked
Medicine	
Surgery	
Pediatrics	
Psychiatry	
Obstetrics	
Newborn	
All inpatient records	
ED records	
General clinic records	
Outpatient/Ambulatory surgery records	

Exercise 9.5

Your physician clinic's chief financial officer has determined that it costs the clinic $3.50 per telephone call for the receptionist to set up an appointment with a physician in the clinic compared with $1.75 per online request to set up an appointment.

1. What would the per-appointment cost savings be if, during one day at the clinic, 250 patient appointments were arranged by online request rather than by telephone?

2. What percentage of savings does this represent?

Exercise 9.6

1. The information services department has requested information about the electronic signature system being used in your facility. They would like to know the locations where physicians are accessing the system. Review the information in the table below and determine the percentage of use from each site. Round to two decimal places.

Community Hospital Electronic Signature System 500 Physicians on Staff; 489 Using the System		
Site	No. of Physicians Using the System at This Site	% of Physicians Using the System at This Site
Medicine, 2 West	54	
Medicine, 2 East	62	
Pediatrics, 3 West	42	
Obstetrics, 1 West	12	
Physician's lounge	87	
HIM department	65	
Personal mobile device	92	
Physician home	75	

2. What is the percentage of physicians not using the electronic signature system? Round to one decimal place.

Exercise 9.7

1. Review the following report and calculate the Unapproved Abbreviations for each physician. Round to two decimal places.

Community Hospital Health Information Services Unapproved Abbreviations List November 20XX			
Physician No.	No. of Discharges	No. of Unapproved Abbreviations	Rate of Unapproved Abbreviations
102	298	34	
237	247	21	
391	110	26	
518	144	22	
637	206	4	
802	82	21	
900	100	12	
Total			

2. Review the following report and calculate the rate of deficiency for each physician. Round to two decimal places.

Community Hospital Health Information Services Physician Documentation Deficiencies January 20XX			
Physician No.	No. of Admissions	No. of H&Ps not Completed within 24 hours of Admission	Rate of Deficiency
102	189	5	
237	234	4	
391	98	8	
518	122	5	
637	178	3	
802	92	7	
900	99	2	
Total			

Productivity

> **Real-World Example:** A health information manager at a small hospital is establishing standards for productivity for a remote employee program. He devised standards in order to monitor the work completed by the remote coding professional. He looked at several months of work performed by the in-house coding professionals and determined the following: Inpatient records at 3 records per hour; outpatient records, 10 per hour; emergency room records, including an evaluation and management review, 5 per hour; outpatient tests only records, 40 per hour; clinic records, 30 per hour. He will be able to select records for the remote coding professional to access through their electronic health record system and then easily monitor the coding professional's productivity.

Productivity is defined as a unit of performance defined by management in quantitative standards. Productivity allows organizations to measure how well the organization converts input into output or labor into a product or service.

Most HIM departments have productivity standards for different areas in the department. For example, in the coding section, a productivity standard may be that employees should code four inpatient records per hour. In a 7.5-hour workday (taking into account breaks the employee will take), 30 inpatient records would be coded per day. But how does the HIM manager or supervisor know how many records should be coded in a day? A number of factors influence this decision. Some things the supervisor should consider are:

- Does the coding professional do anything in addition to coding, such as abstracting, answering the phone, or querying the physician for additional information about the diagnoses and procedures?
- What kinds of records is the coding professional coding? Are they long or short lengths of stay? Are they complex or relatively simple cases to code?

Two simple formulas that accurately calculate labor productivity have been suggested (Miller and Waterstraat 2004):

$$Completed\ work = Total\ work\ output - Defective\ work$$

and

$$Labor\ productivity = \frac{Completed\ work}{Hours\ worked\ to\ produce\ total\ work\ output}$$

Determining the total work output and the hours worked is clear; however, determining the defective work involves auditing the work for any errors. Three ways to audit employees' work output are as follows. First, the manager could perform a review of all the work performed; second, the manager could perform a review of work chosen through a random sample; or third, the manager could use a fixed-percent random sample audit. The last suggestion is the easiest. This method requires the manager to select a fixed percent of an employee's total work for review. The manager also has a predetermined quality standard in mind and then reviews the work and classifies it as completed work or defective work. Additional work could be reviewed if more information is needed to determine the type of defect or until all the work has been reviewed (Miller and Waterstraat 2004).

Table 9.2 shows the calculation for determining inpatient coding productivity for one month. Notice in table 9.2 that Coding Professional D's average work output is 4.69 records per hour ($\frac{work\ output}{total\ hours\ worked} = \frac{375}{80} = 4.69$). However, after auditing the work, it was determined that 240 of those records were coded accurately (completed work output). Coding Professional D's completed work is really 3.00 ($\frac{240}{80} = 3.00$).

Staffing Levels

Healthcare organizations use a variety of methods to determine appropriate staffing levels. For example, many outpatient facilities use patient encounters per **full-time equivalent employee (FTE)** per month. A patient encounter is any personal contact between a patient and a physician or other person authorized to furnish healthcare services for the diagnosis or treatment of the patient. These may include laboratory services, x-ray services, physical therapy, and other ancillary services.

The staffing level is determined by dividing the number of patient encounters by the expected productivity. An FTE is the total number of workers, including part-time, in an area as the equivalent of full-time positions. The number of FTEs does not always equal the actual number of employees because two or more part-time employees might equal one FTE.

$$\frac{Patient\ encounters}{Productivity} = Number\ of\ FTEs\ needed$$

Table 9.2. Inpatient coding productivity calculation for one month

Coding Professional	Work Output (All Records Coded)	Total Hours Worked	Average Work Output per Hour	Completed Work Percentage	Completed Work Output (Records Coded Accurately)	Completed Work per Hours Worked
A	500	140	3.57	91%	455	3.25
B	475	140	3.39	96%	456	3.26
C	300	80	3.75	80%	240	3.00
D	375	80	4.69	64%	240	3.00
Department Average			3.75			3.16

Work Output: number of work units as recorded by the employee or the process
Total Hours Worked: number of hours worked by the employee to produce work, which does not include time for meals, breaks, and meetings
Average Work Output per Hour: work output divided by total hours worked
Completed Work Percentage: percentage of completed work from audit
Completed Work Output: work output multiplied by completed work percentage
Completed Work per Hours Worked: completed work output divided by total hours worked

Example: Community Physician Clinic, a large clinic with 85 providers, experiences 1,500 patient encounters per day. A coding professional is expected to code 150 records per day. To determine the number of coding professionals needed, divide 1,500 by 150. Thus, 10 coding professionals are needed to perform the coding for the physician clinic each day.

Tip: When computing FTE, the manager does not ordinarily round up or down. The reason is that managers must justify the need for any employees. For example, the administration may only want to approve a person working 50% time (0.5 FTE) if a full-time employee is not needed to perform the work.

Hospital HIM departments often use discharges as their method to determine staffing levels.

Example: At Community Hospital, the new HIM director wants to determine the number of employees needed in a coding section. The health information manager first multiplies the average number of inpatient records coded per hour (6) by the number of hours in the workday (7.5), which amounts to 45 records coded per day. Hospital discharges number approximately 65 inpatients per day. Based on this number, the manager then calculates that she needs 1.4 FTEs to accomplish the coding task.

$$\frac{65}{45} = 1.4 \text{ FTE}$$

In this example, the manager would need one full-time employee plus one 0.4 FTE, which is computed as 40 hours per week multiplied by 0.4. Thus, she would need another employee to work 16 hours per week to handle the workload.

Another way to determine the number of employees needed is to calculate how many minutes and hours it would take to perform all the work then divide by the number of productive hours. For example, an HIM director would like to know how many FTEs are needed to analyze the weekly discharges in her facility. There are 350 discharges per week. It takes one employee 15 minutes to code and analyze one record. Using a productive week as 37.5 (7.5 × 5 days) hours, the director determines that she will need 2.3 employees to analyze the week's discharges.

$$15 \text{ minutes} \times 350 \text{ records} = 5{,}250 \text{ minutes}$$

$$\frac{5{,}250 \text{ minutes}}{60 \text{ minutes (in one hour)}} = 87.5 \text{ hours}$$

$$\frac{87.5 \text{ hours}}{37.5 \text{ productive hours}} = 2.3 \text{ FTE}$$

Real-World Example: At a Veteran's Administration Facility, the cancer program manager was able to convince the hospital administration to provide more funding for the cancer registry department by providing a simple graph of the number of new cases, which we will study in Chapter 11. She was able to show that from the previous year there was an increase of about 100 patients and an increase in the number of patients that were being followed-up. The administration had planned to decrease funding to that unit but instead was able to increase the funding in order to provide an additional employee to the cancer registry department (Folkerts 2016).

Exercise 9.8

1. Community Physician's Clinic is a large clinic with 85 physicians. They treat about 9,000 patients each week. Coding professionals are expected to code 100 clinic records each day. How many FTEs are needed to code these records? (Assume a five-day work week and 7.5 hours as a productive day.)

2. Community Physician's Clinic is merging with the Medical Center Physician's Clinic. They will be adding 24 physicians who treat 65,104 patients per year. The coding supervisor at Community Physician's Clinic will be responsible for adding credentialed coding professionals to her current staff. The coding professionals will be expected to code 100 clinical records per day. How many more FTEs will be needed to code these records?

3. Accurate Transcription Company is taking on your hospital as a new client for a one-month trial period. You report that the average number of transcribed lines per month is 142,500. The daily production standard they require is 950 lines per day per transcriptionist. With 20 work days in the month, calculate the number of FTEs needed for this volume.

4. The supervisor over the coding division in the HIM department at Community Hospital reviewed the productivity logs of four newly hired coding professionals after their first month. Using the information below, which employee will require additional assistance in order to meet the standard of 20 medical records coded per day?

Community Hospital Coding Productivity Report Coding Standard: 20 medical records per day				
Coding Professional	Week 1	Week 2	Week 3	Week 4
1	90	105	98	107
2	100	105	105	95
3	75	80	85	105
4	80	95	115	110

5. Using the information below, calculate the labor productivity for the following coding professionals. Round to two decimal places.

	Inpatient coding productivity calculation for September, 20XX					
Coding Professional	Work Output (All Records Coded)	Total Hours Worked	Average Work Output per Hour	Completed Work Percentage	Completed Work Output (Records Coded Accurately)	Completed Work per Hours Worked
1	400	150	2.67	93.75%	375	
2	405	150	2.70	98.77%	400	
3	345	140	1.75	99.13%	342	
4	400	140	2.86	95.00%	380	

Exercise 9.9

1. Community Hospital wants to make the transition to an electronic data management system. The process will involve scanning 7,500 inpatient records, 3,000 outpatient records, and 2,500 ED records into the new system. The hospital estimates that there are 30 pages per inpatient record, 4 pages per outpatient record, and 4 pages per ED record. Assuming that one scanning clerk can scan 7,500 pages per day, how many days will it take to complete the transition?

2. Use the scenario in the question above to answer this question: The HIM department would like to complete this project in 10 days. How many FTEs will the HIM department manager need to hire to complete this in the desired timeframe? Round to one decimal place.

3. Use the information in the table below to answer the following questions. Each employee worked 7.5 hours per day during the 21 workdays in September. Round all answers to two decimal places.

   a. What percentage of the total number of records did each employee code during the month?

   b. How many records is each coding professional coding each workday?

   c. How many records is each coding professional coding per hour? (Use a 7.5-hour workday.)

   d. How many minutes does it take each coding professional to code one record?

   e. What percentage of records is not passing the quality screens for each coding professional?

Community Hospital Health Information Management Department Coding Section—Productive and Quality Audit Reports September 20XX		
Coding Professional	No. of Records Coded	No. of Records Not Passing Quality Screens
A	450	4
B	510	4
C	385	11

Answers:

a. What percentage of the total number of records did each employee code during the month?

Coding Professional A:

Coding Professional B:

Coding Professional C:

b. How many records is each coding professional coding each workday?

Coding Professional A:

Coding Professional B:

Coding Professional C:

c. How many records is each coding professional coding per hour?

Coding Professional A:

Coding Professional B:

Coding Professional C:

(*continued on next page*)

d. On average, how many minutes does it take each coding professional to code one record?

Coding Professional A:

Coding Professional B:

Coding Professional C:

e. What percentage of records are passing the quality screens for each coding professional?

Coding Professional A:

Coding Professional B:

Coding Professional C:

Exercise 9.10

1. An HIM manager must determine the number of FTEs needed to code 750 discharges per week. It takes 20 minutes to code each record. Each coding professional works 37.5 productive hours per week. How many FTEs will the HIM manager need? Round to one decimal place.

2. The coding department at Community Physician's Clinic developed the following report for the denials committee at the clinic. The billing report shows the following information. Calculate the denial rate for each third-party payer category and the total. Round to two decimal places.

Community Physician's Clinic Coding Department Denials–October 20XX			
Payment Source	Number of Claims Sent	Number of Denials	Percentage of Denials
Medicare	460	43	
Medicaid	345	35	
Tricare/Military	182	14	

(continued on next page)

Community Physician's Clinic Coding Department Denials–October 20XX			
Payment Source	Number of Claims Sent	Number of Denials	Percentage of Denials
Commercial payers	1,307	83	
Worker's Compensation	6	1	
Total			

3. Using the information above, how many hours will it take to reconcile these denials if each denial takes 1.5 hours to review and resubmit the bill?

4. The Coding Manager would like these reconciled within one month (20 work days). How many FTEs will the coding manager need?

5. The Coding Manager at Community Physician's Clinic submitted the following report to Administration to explain the charge-lag time experienced. Their goal is to bill the insurance companies within three days of seeing the patient.

Community Physician's Clinic Charge-Lag Report October 20XX Total Claims = 2,300	
Reason Not Billed Within Three Days of Encounter:	
Physician not completed with documentation	120
Physician documentation completed, but record not coded	18
Business Office Hold	32

6. Using the following formula, calculate the percentage of non-billed claims for each category. Round to two decimal places.

$$\frac{Reason\ claim\ not\ billed \times 100}{Total\ number\ of\ claims}$$

Charge-Lag Time Reason Attributed to:	Percentage of Non-Billed Claims
Physician	
Coding Professional	
Business Office	

Budgets

If you are responsible for supervising a group of employees, you will most likely also be responsible for budgeting. Usually health information departments are involved with expense and capital budgets.

A **budget** is a plan that converts the organization's goals and objectives into targets for revenue and spending. Planning for the budget begins several months before the facility's **fiscal year** begins. During the planning process, the HIM supervisor uses skills learned in statistics to help approximate the department's expenses for the coming year. Departmental expenses may include employee wages and benefits, supplies, travel and education, membership dues, subscriptions, postage, copying, and equipment maintenance contracts.

The HIM department may also generate some revenue for the department, for example, if it is responsible for the ROI activity or provides a transcription or coding service for the hospital's physicians.

> **Tip:** A fiscal year is a consecutive 12-month period used by an organization as its accounting period. The fiscal year does not have to be a calendar year. For example, the US government's fiscal year begins October 1 and ends September 30. It can be any 12-month period.

Operational Budget

During the year, usually each month, a department director receives budget reports showing amounts budgeted and actual amounts spent. This report generally alerts the department director as to whether or not he or she is over or under budget. Any differences between the budgeted amount and the amount actually spent are called a **variance**. As will be discussed in chapter 10, a variance is a disagreement between two parts. The variance can be used as a device to monitor the department's activities. Budgets also may be available on the organization's Intranet for viewing at any time. This is an easy way for the manager to stay aware of his or her department's budget. An Intranet is a private network that works like the Internet but can only be accessed by certain individuals, such as employees of a company.

The department director should check the budget report at least monthly to determine whether any adjustments must be made in order to stay within the budget. Often the director may be required to explain why the department is over or under budget. This assessment of a department's financial transactions to identify differences between the budget amount and the actual amount of a line item is called a **variance analysis**.

To determine the variance, subtract the budgeted amount from the actual amount and then divide the difference by the budgeted amount.

Item	Budgeted Amount	Actual Amount	Variance
Supplies	$3,000	$4,000	($1,000)
Education/Training	$1,000	$2,000	($1,000)

Using the information in the preceding table, the variance for supplies is $1,000, or 33.3 percent, over budget.

$$\$4,000 - \$3,000 = \$1,000$$

$$\frac{(\$1,000 \times 100)}{\$3,000} = 33.3\%$$

The variance for education and training is $1,000, or 100 percent, over budget.

$$\$2,000 - \$1,000 = \$1,000$$

$$\frac{(\$1,000 \times 100)}{\$1,000} = 100\%$$

The variances computed above are examples of unfavorable variances, that is, the amounts spent were more than the amounts budgeted.

Favorable variances occur when the amounts actually spent are less than or equal to the amounts budgeted, as shown in the table below.

Item	Budgeted Amount	Actual Amount	Variance
Supplies	$10,000	$8,000	$2,000
Education/Training	$3,500	$2,000	$1,500

In example above, the variance for supplies is $2,000, or 20 percent, under budget.

$$\$10,000 - \$8,000 = \$2,000$$

$$\frac{(\$2,000 \times 100)}{\$10,000} = 20\%$$

The variance for education and training is $1,500, or 42.9 percent, under budget.

$$\$3,500 - \$2,000 = \$1,500$$

$$\frac{(\$1,500 \times 100)}{\$3,500} = 42.9\%$$

Capital Budget

The **capital budget** accounts for the major assets the facility will purchase during the fiscal year, for example, equipment for the HIM department. Capital budget items usually are "high-dollar" purchases. Each facility defines what "high-dollar" means. For example, one facility may consider any assets purchased at a cost of more than $500 to be part of the capital budget.

Moreover, items included in a capital budget usually have a "life" of more than one year; that is, each item's usefulness should last longer than a year. Health information professionals are usually involved in assisting the department director in a cost justification for the capital budget. This is very important because only a certain amount of dollars can be allocated to the facility's departments and supervisors who wish to have their projects approved. The department director may ask the supervisor to calculate the **payback period** of the project. The payback period provides information on how long it will take the project to recover its costs. The formula is

$$\frac{Total\ cost\ of\ project}{Annual\ incremental\ cash\ flow}$$

The annual incremental cash flow refers to the savings that a department realizes from the project. For example, if the HIM department needs a new copy machine, the department director may ask the department supervisor to determine, first, how much a new copy machine costs and, then, what kind of savings would be realized from the purchase of a new machine. The supervisor would investigate the cost from different vendors and then calculate an estimate of the savings. Savings considerations might include the time not spent recopying pages, fixing the copy machine, or releasing papers trapped in the machine, as well as the cost of additional paper.

Example: A new copy machine costs $3,000, and the department will realize a savings of $1,000 per year. The payback period is calculated as $\frac{\$3,000}{\$1,000} = 3$ years. There are some disadvantages to using the payback period because it assumes that there will always be the same amount of savings each year. In this example, it is possible that the savings may be less in the second or third year of use due to the aging of the equipment.

Another useful way that department supervisors determine cost justification is by the **return on investment**, which provides information on the rate at which cash is recovered from an investment project. The formula for computing return on investment is

$$\frac{Average\ annual\ incremental\ cash\ flow}{Total\ cost\ of\ the\ project}$$

Using the figures in the example above, the calculation is

$$\frac{\$1,000 \times 100}{\$3,000} = 33.3\%$$

If 33.3 percent is greater than the facility's required rate of return, the copy machine may be a good investment. Other, more complex formulas are used to determine whether a particular project or major item can be undertaken; however, these formulas are generally performed by the facility's financial department.

Exercise 9.11

Complete the following exercises.

1. In deciding whether to purchase or lease new scanning equipment, the HIM supervisor at Community Hospital calculates the payback period. The hospital's required payback period is three years. If the equipment costs $32,000 and generates $4,500 per year in savings, what would be the payback period for this equipment? Should the department purchase this equipment?

2. The coding section in the HIM department shows its first-quarter budget analysis as having an expected cost of operation of $72,000. However, the actual cost of operation was $76,000. Calculate the budget variance. Round to one decimal place.

3. Administration at Community Hospital System (which includes an inpatient hospital, skilled nursing facility, durable equipment company, mental health facility, and outpatient counseling center) will begin a project of converting from the current EHR to another that will allow all the facilities access to one EHR. The estimated cost of the new EHR is $2,750,000. The savings with the new system is estimated to be $575,000 per year. What is the payback period? Round to two decimal places.

4. The HIM Department shows the following monthly report. Calculate the percentage of variance for each line item and the total. Round to two decimal places.

Community Hospital HIM Department Budget Variance Annual Report, 20XX			
Line Item	**Budgeted Amount**	**Actual Amount**	**Percentage of Variance**
Service Contracts	$2,000	$2,500	
Education/Conferences	$4,500	$2,400	
Travel	$2,000	$1,750	
Dues/Memberships	$720	$545	
Subscriptions/Books	$600	$250	
Supplies	$600	$725	
Total			

5. Your HIM manager has been approved to add $25,000 to the salary budget to pay the coding professionals overtime to catch up on coding records so the claims may be billed. Coding Professional A earns $15.75 per hour, Coding Professional B earns $16.00 per hour, Coding Professional C earns $18.40 per hour, and Coding Professional D earns $17.29 per hour. How many total hours of overtime can be worked if each coding professional works an equal amount of overtime earning time-and-a-half? Round to two decimal places.

Verification of Statistical Reports

Most statistical reports in healthcare settings are computer generated. However, a computer can only calculate statistics from the data that are entered. Standardization of terminology, data elements, and formulas from sources such as those found in appendix A will produce data that are more reliable and useful as well as careful input of data.

When a computerized statistical report is received, the HIM professional should examine it carefully. For example, he or she should verify the total number of discharges listed in a report from coded records and compare it against the total number of discharges according to the census data. Do the totals match? If not, it is important to find out why. Perhaps one of the discharges was not coded. Moreover, computerized statistical reports often give only whole numbers. Thus, the HIM professional may need to calculate certain statistics (for example, death rates) and carry them out to the second decimal place to make the information more valuable to administration or medical staff. Tables or graphs can be created to display a portion of a computerized statistical report; this is discussed further in chapter 11.

Computerized Discharge Reports

Figure 9.1 on shows a sample computerized discharge analysis report indicating that the average length of stay (ALOS) of total patients is 7.25 days. To verify this information, use your knowledge of ALOS and recalculate. The calculation is

$$\frac{4,713}{650} = 7.25$$

Another verification can be done by adding the percentages given for the day-of-the-week admissions and the day-of-the-week discharges to make certain they add up to 100 percent. In the computerized statistical report in figure 9.1, they do add up to 100 percent (13 + 13 + 18 + 15 + 17 + 14 + 10 = 100, and 7 + 12 + 14 + 19 + 14 + 19 + 15 = 100). These data could be presented in the form of a pie chart. (See chapter 11 for more information on pie charts.)

Reports such as the one shown in figure 9.1 are useful to hospital administrators; this type of review can give some insights into the resources and services used in the facility.

Example: The psychiatrists on staff are requesting that a new 15-bed psychiatry wing be built to accommodate their patients. The administrator could look at this report and see that there were only three psychiatry patients in this month. If this is normal for the hospital, then can the administration justify this expense? Most likely not. However, some other questions that could be posed by administration are: Would adding a separate psychiatry wing increase the number of admissions to the hospital? How many psychiatrists are in the community and would they admit their patients to our hospital if there were more beds? Is there something else happening in the community that could increase the number of psychiatry admissions? Are any of the psychiatry physician offices planning to add additional psychiatrists or psychiatric services to the community?

Figure 9.1. Computerized discharge analysis report

* * * YOUR UTILIZATION PROGRAM * * *

	TOTAL			0-13 YEARS		14-64 YEARS		65 AND OVER		PATIENTS OPERATED	EMERGENCY ADMISSIONS	NO. OF PATIENTS	NUMBER RECEIVED
SERVICE	PATIENTS	DAYS	AVG. STAY	PAT.	DAYS	PAT.	DAYS	PAT.	DAYS				
1	2	3	4	5	6	7	8	9	10	11	12	13	14
MEDICINE	204	1880	9.2	1	2	161	1300	42	578	170	3	128	209
CARDIOLOGY	60	626	10.4			43	436	17	190	44	1	17	21
ENDOCRINOLOGY	2	23	11.5			2	23			2		2	3
GASTROENTEROL	13	99	7.6			13	99			13		6	11
ONCOLOGY	17	178	10.5			10	112	7	66	16		8	15
PULMONARY MED	4	40	10.0			4	40			4		1	1
PSYCHIATRY	3	17	5.7			2	14	1	3	1		2	6
OB-LIVE BIR	26	114	4.4			26	114			25		2	3
OB-NOT DELIV	9	23	2.6			9	23			4			
OB-ABOR FETUS	15	26	1.7			15	26			15		1	1
GYNECOLOGY	33	125	3.8			33	125			31		5	11
NEWBORN	25	130	5.2	25	130					6			
PED MED	47	265	5.6	44	217	3	48			30	1	8	11
PED SURG	5	11	2.2	4	9	1	2			5		2	2
PED ORTHO	5	27	5.4	2	10	3	17			5		4	5
PED RHINOLARYN	2	3	1.5	1	1	1	2			1		1	1
PED OPHTH	1	2	2.0	1	2					1		1	1
PED UROL	1	1	1.0	1	1					1			
SURGERY	35	222	6.3	1	2	31	190	3	30	34	2	13	18
CV SURG	7	74	10.6			6	72	1	2	7		4	5
ORTHOPEDICS	77	551	7.2	1	11	73	506	3	34	74	1	51	78
PLAS SURG	4	8	2.0			4	8			4		1	1
PROCTOLOGY	1	5	5.0			1	5			1			
ORAL SURG-ADU	3	6	2.0			3	6			3			
UROLOGY	23	172	7.5			18	131	5	41	22		12	16
OPHTHALMOLOGY	5	18	3.6			3	9	2	9	5		2	2
RHINOLARYNG	5	17	3.4	1	1	3	13	1	3	5		1	1
ADULT T & A	2	4	2.0			2	4			2			
PED T & A	1	1	1.0	1	1					1			
PODIATRY	15	45	3.0			14	41	1	4	15		5	6
TOTALS INC / NB	650			83		484		83		547		277	
		4713	7.3		387		3366		960		8		428
LESS NEWBORNS	25	130											
TOTALS EXC / NB	625	4583											

TOTAL CASES	AVG. STAY	OTHER HOSP.	SNF		HOME CARE		LENGTH OF STAY DISTRIBUTION			
			UNDER 64	65 AND OVER	UNDER 64	65 AND OVER	1-3 DAYS	4-14 DAYS	15-30 DAYS	OVER 30 DAYS
625	7.3	8	1	7			28%	62%	10%	%

% OF PATIENTS OPERATED	% OF EMERG ADM.	% OF PATIENTS W/ CONS	AVG. # OF CONS	TO OTHER HOSP.	TO SNF	TO HOME CARE
84%	01%	43%	2	1.2%	1.2%	

Figure 9.1. Computerized discharge analysis report (*continued*)

HOSP # XXXX   JAN 20XX   PAGE 1

ALIVE STATUS (15)	AMA (16)	TRANSFER (17)	EXP NO AUT (18)	EXP AUT (19)	COR. CASE NO AUT (20)	COR. CASE AUT (21)	COMM. PAT (22)	COMM. DAYS (23)	BLUE CROSS PAT (24)	BLUE CROSS DAYS (25)	MEDICAID PAT (26)	MEDICAID DAYS (27)	MEDICARE PAT (28)	MEDICARE DAYS (29)
184	4	14	2				39	323	72	625	28	172	53	700
56		2	1	1			9	60	20	235	5	43	24	273
2											1	9	1	14
13							3	20	7	54	1	11	2	14
14			3				4	38	4	44	2	30	7	66
4							3	33			1	7		
		3					1	5	1	9			1	3
26							2	14	7	34	2	52		
9							1	1	1	1	6	20		
15							2	4	9	14	2	5		
33							7	22	16	51	10	52		
25							2	11	6	33	13	55		
47							12	73	16	91	18	100		
5							2	3	3	8				
5							3	19	1	7				
2									2	3				
1									1	2				
1											1	1		
33			1		1		11	57	19	107			4	38
6		1					2	22	2	21			3	31
76		1					29	233	20	161	8	21	4	46
4									3	7	1	1		
1							1	5						
3									3	6				
23							5	27	10	73	2	19	5	41
5									3	9			2	9
5							2	3	2	11			1	3
2									2	4				
1							1	1						
15							4	11	7	23	3	7	1	4
616	4	21	7		2		145	985	237	1633	114	605	108	1242

DEATHS						OTHER PAYMENT STATUS							
GROSS DEATH RATE	NET DEATH RATE	GROSS AUT. RATE	NET AUT. RATE	COR CASES	POST-OP	SELF-PAY PAT	SELF-PAY DAYS	WORK-COMP PAT	WORK-COMP DAYS	FREE OTHER – GOV PAT	FREE OTHER – GOV DAYS	UMW PAT	UMW DAYS
01%	01%	22%	22%			26	124	18	107	1	9		

DAY OF WEEK OF ADMISSION							DAY OF WEEK OF DISCHARGE						
SUN	MON	TUES	WED	THURS	FRI	SAT	SUN	MON	TUES	WED	THURS	FRI	SAT
13%	13%	18%	15%	17%	14%	10%	07%	12%	14%	19%	14%	19%	15%

Example: If the cardiologists asked administration to add a new catheterization lab, the administrator can see that 60 patients were seen in this month and they have a fairly high length of stay. Certainly, additional comparison reports, such as checking the operation index, could be reviewed to ascertain the number of patients seen by the cardiologists and the number of cardiac catheterizations performed before a decision is made. Questions administrators might want answered are: Must patients wait to have the procedure performed? How many hours per day is the catheterization lab being used? Are any cardiologists transferring patients to another facility to perform their catheterizations? This information can help administrators decide if another lab is necessary. These types of reports can serve as a baseline to begin collecting other types of data for decision-making projects.

Computerized Financial Statistical Reports

Computers are also used to compile various financial statistical reports. A sample computerized financial report is shown in figure 9.2.

Computerized Readmission Rate Reports

Figure 9.3 shows an example of a computerized readmission rate report. This type of report delineates inpatients by medical service and calculates each medical service's readmission rate. You can use your knowledge of calculating readmission rates to determine if these types of reports are correct.

Case-Mix Index Report

Figure 9.4 shows a sample of a computerized case-mix index report. **Case-mix** is a method of grouping patients according to a predefined set of characteristics. A hospital's **case-mix index (CMI)** is the average relative weight of all cases treated at a given facility or by a given physician, which reflects the resource intensity or clinical severity of a specific group in relation to the other groups in the classification system. Each Medicare severity diagnosis-related group (MS-DRG) has a relative weight assigned by the Centers for Medicare and Medicaid Services (CMS) that reflects the national average resource consumption for that particular MS-DRG. Even though the relative weight is based on resource consumption by Medicare patients, many facilities use this value for all patients. The CMS determines the hospital payment based on the MS-DRG. Each facility has a set dollar amount assigned to it by the CMS, which is based on a number of factors, such as the CMI, geographical area's wage index, type of facility, and so forth. The hospital payment for any discharge is the MS-DRG weight multiplied by the hospital's base rate (Optum 2012).

To determine the total relative weight of an MS-DRG, take the relative rate assigned by CMS and multiply that by the number of patients discharged in that MS-DRG.

For example, the relative weight for MS-DRG 195, Simple pneumonia and pleurisy without CC/MCC is 0.7044. If there were 120 patients discharged in that MS-DRG, the total relative weight would be 84.5280 (0.7044 × 120). Note that case-mix is reported with four decimal places.

Figure 9.2. Computerized financial report

MS-DRG	MS-DRG Title	No. of Pts	No. of Pt. Days	ALOS	Tot. Charges
	Community Hospital Most Frequent MS-DRGs Medicare Patients Only Annual Report 20XX				
293	Heart failure & shock w/o CC/MCC	216	1,252	5.8	$2,125,018.00
066	Intracranial hemorrhage or cerebral infarction w/o CC/MCC	141	1,009	7.2	$1,798,011.89
470	Major joint replacement or reattachment of lower extremity w/o MCC	136	926	6.8	$2,601,090.62
195	Simple pneumonia & pleurisy w/o CC/MCC	117	807	6.9	$1,271,445.45
192	Chronic obstructive pulmonary disease w/o CC/MCC	98	579	5.9	$920,071.41
378	GI hemorrhage w CC	94	487	5.2	$964,597.03
178	Respiratory infections & inflammations w CC	89	905	10.3	$1,656,856.52
330	Major small & large bowel procedures w CC	88	1,092	12.4	$2,493,260.52
391	Esophagitis, gastroent & misc digest disorders w MCC	86	324	3.8	$560,025.93
469	Major joint replacement or reattachment of lower extremity w MCC	81	617	7.6	$1,329,055.73
309	Cardiac arrhythmia & conduction disorders w CC	71	290	4.1	$506,803.44
311	Angina pectoris	70	234	3.3	$466,286.80
872	Septicemia or Severe Sepsis w/o MV 96+ hours w/o MCC	69	619	9.0	$1,209,069.85
640	Misc disorders of nutrition, metabolism, fluids/electrolytes w MCC	63	366	5.8	$532,230.77
286	Circulatory disorders except AMI, w card cath w MCC	56	248	4.4	$687,146.08
068	Nonspecific CVA & precerebral occlusion w/o infarct w/o MCC	52	158	3.0	$336,667.38
280	Acute myocardial infarction, discharged alive w MCC	51	328	6.4	$790,417.76
689	Kidney & urinary tract infections w MCC	47	240	5.1	$367,789.93
189	Pulmonary edema & respiratory failure	43	369	8.6	$707,485.01
839	Chemo w acute leukemia as sdx w/o CC/MCC	41	85	2.1	$198,692.68

(continued on next page)

Figure 9.2. Computerized financial report (*continued*)

	Community Hospital Most Frequent MS-DRGs Medicare Patients Only Annual Report 20XX				
MS-DRG	MS-DRG Title	No. of Pts	No. of Pt. Days	ALOS	Tot. Charges
389	GI obstruction w CC	39	235	6.0	$386,509.40
244	Permanent cardiac pacemaker implant w/o CC/MCC	33	146	4.4	$592,506.88
394	Other digestive system diagnoses w CC	33	218	6.6	$427,499.12
315	Other circulatory system diagnoses w CC	31	189	6.1	$447,102.64
208	Respiratory system diagnosis w ventilator support < 96 hours	31	387	12.5	$1,215,601.28
842	Lymphoma & non-acute leukemia w/o CC/MCC	1	4	4.0	$4,011.41
844	Other myeloprolif dis or poorly diff neopl diag w CC	1	23	23.0	$45,480.70
876	O.R. procedure w principal diagnoses of mental illness	1	20	20.0	$26,289.88
883	Disorders of personality & impulse control	1	19	19.0	$15,508.06
958	Other O.R. procedures for multiple significant trauma w CC	1	14	14.0	$35,775.10
913	Traumatic injury w MCC	1	4	4.0	$5,560.30
916	Allergic reactions w/o MCC	1	5	5.0	$10,687.30
922	Other injury, poisoning & toxic effect diag w MCC	1	2	2.0	$6,522.35
923	Other injury, poisoning & toxic effect diag w/o MCC	1	2	2.0	$3,161.58
941	O.R. proc w diagnoses of other contact w health services w/o CC/MCC	1	3	3.0	$3,302.98
947	Signs & symptoms w MCC	1	6	6.0	$9,279.07
264	Other circulatory system O.R. procedures	1	2	2.0	$23,031.87
956	Limb reattachment, hip & femur proc for multiple significant trauma	1	7	7.0	$21,149.70
959	Other O.R. procedures for multiple significant trauma w/o CC/MCC	1	5	5.0	$14,882.29
977	HIV w or w/o other related condition	1	4	4.0	$7,104.30
837	Other digestive system diagnoses w CC	1	10	10.0	$28,618.33
		1,891	12,240	6.5	$24,851,607.34

Figure 9.3.   Computerized readmission rate report

Community Hospital Readmission Report July–December, 20XX			
Medical Service	No. of Readmissions	No. of Discharges	Readmission Rate (in %)
Cardiology	10	277	3.61
Cardiovascular surgery	10	84	11.90
Family practice	5	75	6.67
Gastroenterology	5	27	18.52
Gynecology	1	68	1.47
Infectious diseases	1	8	12.50
General/Internal medicine	59	611	9.66
Medical oncology	26	67	38.81
Newborn	1	129	0.78
Nephrology	1	162	0.62
Neurology	1	9	11.11
Neurosurgery	2	56	3.57
Obstetrics	3	143	2.10
Oral surgery	2	12	16.67
Organ transplantation	3	45	6.67
Orthopedics	4	84	4.76
Pediatrics	1	55	1.82
Psychiatry	3	22	13.64
Pulmonary Medicine	1	2	50.00
Rehabilitation	3	36	8.33
Renal oncology	2	2	100.00
General surgery	4	71	5.63
Thoracic surgery	3	37	8.11
Urology	1	42	2.38
Vascular surgery	1	26	3.85

To determine the case-mix index, take the sum of all relative weights and divide by the total number of discharges. The formula for computing case-mix is

$$\frac{\textit{Sum of the weights of MS-DRGs (Medicare severity diagnosis-related groups)}}{\textit{for patients discharged during a given period}}$$
$$\textit{Total number of patients discharged}$$

The report in figure 9.4 portrays the facility's case-mix index for all financial classes for the month and the fiscal year to date. It also shows the case-mix index for Medicare-only patients.

Physician Reports

Healthcare organizations have always been interested in finding effective ways of measuring the utilization of services provided by physicians. One approach commonly used to analyze services is profiling. **Profiling** is defined as a measurement of the quality, utilization, and cost of medical resources provided by physicians or groups of physicians that is made by employers, third-party payers, government entities, and other purchasers of healthcare. Managed care providers actively profile physicians for cost containment purposes. Figure 9.5 is a report of a facility's physician profile. This report lists important information about how physicians use the services of the facility. This is important to the organization's administration because they need to know if physician services are increasing or decreasing. If services are increasing,

Figure 9.4. Computerized case-mix index report

Community Hospital Case-Mix Index Report–All Financial Categories Fiscal Year to Date 20XX		
Total Weight	**No. of Discharges**	**Case-Mix Index**
6831.0912	3,230	2.1149
Case-Mix Report–Medicare Cases Only Fiscal Year to Date, 20XX		
Total Weight	**No. of Discharges**	**Case-Mix Index**
2915.2882	1,367	2.1326
Case-Mix Index Report–All Financial Categories October 20XX		
Total Weight	**No. of Discharges**	**Case-Mix Index**
569.2576	269	2.1162
Case-Mix Report–Medicare Cases Only October 20XX		
Total Weight	**No. of Discharges**	**Case-Mix Index**
242.9407	114	2.1311

Figure 9.5. Physician profile

Community Hospital
Physician Profile
Annual Report 20XX

Atten. Phys.	Total						Deaths						Pts. Receiving Consults			
	Cases	Surg Cases	Days	ESD Pts.	ALOS	Preop LOS	TOT	% of Dths	Post Op	W/in 48 hrs	Aut Cas	Cor Cas	Tot Pts.	Cons Rec'd	Avg Cons	Cons Rate
01000	202	18	1,111	69	5.5	3.1	12	5.9	1		1		72	104	1.4	36%
01005	182	21	1,911	49	10.5	5.5	14	7.7		2	1		93	146	1.6	51%
01006	259	42	2,719	88	10.5	4.5	15	5.8	2	2	1		122	175	1.4	47%
01009	242	29	2,250	79	9.3	3.8	18	7.4	1	3	1	1	117	162	1.4	48%
04000	53	6	509	9	9.6	4.0	4	7.5		1			30	43	1.4	57%
10125	1	1	2		2.0	1.0										
15000	3	3	31	1	10.3	1.0							1	1	1.0	33%
15002	76	10	737	19	9.7	4.6	4	5.3		1	1		55	93	1.7	72%
15006	188	18	1,354	64	7.2	5.6	7	3.7	1	1	1	1	77	103	1.3	41%
15007	2		18	2	9.0											
15008	95	5	751	32	7.9	4.0	4	4.2			2		55	76	1.4	58%
Total	**1,303**	**153**	**11,393**	**412**	**8.7**	**3.7**	**78**	**6.0**	**5**	**10**	**8**	**2**	**622**	**903**	**1.4**	**48%**

the question of additional equipment or staff needs to be addressed; if they are decreasing, the question of why becomes paramount. Facilities may also want to add data referencing infection, complication, and readmission rates.

Exercise 9.12

Complete the following exercises using the reports in figures 9.1 through 9.4.

1. The report in figure 9.1 gives the gross death rate (hospital death rate) as 0.01 percent. Recalculate this rate and round to the second decimal place.

2. Recalculate the gross autopsy rate in figure 9.1. Round your answer to the second decimal place.

3. Using the information below, calculate the case-mix index for the following top ten MS-DRGs. Round to four decimal places.

MS-DRG	Title	No. of Disch	Relative Weight	Total Relative Weight
\multicolumn{5}{c}{**Community Hospital** **Top Ten MS-DRGs** **All Financial Categories** **Annual Report 20XX**}
293	Heart failure & shock w/o CC/MCC	216	0.6762	
066	Intracranial hemorrhage or cerebral infarction w/o CC/MCC	141	0.7530	
470	Major joint replacement or reattachment of lower extremity w/o MCC	136	2.1137	
195	Simple pneumonia & pleurisy w/o CC/MCC	117	0.7044	
192	Chronic obstructive pulmonary disease w/o CC/MCC	98	0.7190	
378	GI hemorrhage w CC	94	1.0021	
178	Respiratory infections & inflammations w CC	89	1.3909	
330	Major small & large bowel procedures w CC	88	2.5491	
391	Esophagitis, gastroent & misc digest disorders w MCC	86	1.1976	
469	Major joint replacement or reattachment of lower extremity w MCC	81	3.3905	
Total		**1,146**		

4. Community Hospital reported that their base payment rate from the CMS is $4,000. Calculate the estimated payment for each of the top ten MS-DRGs in the table above using the hospital's base rate.

Answers:

MS-DRG	Relative Weight	Estimated payment
293	0.6762	
066	0.7530	
470	2.1137	
195	0.7044	
192	0.7190	
378	1.0021	
178	1.3909	
330	2.5491	
391	1.1976	
469	3.3905	

5. The medical staff at Community Hospital has determined that the infection rate by physician should be 2 percent or lower. Using the information below, determine which of the following physicians did not meet the goal of an infection rate of 2 percent or less. Round to two decimal places.

Community Hospital Physician Profile January–March 20XX			
Physician No.	No. of Discharges	No. of Infections	Infection Rate
102	298	8	
237	247	4	
391	110	3	
518	144	2	
637	206	5	
802	82	1	
900	100	2	

Spreadsheets

Numerous statistical software packages are available for the creation of spreadsheets. **Spreadsheets**, or worksheets, allow you to enter text, numbers, and formulas to assist in calculations.

A spreadsheet consists of columns lettered across the top of the document and rows numbered down the left side of the document. The intersections of columns and rows form cells, which are the basic units for storing data.

Each software package varies slightly in method. Most packages perform basic arithmetic functions as well as many of the statistical calculations discussed in this book. Various add-in features allow for data sorting, formatting for printing data, and even graphical interface. Most software packages contain a help section and a tutorial to assist the novice. The best way to gain proficiency with any software package is to "just do it" and practice, practice, practice.

Exercise 9.13

Complete the following spreadsheets.

1. Using Worksheet No. 1 in exercise 3.9 on page 43, create a computerized spreadsheet to calculate the patient census.

2. Using the table in exercise 5.4 on pages 76–77, which lists 15 patients by name, age, clinical service, and LOS, create a computerized spreadsheet to calculate the ALOS. Round to one decimal place.

Chapter 9 Matching Quiz

Match the definition with the terms.

Definitions:

a. The financial analysis of the extent of value a major purchase will provide
b. Worksheet into which text, numbers, and formulas are entered to assist with calculations
c. A plan that converts the organization's goals and objectives into targets for revenue and spending
d. The authentication of a computer entry in a health record made by the individual making the entry
e. The total number of workers, including part time, in an area as the equivalent of full-time positions
f. Any consecutive 12-month period an organization uses as its accounting period
g. A financial method used to evaluate the value of a capital expenditure by calculating the time frames that must pass before inflow of cash from a project equals or exceeds outflow of cash
h. A measurement of the quality, utilization, and cost of medical resources provided by physicians that is made by employers, third-party payers, government entities, and other purchasers of healthcare

i. A type of financial plan that allocates and controls resources to meet an organization's goals and objectives for the fiscal year

j. The average relative weight of all cases treated at a given facility, or by a given physician, which reflects the resource intensity or clinical severity of a specific group in relation to the other groups in the classification system.

Terms:

1. _____ Budget
2. _____ Full-time equivalents
3. _____ Payback period
4. _____ Case-mix index
5. _____ Return on investment

6. _____ Spreadsheet
7. _____ Profiling
8. _____ Electronic signature
9. _____ Fiscal year
10. _____ Operational budget

Chapter 9   Review

Complete the following exercises.

1. A coding supervisor must determine the number of FTEs needed to code 600 discharges per week. If it takes an average of 20 minutes to code each record and each coding professional works 7.5 productive hours per day, how many FTEs will the coding supervisor need? Round to one decimal place.

2. The HIM department at Community Hospital will experience a 15 percent increase in the number of discharges coded per day as the result of opening an orthopedic clinic in the facility. The 15 percent increase is projected to be 50 additional records per day. The standard time to code this type of record is 15 minutes. Compute the number of FTEs required to handle this increased volume in coding based on a 7.5-hour productive day. Round to one digit after the decimal.

3. The HIM coding supervisor agrees to pay a new graduate $15.00 per hour. This is a full-time coding position at 2,080 hours per year. The cost for a full-time employee's fringe benefits is 25 percent of the employee's salary. How much must the supervisor budget for the employee's salary and fringe benefits?

4. The same supervisor in the scenario above agreed to increase the salary of the employee to $16.00 per hour once she passed her RHIT exam. Three months after beginning her employment, the employee passed her RHIT exam. What will the new budget be for salary and fringe benefits?

5. The forms used to query physicians in your coding area cost $50.00 per 250 forms for the first 500 and $40 for every 100 thereafter. If you need to order 850 forms, what is the total cost to be budgeted?

6. You currently lease scanning equipment at a cost of $2,750 per quarter and two copy machines at $150 each per month plus $0.01 per page copied. You estimate you will copy a total of 30,000 pages a year per copier. What will you need to budget annually for this leased equipment?

7. What is the variance and percent of variance for each item listed in the HIM department budget shown in the table below? Round to two decimal points.

Community Hospital Health Information Department Fiscal Year 20XX			
Item	**Budget Amount**	**Actual Amount**	**Variance/% of Variance**
Supplies	$1,500	$1,495	
Outside temp service	$10,500	$8,500	
Travel	$2,500	$2,575	
Conference fees	$750	$800	
Postage	$2,000	$1,035	
Subscriptions	$325	$320	
Maintenance contracts	$6,000	$3,525	

8. All the patients who present to the emergency services department with a suspected acute myocardial infarction (AMI) are expected to receive an electrocardiogram (ECG) within 10 minutes of their arrival. Of the 45 patients who had a suspected AMI during the last quarter, 33 had an ECG within the specified time frame. What was the rate of compliance? Round to two decimal places.

9. Last month, the ROI specialist received 580 requests for information. He was able to answer 307 within the specified time frame of three working days. What is the rate of compliance in answering requests within the specified time frame? Round to two decimal places.

10. Estimate the hospital charges for the patients listed in the table below based on an average cost of $1,500 per day.

Community Hospital		
Patient Number	**LOS**	**Estimated Charges**
126745	4	
853275	6	
903629	2	
956825	7	
957032	10	
903412	8	
934818	11	
563498	9	
985476	5	
894532	3	

11. Last year, Community Hospital had 32,687 discharges. Of these, 1,789 were readmissions. What is the hospital's readmission rate? Round to two decimal places.

12. In September, the hospital had three coding professionals who coded 1,500 inpatient records, and 22 of the records failed the quality screens.

   a. What is the average number of records coded by each coding professional?

   b. What was the average number of records coded each working day (Monday through Friday at 21 workdays) in September? Round to two decimal places.

   c. What percentage of records passed the quality screens? Round to two decimal places.

13. At Community Hospital each full-time employee is required to work 2,080 hours annually. The table below shows the amount of time that five employees were absent from work over the past year. Use this information to answer the following questions. Round all answers to two decimal places.

Community Hospital Health Information Management Department Coding Section Absentee Report Annual Statistics 20XX		
Employee Name	**Vacation Hours Used**	**Sick Leave Hours Used**
A	40	6
B	22	16
C	36	8
D	80	32
E	16	40

   a. What is the total absentee rate for each employee?

   b. What is the sick leave rate for each employee?

   c. What is the total sick leave rate for this group of employees for the year?

14. The coding department of Community Physician's Clinic is interested in purchasing a software program that will edit claims before they are sent to the Billing Office. The license fee for the software is $60,000 per year. The software is expected to reduce the number of errors on claims and thus reduce the number of claims (denials) returned to the clinic for recoding. Currently, the department codes 47,600 provider visits per month and 500 claims are returned each month for recoding. The facility pays two FTEs in the Billing Office $14.00 per hour each plus 25 percent in benefits to refile the returned claims. The software company promises that its software will reduce the number of returned claims by 90 percent.

   a. What is the rate of claims that are currently being returned for recoding each month? Round to two decimal places.

   b. How many claims are estimated to be returned after the installation of the software?

    c. If the clinic eliminated the two FTEs that handle the returned claims, what savings would it realize after installation of the software?

    d. What is the payback period?

    e. What is the return on investment? Round to two decimal places.

15. Using the information in the table below, calculate the case-mix index for each month in the first quarter at Community Hospital. Round to four decimal places.

Community Hospital First Quarter Statistics 20XX Case-Mix Report			
	January	**February**	**March**
Total discharges	3,213	2,456	3,167
Total weight	7,245.2785	7,458.7499	8,917.4576
Case-mix index			

CHAPTER 10

Descriptive Statistics in Healthcare

Learning Objectives

At the conclusion of this chapter, you should be able to

- Explain how and why percentiles are used
- Compute the percentile from an ungrouped distribution
- Differentiate among range, variance, and standard deviation
- Calculate range, variance, standard deviation, and correlation

Key Terms

Decile	Median	Skewness
Descriptive statistics	Mode	Standard deviation (SD)
Frequency distribution	Normal distribution of data	Variability
Measurements	Outlier	Variable
Measures of central tendency	Quartile	Variance
Mean	Range	

Descriptive statistics are used to describe data in ways that are manageable and easily understood. They describe a population. They also summarize data and we can easily get a sense of the data. The following sections discuss the basic concepts of rank, quartile, decile, percentile, measures of central tendency (mean, median, mode), measures of variation (range, variance, standard deviation), and correlation.

Concepts in Descriptive Statistics

Health information professionals use descriptive statistics in many aspects of their day-to-day work. For example, they determine the number of patients in certain payment categories and review the top ten DRGs for medical staff committee reports. The concepts covered in this chapter will help health information professionals simplify large amounts of data with ease.

Frequency Distribution

Before studying measures in descriptive statistics, it would be useful to briefly cover two concepts: variable and frequency distribution. A **variable** is a characteristic that can have different values. For example, a person may be HIV negative or positive. The characteristic or variable is HIV status and the values are negative and positive. Third-party payers, race, length of stay (LOS), and services are examples of variables. Within each variable, there is more than one possible value. For example, third-party payers include numerous insurance companies. The variable is "third-party payer" while the values are the names of the organizations paying for services.

Because it is difficult to draw conclusions from data in raw form, they are often summarized into frequency distributions. A **frequency distribution** shows the values that a variable can take and the number of observations associated with each value. In the previous example, a facility conducting HIV testing may be interested in the number or frequency of HIV negative and positive individuals using their services. This information is valuable when seeking funding.

Example: Table 10.1 provides an example of a frequency distribution in which types of third-party payers are identified, along with the number of patients in an organization associated with each payer.

Table 10.1. Example of a frequency distribution of number of patients discharged by third-party payer

Community Hospital Patients Discharged by Payer June 20XX	
Third-Party Payer	**No. of Patients**
Medicare	98
Medicaid	56
Tri-Care	23
Blue Cross	85
Mutual of Omaha	67
Other Private Payer	76
Total	**405**

Rank

Rank denotes a value's position in a group relative to other values organized in order of magnitude. For example, a rank of 50 means that a value or score is 50th from the beginning (or end) of a series. The number of scores in a sequence is important in determining the significance of a rank. If there are only 60 scores, a rank of 50th is interpreted much differently than if there are 1,000 scores. For this reason, it may be more useful to express data as percentiles.

In ranked data, the position of the observation is more important than the number associated with it. For example, it is possible to list the major causes of death in the United States, along with the number of lives that each cause claimed. If the causes of death were ordered starting with the one that resulted in the greatest number of deaths and ending with the one that caused the fewest, and these were assigned consecutive integers, the data are said to be ranked.

Table 10.2 shows a report listing the top ten leading causes of death in the United States for the latest data available (2013). Note that cerebrovascular disease would be ranked fifth regardless of whether it caused 130,556 or 84,768 deaths.

Quartile

In addition to determining the rank of the score in a group, it can be helpful to divide data into parts to better understand the relationship among scores. Data organized in order of magnitude can be divided into four equal parts, or **quartiles**. The first quartile corresponds to the 25th percentile and includes the first 25 percent of the data, the second quartile corresponds to the 50th percentile and includes 50 percent of the data, and so on.

Table 10.2. Top Ten Leading Causes of Death in the United States in 2013

Rank	Causes of Death	Total Deaths
1	Heart disease	611,105
2	Cancer	584,881
3	Chronic lower respiratory diseases	149,205
4	Accidents (unintentional injuries)	130,557
5	Stroke (cerebrovascular diseases)	128,978
6	Alzheimer's disease	84,767
7	Diabetes mellitus	75,578
8	Influenza and pneumonia	56,979
9	Nephritis, nephritic syndrome, and nephrosis	7,112
10	Intentional self-harm (suicide)	41,149

Source: Centers for Disease Control 2015a.

Example: The following birth weights were recorded as: 7.8, 5.6, 8.9, 9.10, 5.7, 4.8, 8.1, 9.2, 9.1, 9.4, and 7.6.

Write the data in increasing order: 4.8, 5.6, 5.7, 7.6, 7.8, 8.1, 8.9, 9.1, 9.2, 9.4, 9.10

Find the median = 8.1

The lower half of the data is 4.8, 5.6, 5.7, 7.6, 7.8,

   Q_1 = 5.7 (the middle value)

The upper half of the data is 8.9, 9.1, 9.2, 9.4, 9.10

   Q_3 = 9.2 (the middle value)

Decile

In similar fashion deciles represent data divided into 10 equal parts. The first decile corresponds to the 10th percentile and includes the first 10 percent of the scores, the second decile corresponds to the 20th percentile and includes the second 10 percent of the data, and so on (IIST 2015).

Example: Community Physician's Clinic recorded the wait times for 20 patients. The wait times were (in minutes): 13, 3, 5, 12, 16, 7, 24, 6, 18, 14, 17, 4, 11, 8, 9, 15, 23, 10, 22, 19.

Place the times in order:

   3, 4, 5, 6, 7, 8, 9, 10, 11, 12, 13, 14, 15, 16, 17, 18, 19, 22, 23, 24

   10% of 20 = 2—every two values is a decile.

Percentile

As quartiles divide scores into four equal parts and deciles into 10, percentiles separate the scores into 100 equal parts. If a person scores at the 54th percentile, his score is greater than or equal to 54 percent of all the scores in the group. This is called a percentile rank.

How and Why Percentiles Are Used

Percentiles help people understand their score relative to all scores from a group. If a student is told that she received a score of 34 on a test and she did not know how many points were possible, the 34 has no meaning to her. However, if she is told that the score was in the 95th percentile, this would give a better understanding of the score compared with her peers; that is, only five percent of the class received a higher score.

To find the score that falls within a given percentile in a group of data arranged in order of magnitude:

1. Multiply the desired percentile's percentage by the total number of scores in the given group of scores (*N*). For example, the 38th percentile's percentage would be 38 percent. Likewise, the 90th percentile's percentage would be 90 percent.

2. This number indicates the rank of the score in the group that represents the desired percentile.

Example: The following numbers represent lengths of newborns in inches.

$$12, 12, 12, 13, 13, 15, 15, 16, 17, 18, 19, 20, 21, 21, 22, 22, 23, 23, 24, 25$$

$$N = 20$$

To find the 60th percentile:

1. Multiply 60 percent by 20 (*N*) = 12

2. Count up to the 12th score

3. The 60th percentile is 20

This means that 40 percent of the newborns were over 20 inches in length at birth.

On the other hand, if you want to know in what percentile a score is, take that score and divide the number of scores that are equal to and less than your score by the total number of scores and then multiply by 100.

Example: For instance, in the example above, suppose you want to find the percentile of the newborns that are over 17 inches in length. Take 9 (17 is the ninth score) divided by 20 (the *N*) × 100.

$$\left(\frac{9}{20}\right) \times 100 = 45\text{th percentile}$$

Seventeen falls in the 45th percentile. This means that 45 percent of the newborns were 17 inches or less in length at birth and 55 percent (100 percent − 45 percent) were over 17 inches in length at birth.

Exercise 10.1

1. A pediatrician at the Community Physicians Clinic told a mother that her six-month old child is in the 54th percentile in weight. This means that her child's weight is greater than or equal to 54 percent of all six-month old children. True or false?

2. Use the information below to find your percentile. Your score is 86.

Test Scores out of 100 Points	
95	97
99	74
84	91
65	94
54	89
35	88
86	56
77	96
76	27
100	75
92	93

3. Using the information below for University Hospital, answer the following questions.

University Hospital C-sections by Physician January–December 20XX	
Physician Number	**Number of C-sections**
101	3
202	7
303	27
305	33
401	5
407	8
508	1
518	12
629	9
710	2
911	4
912	18
933	22
944	15
975	20

a. Which percentile is Dr. 975?

b. Find the 60th percentile

4. Dr. Sullivan, a new physician at Community Physician's Clinic has acquired twenty new patients in the first month of his practice. He wants to offer free diet counseling to be given by a new dietician at the clinic to all his new patients whose weight is over the 85th percentile. He asks the health information management (HIM) professional to determine who these patients would be.

New Patients seen by Dr. Sullivan October 20XX	
Patient Number	**Weight**
892345	196
877654	207
764309	155
753254	185
912356	186
455656	192
232323	147
567815	209
875408	242
543465	307
872345	245
925627	232
647382	222
980753	150
765497	189
743952	195
867342	180
142849	175
745261	172
654811	165

a. Using the information above, determine the patients who would be included for the free diet counseling.

b. Dr. Sullivan determines that weight is not low enough to include patients he believes should be included for free counseling and asks you to determine the percentile for 172 lbs., which he believes is a more realistic weight to have to begin counseling.

5. Dr. Davis, a new endocrinologist at the Community Physician's Clinic, acquired 20 new diabetic patients during his first month of practice. Their A1C results are listed below.

New patients seen by Dr. Davis October 20XX	
Patient Number	**A1C result**
893245	5.7
879554	5.8
766509	6.2
752354	6.1
918756	6.8
457656	11.5
235423	10.7
561115	6.7
872208	6.8
544565	9.2
876745	8.4
929827	7.2
648382	6.9
980053	5.5
768997	5.7
741452	6.7
861942	10.4
146349	8.5
749961	9.6
656511	6.0

a. Dr. Davis would like to offer a weight-loss clinic to the patients who are above the 40th percentile of the results. Which patients would that be? List by patient number.

Measures of Central Tendency

In summarizing data, it is often useful to have a single number that is representative of the entire collection of data or specific population. Such numbers are customarily referred to as **measures of central tendency** A common measure of central tendency is average or mean. It is the sum of a set of numbers divided by the number of data points. One of the most common examples of a mean or average in a healthcare facility involves average length of stay, or ALOS (average number of days from admission to discharge that patients stay in the hospital). The ALOS was discussed in detail in chapter 5 and is discussed briefly in this chapter.

Three measures of central tendency are frequently used: mean, median, and mode. Each measure has advantages and disadvantages in describing a typical value.

Mean

The **mean** is a measure of central tendency that is determined by calculating the arithmetic average of the observations in a frequency distribution. It is common to use the term average to designate mean. It is computed by dividing the sum of all the scores (Σ) by the total number of scores (N).

> **Example:** Seven hospital inpatients have the following lengths of stay: 2, 3, 4, 3, 5, 1, and 3 days. To construct a frequency distribution, all the values that the LOS can take are listed in ascending order (in this example, 1, 2, 3, 4, and 5) and the number of times a discharged patient had each LOS is entered. Table 10.3 shows the frequency distribution for this example. As the table shows, three patients were discharged with an LOS of three days each and the remaining four patients were discharged with an LOS of one, two, four, and five days each.
>
> To obtain the mean, divide the total number of inpatient days ($1 + 2 + 3 + 3 + 3 + 4 + 5 = 21$) by the number of values (or frequency distribution), in this case, seven inpatients. This gives a mean of three days. This may also be written as mean ($\bar{X}$) = 3 days.
>
> The symbol $\bar{X}$ (pronounced "ex bar") is used to represent the mean in this formula
>
> $$\frac{Total\ sum\ of\ all\ the\ values}{Number\ of\ the\ values\ involved} = \bar{X}$$
>
> or
>
> $$\frac{\Sigma\ scores}{N} = \frac{Sum\ of\ all\ scores}{Total\ number\ of\ scores}$$

> **Tip:** You may hear individuals refer to the average or mean as "The average age is 10 to 20." This is the wrong use of this statistic. In this example, they are referring to a range of ages, which may be the desired expression in some instances. However, the average is only one value.

Table 10.3. Frequency distribution of seven hospital inpatients

LOS	No. of Patients Discharged
1	1
2	1
3	3
4	1
5	1

The mean is the most common measure of central tendency. One of its advantages is that it is easy to compute. It is used as the basis for a large proportion of statistical tests. One disadvantage of the mean is that it is sensitive to **outliers**, extreme statistical values that fall outside the normal range and may distort its representation of the central tendency of a set of numbers. For example, if six women in a group weighed 110, 115, 120, 122, 125, and 227 pounds, the mean weight of the group would be 819/6, or 136.5 pounds. However, given that five of the women weigh 125 pounds or less, the mean of this sample is not a very good indication of central tendency. Thus, the more asymmetric or unequal the distribution, the less desirable it is to summarize the observations by using the mean.

Median

The **median** is the midpoint (center) of the distribution of values, or the point above and below which 50 percent of the values fall. The median value is obtained by arranging the numerical observations in ascending or descending order and then determining the middle value. This may be the middle observation (if there is an odd number of values) or a point halfway between the two middle values (if there is an even number of values).

To arrive at the median in an even-numbered distribution, add the two middle values together and divide by 2. When the two middle values are the same, the median is that value.

Example: The numbers in the LOS example used earlier are sequenced as follows:

1

2

3

3 ← median (midpoint)

3

4

5

The median is 3.

Example: The median weight of the women who weighed 110, 115, 120, 122, 125, and 227 pounds is shown as follows:

110

115

120

$\leftarrow$ median $\left(120 + 122 = \dfrac{242}{2} = 121\right)$

122

125

227

The median is 121.

> **Tip:** The advantage to using the median as a measure of central tendency is that it is unaffected by outliers. The value of 121 pounds is much more representative of the fact that five out of the six women weigh 125 pounds or less than the mean value of 136.5 as seen in the previous example.

The median is also often used in calculating LOS in long-term care cases. As discussed in chapter 5, a long-stay patient's discharge days are allocated to the period in which he or she is discharged. Sometimes this can give a distorted average, especially on a monthly (rather than annual) basis.

> **Example:** In March, a long-term care facility discharged 130 patients with a total LOS of 1,267 days. The LOS for one of the patients was 365 days. The ALOS for all 130 patients was 9.8 days ($\frac{1,267}{130} = 9.75$). If the stay of the one patient is removed from the total LOS, the ALOS becomes 6.99 or 7.0 days ($1,267 - 365 = \frac{902}{129} = 6.99$). Should one patient or a few patients in a population affect the average to this degree? Is the statistical computation meaningful for decision-making purposes? In this situation, the facility has two options:
>
> - First, a notation can be made on the report that either the ALOS of 9.8 includes one patient who stayed 365 days or the ALOS of 7.0 excludes one patient who stayed 365 days. Both calculations can be made. Appropriate notes should be attached to the report to indicate the difference.
> - Second, the computation using the median rather than the mean can be used. The individual LOSs would be arranged in numerical order from highest to lowest or vice versa.

Median Used to Describe Length of Stay

The list in table 10.4 includes the LOS of 15 discharged patients.

These numbers placed in order from highest to lowest are: 28, 21, 9, 8, 5, 5, 4, 4, 4, 4, 3, 2, 2, 2, and 1. The midpoint falls at 4. Note that, regardless of value, 50 percent of the total numbers fall above this point and 50 percent fall below. The median provides a more revealing representation of the ALOS when one or a few long-stay patients would otherwise distort the arithmetic mean. The median is not sensitive to outliers as is the mean. However, one disadvantage of using the median is that manual computation is much more time-consuming than computation of the mean. Moreover, it would be impractical with a large number of discharged patients. If the statistical computation is manual, it would be better to use the mean. However, if the statistical computation is computerized, it would be better to use the median.

According to table 10.4, patients on the clinical medicine service stayed 28, 8, 5, 5, 4, 4 and 2 days for a total of 56 days. Using the formula, the ALOS for medicine patients is 8.0 days. The median, or midpoint, is 5. One patient had a long stay of 28 days. If that patient is removed from the calculation, the ALOS for medicine patients would be 4.7 days. In this case, the median would be a better choice to show the ALOS for these patients.

Table 10.4.   LOS of 15 discharged patients

Name	Age	Clinical Service	Admission Date	Length of Stay
Bertram	32	Medicine	6/01	4
Williams	22	Medicine	5/28	8
Capney	47	Medicine	6/01	4
Darcy	27	Medicine	5/08	28
Ediger	62	Surgery	6/01	4
Fitzroy	53	Medicine	5/31	5
Guilford	21	Obstetrics	6/03	2
Hansen	30	Obstetrics	6/01	4
Isaacs	76	Medicine	6/03	2
Jamison	35	Surgery	5/15	21
Kapowski	20	Obstetrics	6/03	2
Lawrence	50	Medicine	5/31	5
Bennett	41	Obstetrics	6/02	3
Oswald	14	Obstetrics	6/04	1
Petersen	48	Surgery	5/27	9
Total				**102**

Mode

Mode is the third measure of central tendency and is the value that occurs most frequently in the data. In this sense, it is the value that is most typical. Its advantage is that it is the simplest of the measures of central tendency because it does not require any calculations. The example in table 10.4 shows that the mode is 4 because 4 is the most frequent value in the set.

While the mode is simple to use, there are disadvantages to using it. In the case of a small number of values, each value could occur only once and there will be no mode. Or, two values may be more common than others and you could have two or more modes.

> **Tip:** The mode does not have to be numerical. If you ask every person in your class what his or her favorite food is and tally the answers, you will most likely find a mode.

Example: Add another patient's LOS of 35 to the LOS example on page 177 to illustrate the mean and the median. The values would now total 56 ($1 + 2 + 3 + 3 + 3 + 4 + 5 + 35$). Divide 56 by the number of values involved (8) to calculate the mean of 7, or $\frac{56}{8} = 7$.

The median would be calculated as follows:

1

2

3

3

$\leftarrow$ median $\left(3+3=\dfrac{6}{2}=3\right)$

3

4

5

35

The median is 3, and the mode remains at 3.

This example shows that the median and the mode can be unaffected by extreme values.

The mode is rarely used as a sole descriptive measure of central tendency because it may not be unique; there may be two or more modes. These are called bimodal (two modes) or multimodal (several modes) distributions.

Example: The following represents a collection of values of LOSs:

1

1

1

2

2

3

3

3

4

5

5

5

7

9

In this group of patients, the modes for the LOS are 1, 3, and 5. The mode is the score that occurs most frequently; in this example, it occurred three times in 1, 3, and 5.

The choice of a measure of central tendency depends on the number of values and the nature of their distribution. Occasionally the mean, median, and mode are identical. For statistical analyses, however, the mean is preferable, whenever possible, because it includes information from all observations. However, if the series of values contains a few that are unusually high or low, the median may represent the series better than the mean. The mode is often used in samples where the most typical value is preferred.

Exercise 10.2

Complete the following exercises.

1. Fourteen patients have the following LOS: 2, 6, 6, 4, 7, 18, 5, 5, 3, 8, 6, 7, 9, and 4. Compute the mean, median, and mode. Round the mean to two decimal places.

2. A student's 10 scores on 10-point class quizzes include a 5, an 8, a 3, five 9s, a 7, and a 10. The student claims that her average grade on quizzes is 9 because most of her scores are 9s. Is this correct? Explain. Round the mean to one decimal place.

3. Fourteen patients have the following LOS: 3, 4, 5, 2, 5, 17, 5, 3, 2, 6, 5, 4, 7, and 2. Calculate the mean, median, and mode. Round the mean to one decimal place.

4. An HIM supervisor timed his staff for eight hours during the workday to determine the average number of inpatient records coded in one hour. Using the findings listed below, what were the mean, median, and mode for each coding professional? What were the overall mean, median, and mode for the coding section? Round the mean to one decimal place.

Community Hospital HIM Department Number of Records Coded							
Coding Professional A		**Coding Professional B**		**Coding Professional C**		**Coding Professional D**	
Hour 1	3	Hour 1	3	Hour 1	5	Hour 1	4
Hour 2	4	Hour 2	4	Hour 2	6	Hour 2	4
Hour 3	6	Hour 3	6	Hour 3	3	Hour 3	3
Hour 4	3	Hour 4	1	Hour 4	5	Hour 4	4
Hour 5	2	Hour 5	4	Hour 5	4	Hour 5	5
Hour 6	5	Hour 6	6	Hour 6	4	Hour 6	6
Hour 7	4	Hour 7	3	Hour 7	2	Hour 7	2
Hour 8	4	Hour 8	4	Hour 8	5	Hour 8	1

(continued on next page)

Community Hospital HIM Department Number of Records Coded
Answers: Coding Professional A:
Coding Professional B:
Coding Professional C:
Coding Professional D:
Overall:

5. The quality manager at Community Physician's Clinic is investigating a complaint that the wait times are too long at the clinic. She wishes to use the median to determine the wait times. Calculate the median and mean of the following wait times. Round the mean to one decimal place.

(In minutes): 12, 17, 11, 10, 9, 22, 18, 20, 8, 7, 6, 12, 12, 13

Measures of Variation

Measures of central tendency are not the only statistics used to summarize a frequency distribution. A facility also may want to consider the spread of the distribution, also called the measure of variation. The measure of variation shows how widely the observations are spread out around the measure of central tendency. The mean gives a measure of central tendency of a list of numbers but tells nothing about the spread of the numbers in the list.

Example: Review the following three groups:

Group A	3	5	6	3	3
Group B	4	4	4	4	4
Group C	10	1	0	0	9

Each of these groups has a mean of 4 ($\frac{20}{5}$), and yet it is clear that the amount of dispersion or variation within the groups is different. The measures of spread increase with greater variation in the values in the frequency distribution. The spread is equal to zero when there is no variation, for example, when all the values in a frequency distribution are the same, as shown in group B.

Variability

Variability refers to the difference between each score and every other score in a frequency distribution. For example, if there are 100 scores, you would have to compute the difference between the first score and each of the 99 other scores, and then compute the difference between the second score and each of the 98 remaining scores, and so on. There would be 4,950 differences in all. A more feasible approach, which serves the purpose equally well, is to define the differences or deviations for all the scores in terms of how far each is from the average or the mean.

Range

The **range** is the simplest measure of spread. It indicates the difference between the largest and smallest values in a frequency distribution. In reviewing the three groups in the previous section on variability, the largest number in group A is 6 and the smallest is 3, a difference of 3. In group B, the difference is 0, and in group C, the difference is 10. Therefore, the range for group A is 3, the range for group B is 0, and the range for group C is 10.

Range has the advantage of being easy to compute. It is the simplest order-based measure of spread, but it is far from optimal as a measure of variability for two reasons. First, as the sample size increases, the range also tends to increase. Second, it is obviously affected by extreme values that are very different from other values in the data.

Exercise 10.3

Complete the following exercises.

1. Fourteen patients have the following LOS: 3, 4, 5, 7, 19, 3, 2, 3, 1, 5, 3, 4, 7, and 2. What is the range of this distribution of numbers?

2. Find the range in the following sets:
   a. 2, 3, 7, 20, 6, 8
   b. 0, 1, 8, 20, 4, 7.65
   c. 85, 91, 132, 76, 35, 47

3. The range in a frequency distribution is 20. If the lowest value is 2, what is the highest value?

4. The range in a frequency distribution is 45. If the highest value is 109, what is the lowest value?

5. A group of women seen at a diabetes clinic weighed 140, 125, 210, 245, 202, 199, 173, and 197 pounds. What is the range?

Because the range is determined by the two extremes only, a preferable measure of variability would include the distribution of all the values, not just those at the extremes. More informative measures of variation are variance and standard deviation (SD).

Variance

The **variance** of a frequency distribution is the average of the SDs from the mean. The symbol s^2 is used to show the variance of a sample. "The variance of a distribution is larger when the observations are widely spread" (Horton 2013, 541). The formula for calculating the variance is:

$$s^2 = \frac{(X_1 - \bar{X})^2 + (X_2 - \bar{X})^2 + (X_3 - \bar{X})^2 \text{ and so on}}{N - 1}$$

Or you could use the notation of

$$s^2 = \frac{\Sigma(X - \bar{X})^2}{N - 1}$$

To calculate the variance, first determine the mean. Then, the squared deviations from the mean are calculated by subtracting the mean from each value in the distribution. The difference between the two values is squared $(X - \bar{X})^2$. The squared differences are summed and divided by $N - 1$.

s^2 = variance

Σ = sum

X = value of a measure or observation

$\bar{X}$ = mean

N = number of values or observations

$N - 1$ is used in the denominator instead of N to adjust for the fact that the mean of the sample is used as an estimate of the mean of the underlying population.

The more the values in a distribution are different from one another, the greater the variance and SD. On page 181, the variance in group B equals 0 because all the values are the same. Measures of variation equal zero when there is no variation.

Example: Calculate the variance using the previous data: a sample of 14 patients has the following LOS: 2, 3, 3, 1, 4, 18, 3, 2, 1, 5, 4, 3, 6, and 1. In the next computation, $\bar{X}$ is the actual LOS per patient. The mean LOS is calculated as follows:

$$\frac{56}{14} = 4 \text{ days}$$

The order of this computation is as follows:

1. Subtract the mean from each LOS score (enter result in column 3).

2. Square each result (enter result in column 4).

3. Add columns 3 and 4.

4. Divide column 4 by $(N - 1)$.

The variance is computed as follows:

$$s^2 = \frac{(2-4)^2 + (3-4)^2 + (3-4)^2 + (1-4)^2 + (4-4)^2 \ and \ so \ on}{(14-1)} = \frac{240}{13} = 18.46$$

Column 1	Column 2	Column 3	Column 4
		LOS − Mean (4) $(X - \bar{X})$	(LOS − Mean)^2 $(X - \bar{X})^2$
Patient	Length of Stay		
1	2	−2	4
2	3	−1	1
3	3	−1	1
4	1	−3	9
5	4	0	0
6	18	14	196
7	3	−1	1
8	2	−2	4
9	1	−3	9
10	5	1	1
11	4	0	0
12	3	−1	1
13	6	2	4
14	1	−3	9
Total	**56**	**0**	**240**

In this example, the size of the variance is influenced by the one LOS of 18 days. The more the values in a distribution are different from each other, the greater the variance and SD.

> **Tip:** The sum of the deviations from the mean is always equal to zero. Therefore, by squaring the differences from the mean, the negative and positive deviations do not cancel each other out. When they are squared, negative as well as positive values become positive.

Standard Deviation

The **standard deviation (SD)** is the square root of the variance. As such, it can be more easily interpreted as a measure of variation. If the SD is small, there is less dispersion around the mean. If the SD is large, there is greater dispersion around the mean.

> **Tip:** The square root of a number is that number whose square is the number. The square of a number is that number multiplied by itself. For example, the square root of 9 is 3 $(3 \times 3 = 9)$.

To understand this concept, it is helpful to learn about what mathematicians call normal distribution of data. A **normal distribution of data** means that most of the values in a set of data are close to the "average" and relatively few values tend to one extreme or the other, creating a bell-shaped distribution curve.

The SD is a statistic that tells how closely all the observations are clustered around the mean in a set of data. When the examples are closely gathered and the bell-shaped curve is steep, the SD is small. When the examples are spread apart and the bell-shaped curve is relatively flat, the SD is relatively large.

Therefore, normal distribution means that if the variable of a particular characteristic for every member of the population were measured, the frequency distribution would display a normal pattern, with most of the **measurements** near the center of the frequency. It also would be possible to accurately describe the population, with respect to a variable, by calculating the mean, variance, and SD of the values.

Example: Computing the value of a SD can be complicated. Figure 10.1 shows an example of a normal distribution. The center, or mean, is at 6. The SD in this example is 2.45. This means that about 68 percent of the observations in the frequency distribution fall within 2.45 SDs of 6 (6 $\pm$ 2.45). Thus, 68 percent fall between 3.55 and 8.45; approximately 95 percent fall between 1.1 and 10.9; and 99.7 percent fall between -1.35 and 13.35.

The formula for calculating SD is

$$SD = \sqrt{\frac{\Sigma(X - \bar{X})^2}{(N - 1)}}$$

Example: Continuing with the LOS example on page 229, the mean is 4 and the variance is 18.46. Thus, the SD is 4.3 (the square root of 18.46 = 4.30).

This means that ± 1 SD contains values ranging from -0.3 to 8.3 (to get these figures add 1 SD to the mean of 4 so ± 1 SD = 4 $-$ 4.3 to 4 + 4.3 = -0.3 to 8.3).

± 2 SD includes values ranging from -4.6 to 12.6 (to get these figures add 2 SD to the mean of 4 so ± 2 SD = 4 $-$ 8.6 to 4 + 8.6 = -4.6 to 12.6).

And ± 3 SD includes all values ranging from -8.9 to 16.9.

Figure 10.2 shows a graph of SD of the LOS example.

Figure 10.1.   Example of normal distribution

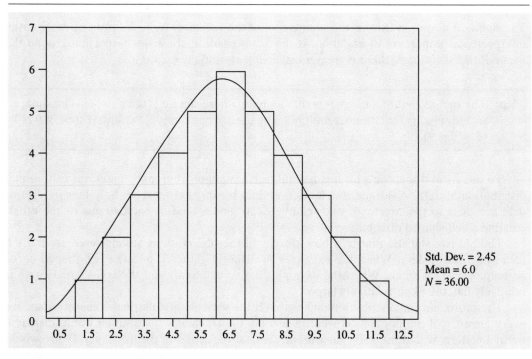

Std. Dev. = 2.45
Mean = 6.0
N = 36.00

Figure 10.2.   Example of standard deviation

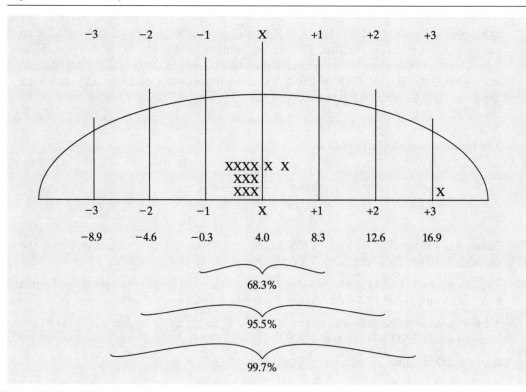

Source: Huffman 1994.

Example: In evaluating the LOS data, one can conclude that 13 out of 14 (92.9%) LOS fell within ± 1 SD from the mean. The remaining value, 18, falls outside the ± 3 SD from the mean and is called an outlier.

It should be noted that the distribution in figure 10.2 is not a normal distribution. As stated earlier, in a normal distribution, one SD in both directions from the mean contains 68.3 percent of all values. In this data set, approximately 93 percent of the scores fall between ± 1 SD from the mean. Visual inspection of the data in the LOS example reveals a fairly homogeneous data set despite the large SD. This emphasizes the importance of visual inspection of the data set when making decisions based on statistical calculations.

Exercise 10.4

The following sample report from a cancer registry shows the SDs of weights for 20 males with adenocarcinoma of the rectum. Validate the calculations used in the report.

Weights of Males with Adenocarcinoma of Rectum			
Patient	**Weight lbs. (X)**	$(X - \bar{X})$	$(X - \bar{X})^2$
1	142	−30	900
2	148	−24	576
3	151	−21	441
4	155	−17	289
5	155	−17	289
6	158	−14	196
7	164	−8	64
8	165	−7	49
9	170	−2	4
10	173	1	1
11	175	3	9
12	175	3	9
13	175	3	9
14	183	11	121
15	185	13	169
16	186	14	196
17	189	17	289

(*continued on next page*)

Weights of Males with Adenocarcinoma of Rectum			
Patient	Weight lbs. (X)	($X - \bar{X}$)	($X - \bar{X})^2$
18	193	21	441
19	198	26	676
20	200	28	784
Total	**20**	**3,440**	**0**	**5,512**

$*SD = 17.0; s^2 = \frac{5,512}{19} = 290.1;$ mean $= 172;$ and $N - 1 = 19$

Not all distributions are symmetrical or have the usual bell-shaped curve. Some curves are skewed; that is, their numbers do not fall in the middle but, rather, on one end of the curve. **Skewness** is the horizontal stretching of a frequency distribution to one side or the other so that one tail is longer than the other. The direction of skewness is on the side of the long tail. Thus, if the longer tail is on the right, the curve is skewed to the right. If the longer tail is on the left, the curve is skewed to the left. (See figures 10.3 and 10.4.)

An example of skewness may occur in LOSs when one or more of a group of patients has an unusually long LOS. An unusually long LOS would raise the mean and thus result in a positive skewness.

Other Curves

Although less common than the normal, positive, and negative skewed curves, you may come across other types of curves in the graphical representation of data. Some examples of the other types of curves include a bimodal distribution, multimodal distribution, a J-shaped curve, and a reverse J-shaped curve, which are shown in figures 10.5–10.8.

Figure 10.3.   Example of a curve skewed to the right (positive skew)

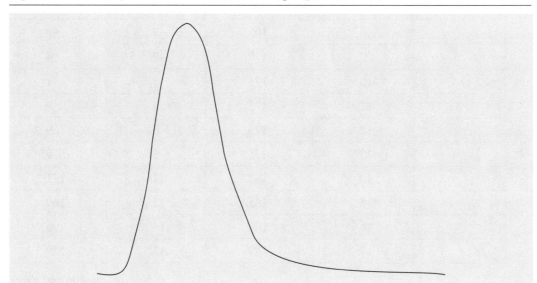

Figure 10.4.   Example of a curve skewed to the left (negative skew)

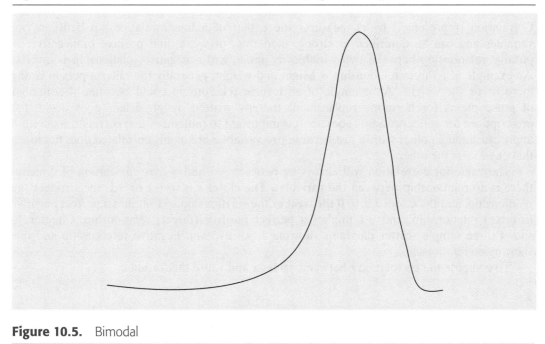

Figure 10.5.   Bimodal

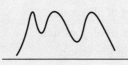

Figure 10.6.   Multimodal

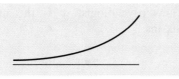

Figure 10.7.   J-shaped

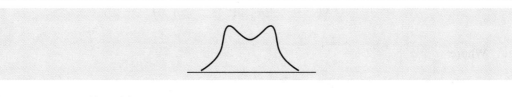

Figure 10.8.   Reverse J-shaped

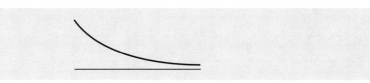

Correlation

Correlation (represented by *r*) measures the extent of a linear relationship between two variables and can be described as strong, moderate, or weak, and positive or negative. A positive relationship between two variables is direct, and a negative relationship is inverse. An example of a direct relationship is height and weight; generally the taller a person is, the more he or she weighs. An example of an inverse relationship could be when the number of prescriptions for hormone replacement therapy written by physicians goes down, the prescriptions for antidepressants goes up. It is important to remember that correlation does not imply causation; in other words, just because two variables are highly correlated does not mean that one *causes* the other.

The value for correlation will always be between −1 and +1. A correlation of 0 means there is no relationship between the variables. The closer *r* is to −1 or +1, the stronger the relationship, and the closer *r* is to 0 the weaker the relationship. −1 implies a perfect negative (inverse) relationship, and +1 implies a perfect positive (direct) relationship. Chapter 11 shows three sample scatter diagrams showing a positive and negative relationship and one showing no relationship.

To compute the correlation *r* between values *x* and *y,* use the formula:

$$ r = \frac{\Sigma xy - \dfrac{\Sigma x \Sigma y}{n}}{\sqrt{\left(\Sigma x^2 - \dfrac{(\Sigma x)^2}{n}\right)\left(\Sigma y^2 - \dfrac{(\Sigma y)^2}{n}\right)}} $$

Where:

Σx is the sum of all the *x* values.

Σy is the sum of all the *y* values.

Σxy is the sum of all the *x* values multiplied by the *y* values.

Σx^2 is the sum of the squares of all *x* values.

Σy^2 is the sum of the squares of all *y* values.

n is the number of subjects in the group.

Example: In this example, *x* = the number of phone calls per week to make an appointment to see a new psychologist; *y* = the number of actual visits to the psychologist plus any walk-ins.

Raw Values	
$\bar{x}$	$\bar{y}$
5	1
6	4
9	8

(continued on next page)

Raw Values	
$\bar{x}$	$\bar{y}$
11	9
14	14
15	16
21	18
$\bar{x} = 11.57$	$\bar{y} = 10$
$\Sigma x = 81$	$\Sigma y = 70$
$\Sigma x^2 = 1{,}125$	$\Sigma y^2 = 938$
$(\Sigma x)^2 = 6{,}561$	$(\Sigma y)^2 = 4{,}900$
$n = 7$	$n = 7$
$xy = 1{,}014$	

In this example, the values for Σx, Σy, Σx^2, Σy^2, $(\Sigma x)^2$, $(\Sigma y)^2$ and Σxy are computed as follows:

$\Sigma x = (5 + 6 + 9 + 11 + 14 + 15 + 21)$
$\Sigma x = 81$

$\Sigma y = (1 + 4 + 8 + 9 + 14 + 16 + 18)$
$\Sigma y = 70$

$\Sigma x^2 = (5^2 + 6^2 + 9^2 + 11^2 + 14^2 + 15^2 + 21^2)$
$\Sigma x^2 = 1{,}125$

$\Sigma y^2 = (1^2 + 4^2 + 8^2 + 9^2 + 14^2 + 16^2 + 18^2)$
$\Sigma y^2 = 938$

$\Sigma(x)^2 = (81)^2$
$\Sigma(x)^2 = 6{,}561$

$\Sigma(y)^2 = (70)^2$
$\Sigma(y)^2 = 4{,}900$

$\Sigma xy = (5 \times 1) + (6 \times 4) + (9 \times 8) + (11 \times 9) + (14 \times 14) + (15 \times 16) + (21 \times 18)$
$\Sigma xy = 1{,}014$

Next, plug these values into the formula for r.

$$r = \frac{1{,}014 - \dfrac{(81)(70)}{7}}{\sqrt{\left(1{,}125 - \dfrac{6{,}561}{7}\right)\left(938 - \dfrac{4{,}900}{7}\right)}}$$

$$r = \frac{1,014 - 810}{\sqrt{(1,125 - 937.29)(938 - 700)}}$$

$$r = \frac{204}{\sqrt{(187.71)(238)}}$$

$$r = .97$$

In this example, $r = 0.97$ is a very strong positive correlation. Although causation cannot be implied, it can still be said that there is a strong direct relationship between x and y. In this case, there is a very strong correlation between the number of appointments made and the number of actual visits made with the psychologist.

Calculating the correlation can be a lengthy process, especially if there are a large number of subjects. Therefore, after learning how to do the process by hand, it is best to use computer software or a calculator that is capable of computing r from keying in the values of x and y; in this way, your answer will be accurate.

Calculations for variance, SD, and correlation are not usually part of the health information technician's day-to-day activities; however, it is important to be familiar with these concepts. For example, you may pick up a journal article, listen to a speaker who is discussing these calculations, or be asked to validate the data. An understanding of them may be necessary in order to communicate this information with others.

Chapter 10   Matching Quiz

Match the definition with the terms.

Definitions:

a. The horizontal stretching of a frequency distribution to one side or the other so that one tail is longer than the other

b. The midpoint (center) of the distribution of values, or the point above and below which 50 percent of the values fall

c. These describe a population.

d. The difference between each score and every other score in a frequency distribution

e. An extreme statistical value that falls outside the normal range

f. A measure of central tendency that is determined by calculating the arithmetic average of the observations in a frequency distribution

g. The fourth equal part of a distribution

h. Distance or extent between possible extremes

i. A characteristic or property that may take on different values

j. A measure of central tendency that consists of the most frequent observation in a frequency distribution

Terms:

1. _____ Median
2. _____ Mean
3. _____ Mode
4. _____ Range
5. _____ Variability

6. _____ Descriptive statistics
7. _____ Quartile
8. _____ Variable
9. _____ Outlier
10. _____ Skewness

Chapter 10   Review

1. Your medical terminology instructor listed the following grades for the class out of a 75-point test:

   34, 36, 41, 43, 44, 49, 50, 55, 57, 60, 64, 66, 67, 67, 67, 68, 68, 69, 70, 73

   a. Find the 90th percentile.
   b. Your score was 64; what is your percentile?

2. From the following list of number of discharges each day in September, compute the mean, median, mode, and range. Round the mean and median to one decimal point.

University Hospital Number of Discharge Days June 20XX					
Day	No. of Discharges	Day	No. of Discharges	Day	No. of Discharges
1	33	11	63	21	54
2	21	12	70	22	57
3	42	13	62	23	22
4	40	14	70	24	27
5	43	15	44	25	43
6	50	16	40	26	44
7	62	17	28	27	61
8	56	18	43	28	63
9	62	19	51	29	67
10	53	20	35	30	56

3. Use the following information to compute the ALOS and median LOS and range for Community Nursing Center. The discharge date is June 2, 20XX (a non-leap year). Round the ALOS to one decimal place.

Community Nursing Center Discharge Report June 2, 20XX		
Patients	**Admission Date**	**LOS**
1	January 2, 20XX	
2	January 10, 20XX	
3	February 8, 20XX	
4	February 10, 20XX	
5	February 26, 20XX	
6	March 1, 20XX	
7	March 6, 20XX	
8	March 12, 20XX	
9	March 15, 20XX	
10	April 1, 20XX	
11	April 15, 20XX	
12	May 3, 20XX	
13	May 5, 20XX	
14	May 6, 20XX	
15	May 18, 20XX	

4. The following table shows the LOS for a sample of 11 discharged patients. Using the data in the table, calculate the mean, range, variance, and standard deviation, and then answer questions e and f. Round the variance and standard deviation to one decimal place.

   a. Mean

   b. Range

   c. Variance

   d. Standard deviation

   e. What value is affecting the mean and standard deviation of this distribution?

   f. Does the mean adequately represent this distribution? If not, what would be a better measure of central tendency for this data set?

Patient	Length of Stay	LOS − Mean (5) $(X - \bar{X})$	(LOS − Mean)^2 $(X - \bar{X})^2$
1	1		
2	3		
3	5		
4	3		
5	2		
6	29		
7	3		
8	4		
9	2		
10	1		
11	2		

5. When two variables are correlated, it means that one is the cause of the other. True or false?

6. Dr. Anderson, a new pediatrician at Community Physician's Clinic, wants to study his new patient's growth charts to determine if they are within the guidelines for weight for age. His last ten six-month-old male infants showed weights of 13.2, 14.6, 15.8, 16.5, 18.5, 12.1, 15.4, 16.1, 18.0, 13.2. What is the mean, median, and range of infant weights he is seeing? Round to one decimal place.

7. Dr. Anderson wants to follow the guidelines that recommend a six-month-old infants should weigh 16.5 pounds. In what percentile is the 12.1-pound-infant?

8. A coding supervisor recorded the following salaries for the seven coding professionals in her HIM department section as $15.25, $16.72, $17.23, $15.34, $15.93, $17.05, and $16.21. Find the first and third quartile (Q_1 and Q_3).

9. Last month, 10 patients between the ages of 11 and 13 were seen in their pediatrician's clinic. Their heights were recorded as 51, 57, 60, 51, 52, 49, 53, 57, 61, and 50 inches. Determine the mean, median, and mode. Round to one decimal place.

10. Community Physician's Clinic is examining the number of patients who make appointments by emails and if they actually keep the appointment date and time. They collected the following information for the past month:

Week 1	Number of Appointments Made by Email	Number of Appointments Kept
1	10	9
2	8	8
3	6	6
4	12	11

Determine if there is a correlation between these using the formula for a correlation. Round to two decimal places.

11. Using the information in the question above, the Administrator of the Clinic wants to have everyone make appointments by email instead of by telephone. However, the HIM professional tells him _____.

    a. This is a causal relationship and proves that patients who make appointments by email are more likely to keep the appointment.

    b. This is not a causal relationship; there is only a positive relationship between making the appointment by email and keeping the appointment.

    c. This is just a somewhat good correlation and may not be positive.

    d. This is a poor correlation and does not necessarily mean that appointments will kept in the future.

12. A graph with a bell-shaped curve is referred to as having a _____.
    a. Normal distribution
    b. Bimodal distribution
    c. Binomial distribution
    d. Multimodal distribution

13. When a distribution is skewed to the right, this means it has (a) _____.
    a. Positive skew
    b. Negative skew
    c. No skew
    d. Multiskewed

14. Using the information below, determine the mean and median age and range of ages of the patients discharged. Round mean to one decimal place.

LOS of 15 discharged patients				
Name	Age	Clinical Service	Admission Date	LOS
Bertram	32	Medicine	6/01	4
Williams	22	Medicine	5/28	8
Capney	47	Medicine	6/01	4
Darcy	27	Medicine	5/08	28
Ediger	62	Surgery	6/01	4
Fitzroy	53	Medicine	5/31	5
Guilford	21	Obstetrics	6/03	2
Hansen	30	Obstetrics	6/01	4
Isaacs	76	Medicine	6/03	2
Jamison	35	Surgery	5/15	21

(continued on next page)

LOS of 15 discharged patients				
Name	**Age**	**Clinical Service**	**Admission Date**	**LOS**
Kapowski	20	Obstetrics	6/03	2
Lawrence	50	Medicine	5/31	5
Bennett	41	Obstetrics	6/02	3
Oswald	14	Obstetrics	6/04	1
Petersen	48	Surgery	5/27	9
Total				**102**

15. Decide whether the following statements have a positive or negative correlation:

   1. Positive correlation
   2. Negative correlation

   a. _____ People who suffer from depression have higher rates of suicide than those who do not.
   b. _____ The more absences you have in class, the more your grades will decrease.
   c. _____ The more you exercise your muscles, the stronger they become.
   d. _____ The more iron that an anemic patient takes, the less tired he will be.
   e. _____ As your attendance to your studies decrease, your achievement drops

CHAPTER 11

Presentation of Data

Learning Objectives

At the conclusion of this chapter, you should be able to

- Explain, differentiate, and apply the following terms: nominal, ordinal, interval, and ratio, and discrete and continuous data
- Differentiate between tables and the following graphs: bar graphs, pie charts, line graphs, histograms, frequency polygons, pictograms, and scatter diagrams and choose the appropriate graph to use
- Create tables and graphs to display statistical information
- Prepare the basic elements of a report

Key Terms

Bar chart	Interval data	Ratio data
Bar graph	Line graph	Run chart
Categorical data	Nominal data	Scales of measurement
Continuous data	Ordinal data	Scatter diagram
Discrete data	Pictogram	Table
Frequency polygon	Pie chart	
Histogram	Pie graph	

Types of Data

A set of raw data may not necessarily provide a user (such as an administrator, a physician, or a health information management [HIM] professional) with information that can be easily interpreted. Descriptive statistics are the most common type of statistics that the health information technician will encounter or be responsible for producing. Descriptive statistics describe populations, which can refer to patients, medical services, nursing units, or hospital departments. As mentioned in chapter 10, these statistics provide an overview of the general features of a set of data. The statistics can assume a number of different forms, the most common being tables and graphs. However, before choosing the appropriate method for displaying a set of data, it is important to determine whether the data are categorical or numerical.

Categorical Data

Categorical data are data that are collected and then sorted or divided into groups. There are four types or **scales of measurement** of categorical data: nominal, ordinal, ratio, and interval. Ratio and interval data are considered metric variables. Metric variables are numeric variables that answer questions of how much or how many.

Nominal Data

Nominal data are the lowest level of measurement. The word *nominal* means "pertaining to a name." In the nominal scale, observations are organized into categories in which there is no recognition of order. Examples of nominal data include true/false, male/female, types of insurance carriers, or patient occupations. Often numbers are used to represent categories. For example, male may be listed as 1 and female as 2; or persons may be grouped according to blood type, where 1 represents type A; 2, type B; 3, type AB; and 4, type O. The sequence of the values is not important. The numbers simply serve as labels for some piece of information and are used for convenience only.

Averages cannot be computed on nominal-level data. Nominal items may have numbers assigned to them and may appear to be a higher level; however, they are not. Nominal data is used to reference items. For example, an average blood type of 2.3 for a given population is meaningless. Instead of calculating the mean for nominal data, the proportion (or "how many") that falls into each category is reported.

The following types of healthcare payment categories are an example of nominal data.

Payment Categories

1   Medicare
2   Medicaid
3   Blue Cross
4   Other Commercial Insurance
5   Self-pay
6   Other

Ordinal Data

Ordinal data are types of data where the values are in ordered categories. The word *ordinal* means "to put something in order." On the ordinal scale, only the order of the numbers is meaningful, not the numbers themselves. This is because the intervals or distances between categories are not necessarily equal. For example, head injuries may be classified according to level of severity, where 4 is fatal; 3, severe; 2, moderate; and 1, minor.

A natural order exists among the groupings, with the largest number representing the most serious level of injury. However, the order could be reversed; there is no hard-and-fast rule. There is no reason why 1 could not represent the fatal injury and 4, the minor injury. In addition, the distance between a fatal and a severe injury may not necessarily be the same as the distance between a moderate and a minor injury. The following list shows how this works in a classification of brain injury.

1 Minor

2 Moderate

3 Severe

4 Fatal

Another good example of ordinal data is the Likert scale used in many surveys: 1 = strongly disagree; 2 = disagree; 3 = neither agree nor disagree; 4 = agree; 5 = strongly agree. In this example, there is a natural order 1 through 5; however, 1 could just as easily be "strongly agree" and 5, "strongly disagree."

Interval Data

Interval data include units of equal size, such as intelligence quotient (IQ) results. There is no zero point. The most important characteristic is that the intervals between values are equal. An example of interval scale is time. Time is measured in terms of 24 hours in a day. The time between each hour is the same. For example, there are 60 minutes between 1:00 a.m. and 2:00 a.m. and between 5:00 p.m. and 6:00 p.m.

Ratio Data

Ratio data or scale is the highest level of measurement. On the ratio scale, there is a defined unit of measure, a real zero point, and the intervals between successive values are equal. Ratio data may be displayed by units of equal size placed on a scale starting with zero and thus can be manipulated mathematically, such as 0, 5, 10, 15, and 20.

Example: An example of the ratio scale is age. The difference between two consecutive years would be the same (the difference between age 1 and 2 is one year; the difference between age 55 and 56 is one year, and so on). There is a "zero point" in that zero would mean an absence of age or birth; and someone who is 100 years old is twice as old as someone who is 50 years old.

Exercise 11.1

Review the following table and answer the questions below.

Community Hospital Discharges by Gender Annual Statistics, 20XX	
Male patients	1,203
Female patients	1,235

1. What example of scales of measurement is depicted in the table?

2. Is it accurate to state that a temperature of 80 degrees Fahrenheit is twice as hot as 40 degrees Fahrenheit?

3. If a physician's office saw 50 patients yesterday and 100 patients today, is it correct to state that twice as many patients were seen today as yesterday?

4. Your health information instructor reported that on the last test given, 5 students received an A, 10 received a B, 3 received a C, 1 received a D, and no one received an F. What example of scales of measurement was given?

5. A physician's clinic conducted a survey to determine the level of patient satisfaction with various departments in the clinic. What type of scale is the following survey item?

> The information clerk at the clinic gave me the correct directions to find the department I was looking for.
>
> Please answer this question on a scale from 1 to 5 where 1 = strongly disagree and 5 = strongly agree.

Numerical Data

There are two types of numerical statistical data: discrete data and continuous data.

Discrete Data

Discrete data are finite numbers. That is, they can have only specified values. The number of children in a family is an example of discrete data. A family can have two or three children but cannot have 2.25 or 3.5 children. The numbers represent actual measurable quantities rather than labels.

Other examples of discrete data include the number of motor vehicle accidents in a particular community, the number of times a woman has given birth, the number of new cases of cancer in your state within the past five years, and the number of beds available in your hospital.

In discrete data, a natural order exists among the possible data values. In the example of the number of times a woman has given birth, a larger number indicates that she has had more children; the difference between one and two births is the same as the difference between four and five; and the number of births is restricted to whole numbers (a woman cannot give birth 2.3 times). For the most part, measurements on the nominal and ordinal scales are discrete.

Continuous Data

Continuous data represent measurable quantities but are not restricted to certain specified values. A variable that is continuous can take on a fractional value. For example, a patient's temperature may be 102.6° F. Another example is height. One could say that someone is approximately 6 feet tall, refine it to 5 feet 10 inches, and refine it still further to 5 feet 10 inches. Age is yet another example. A person may have been 20 years old on your last birthday, but now the person would be 20 plus some part of another year.

The only limiting factor for a continuous observation is the degree of accuracy with which it can be measured. For analysis, continuous data often are converted to a range that acts as a category. For example, age can be categorized in ranges (0–20, 21–40, and so on). Measurements on the interval and ratio scales can be grouped; interval and ratio variables are continuous.

Data Display

Data display is critical to data analysis because it reveals patterns and behaviors. When preparing a statistical report, the user must define its objectives and scope:

- What information is needed?
- What information do you want your audience to know?
- What information is available?
- Are the data collected routinely by the facility, or must additional data be collected?

If the purpose requires frequencies, percentages, or relationships among variables, the data may be presented in the form of a table or a graph. Basically, statistical tables are used for summarizing data; they simply list values into rows and columns and do not easily capture the audience's attention. On the other hand, graphs and charts can present data for quick visualization of relationships.

Tables

A table is an orderly arrangement of values that groups data into rows and columns. Almost any type of quantitative information can be grouped into tables. Columns allow you to read data up and down, and rows allow you to read data across. The columns and rows should be labeled. Many word-processing, spreadsheet, and database software programs offer assistance in the creation of tables. In table 11.1, variables arranged in columns across the page identify the individual patient name, age, clinical service, and length of stay. Each row represents one patient.

Table 11.1. Community Medical Center analysis showing patients discharged

Community Hospital Discharges 12/1/20XX			
Name	Age	Clinical Service	Length of Stay
Smith	5	Surgical	1
Valdez	22	Obstetrical	1
Chu	26	Obstetrical	2
MacDuff	18	Obstetrical	3
Johnson	10	Surgical	7
O'Brien	80	Surgical	8
Lewandowski	35	Surgical	11
Jones	52	Medical	15
Shultz	69	Medical	37
Martini	49	Medical	42
Source: Community Medical Center.			

There are a number of advantages to using tables, including:

- More information can be presented.
- Exact values can be included to retain precision.
- Supportive details can be provided.
- Less work and fewer costs are required in the preparation.
- Flexibility is maintained without distortion of data.

The essential components of a table include:

- **Table number:** Use table numbers in a professional report in order to identify the table referenced in the body of the report.
- **Title:** The title must explain as simply as possible what is contained in the table. The title should answer the questions:
  ○ What are the data? For example, are these percentages or frequencies?
  ○ Who? Whom is the table about? For instance, are these male or female patients, a certain service, or a type of disease?
  ○ Where? For example, is this your hospital, the United States, or your state?
  ○ When? What is the time period?
- **Headnote:** A headnote is a short explanatory note that applies to the values in the table, just under the title. Use a smaller print for this value. For example, if you were reporting data that was in the millions, you could place this in the headnote as "In Millions" unless you include it in the title.
- **Caption:** This refers to the headings of the columns. They should be brief and self-explanatory.
- **Stubs:** The categories (the left-hand column of a table).
- **Body or Cells:** The information formed by intersecting columns and rows. Data are entered into the cells.
- **Source footnote:** Located at the bottom of a table. This may include the source for any factual data or contain explanatory notes.

Table 11.2 illustrates the essential components of a table.
Table 11.3 shows a sample table with completed components.

Table 11.2.   Essential components of a table

Title (Headnote)			
	Caption	**Caption**	**Caption**
Stub	Cell	Cell	Cell
Stub	Cell	Cell	Cell
Stub	Cell	Cell	Cell
Source:			

Table 11.3. Lung cancer by age and gender at Community Hospital, 20XX

Community Hospital Lung Cancer by Age and Gender Annual Statistics, 20XX		
Age, years	**Male**	**Female**
≤ 30	1	0
31–40	2	1
41–50	2	1
51–60	10	10
61–70	42	44
71+	29	27
Total	**86**	**83**

Although these rules are important in the construction of tables, it is more important to use good judgment. Check the table to be sure that it is logical and self-explanatory. Are headings specific and understandable for every column and row? Are sources identified, if appropriate? Do totals add up in columns and rows? Is the table easy to read? Remember to present the data in a format that illustrates a specific idea.

Frequency Distribution Tables

As discussed in chapter 10, a frequency distribution shows the values that a variable can take and the number of observations associated with each value. A variable is a characteristic or property that may take on different values. For example, third-party payers, discharge service, and admission day are examples of variables.

Example: The Utilization Resource Committee is interested in knowing the admission days for patients in your hospital. To construct a frequency distribution, you would list the days of the week and then enter the observations or number of patients admitted on the corresponding day of the week. Table 11.4 illustrates what this would look like.

A frequency distribution table also may show the proportion, that is, the proportion of patients admitted on any of the days. To determine this, the value is divided by the total. The total should always equal 1.00.

Table 11.5 shows the same frequency distribution as in the example in table 11.4 but with the proportion added. Notice that to arrive at the proportion, the student should divide the number of patients admitted by the total. For example, Sunday shows 20 admissions of the 132 total.

$$\frac{20}{132} = 0.15$$

Table 11.4.   Report illustrating sample frequency distribution table

Sample Frequency Distribution for Admission Day June 20XX	
Day of the Week	**No. of Patients Admitted**
Sunday	20
Monday	29
Tuesday	28
Wednesday	12
Thursday	13
Friday	22
Saturday	8
Total	**132**

Table 11.6 shows a frequency distribution table of adult cigarette consumption from 2000 to 2011. Additionally, you see the total consumption of cigarettes and the per capita consumption along with all types of combustible and noncombustible tobacco and noncigarette combustible tobacco.

In this table you can clearly see that there is a decrease in the amount of per capita cigarette consumption, but also take note of the increase in noncigarette combustible tobacco. This includes all combustible products other than cigarettes including chewing tobacco, snuff, and e-cigarettes.

Table 11.5.   Report illustrating sample frequency distribution with proportion

Sample Frequency Distribution for Admission Day June 20XX		
Day of the Week	**No. of Patients Admitted**	**Proportion**
Sunday	20	0.15
Monday	29	0.22
Tuesday	28	0.21
Wednesday	12	0.09
Thursday	13	0.10
Friday	22	0.17
Saturday	8	0.06
Total	**132**	**1.00**

Table 11.6.   Report illustrating frequency distribution

Year	Cigarettes		All combustible tobacco		Noncigarette combustible tobacco	
	Total consumption (in millions)	Adult per capita consumption	Total consumption (in millions)	Adult per capita consumption	Total consumption (in millions)	Adult per capita consumption
2000	435,570	2,076	450,725	2,148	15,155	72
2001	426,720	2,010	440,693	2,075	13,973	66
2002	415,724	1,936	430,763	2,006	15,040	70
2003	400,327	1,844	415,930	1,916	15,603	72
2004	397,655	1,811	414,421	1,888	16,766	76
2005	381,098	1,717	401,187	1,807	20,089	90
2006	380,594	1,695	401,241	1,787	20,648	92
2007	361,590	1,591	384,087	1,690	22,497	99
2008	346,419	1,507	371,264	1,615	24,845	108
2009	317,736	1,367	342,124	1,472	24,388	105
2010	300,451	1,278	329,239	1,400	28,788	1222
2011	292,769	1,232	326,577	1,374	33,808	142

Source: Centers for Disease Control and Prevention 2012.

Table 11.7 shows a frequency distribution table of deaths attributed to smoking by gender in the United States from 1965 to 2013.

To display discrete or continuous data in the form of a frequency distribution table, the range of values of the observations must be broken down into a series of distinct groups that do not overlap. For example, when arranging a frequency distribution table by patient age, age ranges should not be listed as 1–10, 10–20, 20–30, 30–40, and so on because a patient could be placed in two categories if he were age 20: the 10-to-20 age range and the 20-to-30 age range. Thus, age ranges should be listed as 1–10, 11–20, 21–30, 31–40, and so on.

Notice the years in table 11.7. They do not overlap each other; 1965–1999, then the next group is 2000–2004, and so on.

Summarizing the data involves setting up categories and counting the number of cases that fall into each category, thereby creating a frequency distribution. Following are some general rules for choosing the classes or categories into which the data are to be grouped and the range of each:

- Do not use fewer than 5 or more than 15 categories. However, the choice depends mostly on the number of values to be grouped.

Table 11.7. Report illustrating frequency distribution

2014 Surgeon General's Report
Smoking-attributable mortality by gender, United States, 1965–2014

Disease	Males				Females			
	1965–1999	2000–2004	2005–2009	2010–2014	1965–1999	2000–2004	2005–2009	2010–2014
Total cancers	3,091,600	522,360	501,500	501,500	1,053,700	281,880	317,000	317,000
Total cardiovascular and metabolic diseases	3,853,200	395,700	478,000	478,000	1,685,800	246,790	325,000	325,000
Total pulmonary diseases	1,440,700	268,980	291,000	291,000	715,800	247,720	274,500	274,500
Perinatal conditions	54,200	2,230	2,910	2,910	40,200	1,660	2,160	2,160
Residential fires	41,930	2,080	1,680	1,680	33,280	1,600	1,420	1,420
Total secondhand smoke	853,690	156,940	117,630	117,630	490,310	90,060	88,790	88,790

Source: Department of Health and Human Services 2014.

- Categories should be well defined. Choose categories that cover the smallest and largest values and do not produce gaps between categories.
- The categories should be mutually exclusive where each observation is grouped into one— and only one—category. Avoid successive classes that overlap or have common values.
- Whenever possible, make the classes cover equal ranges (or intervals) of values. These ranges also should be made up of numbers that are easy to work with.
- A table should be able to stand alone; that is, the audience should be able to review the table and understand it without supporting information.

Exercise 11.2

The table below lists the patients seen last month at Community Hospital with their age and cholesterol reading. Create a table using common age categories and these ranges for cholesterol.

Community Hospital Cholesterol Readings, October, 20XX Desirable ≤ 199 Borderline High 200–239 High ≥ 240							
Age	Cholesterol	Age	Cholesterol	Age	Cholesterol	Age	Cholesterol
14	118	44	138	38	165	56	185
80	139	47	204	18	142	20	200
42	187	48	236	62	139	45	241
37	201	25	186	37	202	63	175
23	107	56	201	32	207	70	188
24	109	47	198	17	157	42	239
67	132	20	210	55	238	55	175
55	235	43	248	13	134	61	168
52	185	50	137	44	239	53	173
52	192	34	188	64	165	41	238
47	144	38	245	70	172	60	180
42	158	75	175	44	245	30	207
37	160	55	207	65	187	62	185
33	155	69	192	51	248	49	207

(continued on next page)

Community Hospital Cholesterol Readings, October, 20XX Desirable ≤ 199 Borderline High 200–239 High ≥ 240							
Age	Cholesterol	Age	Cholesterol	Age	Cholesterol	Age	Cholesterol
39	221	31	196	43	240	39	147
34	244	51	147	51	188	53	155
75	186	63	200	50	203	46	246
81	160	18	137	20	145	43	222
79	154	37	245	72	175	26	147
67	154	43	256	39	200	46	201
50	192	44	188	19	145	60	152
53	188	52	200	63	145	35	150
26	137	51	147	36	176	53	215
24	140	19	132	33	185	60	165
22	138	73	147	16	137	63	168

Exercise 11.3

The following table shows a frequency distribution of patients with colon cancer treated at Community Hospital. Compute the proportion of patients in each category. Round to two decimal places.

Community Hospital Ages of Patients with Colon Cancer Annual Statistics, 20XX		
Age	No. of Patients	Proportion
≤ 30	3	
31–40	12	
41–50	18	
51–60	60	
61–70	65	
71+	48	

Graphs

Graphs of various types are the best means for presenting data for quick visualization of relationships. They often supply a lesser degree of detail than tables. However, data presented in a graph can be helpful in displaying statistics in a concise manner. There are advantages to using graphs. They grab the audience's attention. They are not meant to entertain the audience but rather present an easy-to-understand version of the data. The visual perception is more immediate when looking at the data rather than reading it. It is easier to see trends and comparisons with graphs.

Graphs should be easy to read, simple in content, and correctly labeled. The presentation of data in the form of a graph is an excellent way to convey the message you want to get across. Instead of presenting an entire statistical report in a table to a group, such as the medical staff or administration, you can create a graph to depict certain data. Many computer software programs are available that convert data into graphic form automatically and attractively.

When creating graphs, follow these general guidelines:

- The title must relate to what the graph is displaying. Follow the same general guidelines for the title in graphs as given in tables, including what are the data, what is the graph about, to whom it refers, and the time period.
- When several variables are included on the same graph (for example, males and females), each should be identified by using a legend or key.
- Categories should be natural; that is, the vertical axis should always start with zero. The scale of values for the x-axis reads from the lowest value on the left to the highest on the right. The scale of values for the y-axis extends from the lowest value at the bottom of the graph to the highest at the top.
- Scale captions are placed on both axes to identify the values clearly. These are simply titles placed on each axis to identify the values. (See figure 11.1.)
- Graphs should emphasize the horizontal. It is easier for the eye to read along the horizontal axis from left to right. Also, graphs should be greater in length than in height. A useful guideline is to follow the three-quarter-high rule, which states that the graph's height (y-axis) should be three-fourths of its length (x-axis).
- The exact reference to an outside source should be given.

Tip: Selecting the most appropriate graph to accompany your data adds a great deal to the effectiveness of your presentation. High-resolution photographs, maps, flowcharts, and other images may be used as figures (Jacobsen 2012).

Tip: Many software programs give presenters the opportunity to create three-dimensional graphs; however, it is recommended to not use these in presentations because they may be difficult to read.

Bar Graphs

Bar graphs, also called **bar charts**, are appropriate for displaying categorical data. The simplest bar graph is a one-variable bar graph. In this type of graph, the various categories

Figure 11.1. Cigarette Consumption United States 2000–2011

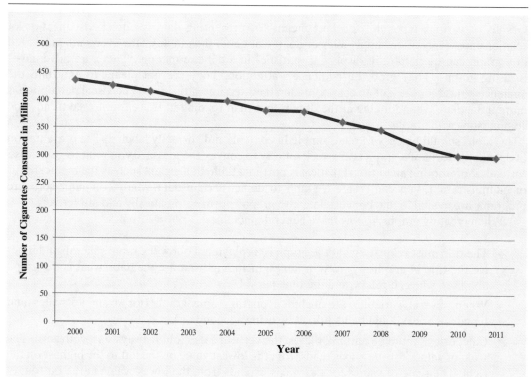

Source: Centers for Disease Control and Prevention 2012.

of observations are presented along a horizontal axis, called the x-axis. (See figures 11.2 and 11.3.) The vertical axis, called the y-axis, displays the frequency of the data. Data representing frequencies, proportions, or percentages of categories are often displayed by using bar graphs. A grouped bar chart is used to display information from tables containing two or three variables. Figure 11.4 shows an example of a three-variable bar graph.

Pie Charts

A **pie chart**, also called a **pie graph**, is a method of displaying data as component parts of a whole. It is an easily understood chart in which the sizes of the slices of the pie show the proportional contribution of each part. Pie charts are best to use when you want to show each category's percentage of the total. They do not show changes over time. A circle is divided into sections such as wedges or slices. These represent percentages of the total (100 percent). To make a pie chart, include all the categories that make up a whole. Therefore, data must be converted into percentages unless you are working with computer software that converts your numbers into percentages. Pie chart wedges may be shaded or colored to help differentiate the sections. In addition, they can be cut out of the pie to help emphasize a percentage. Computer software programs are extremely useful when creating pie graphs. (See figures 11.5 and 11.6 for examples of pie charts.)

Figure 11.2.   Example of a one-variable bar graph

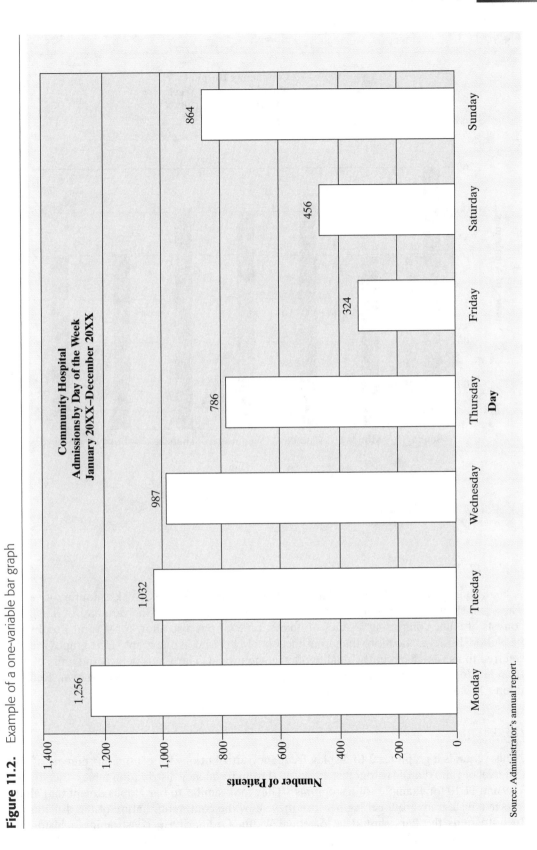

Community Hospital
Admissions by Day of the Week
January 20XX–December 20XX

Number of Patients

Day

1,256   1,032   987   786   324   456   864

Monday   Tuesday   Wednesday   Thursday   Friday   Saturday   Sunday

1,400   1,200   1,000   800   600   400   200   0

Source: Administrator's annual report.

Figure 11.3. Example of a two-variable bar graph

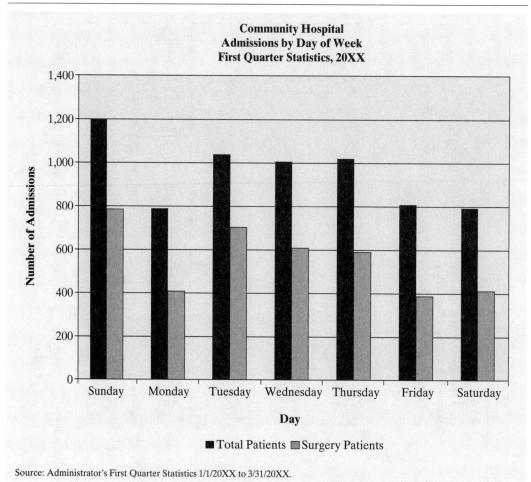

Community Hospital
Admissions by Day of Week
First Quarter Statistics, 20XX

■ Total Patients ■ Surgery Patients

Source: Administrator's First Quarter Statistics 1/1/20XX to 3/31/20XX.

Line Graphs

A **line graph** is often used to show data over time (for example, days, weeks, months, or years). The x-axis shows the time period, and the y-axis shows the values of the variables. A line graph consists of a line connecting a series of points. Line graphs also allow for several variables to be plotted; however, no more than four lines should be used in one graph. Line graphs are also referred to as **run charts** in the quality management field. The x-axis depicts the units of time from left to right, and the y-axis measures the values of the variable being shown. Refer to figures 11.7 and 11.8 for examples of line graphs.

Histograms

A **histogram** is a graph used to display frequency distributions for continuous numerical data (interval or ratio data). Histograms are created from frequency distribution tables. (See figures 11.9 and 11.10 for examples of histograms.) They look similar to bar graphs except that all the bars in a histogram are touching because they show the continuous nature of the distribution. In histograms the bars should be of equal width. Ordinarily in constructing a histogram,

Figure 11.4. Example of a three-variable bar graph

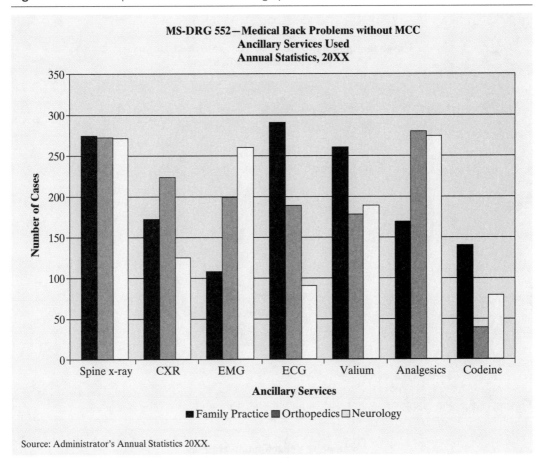

MS-DRG 552—Medical Back Problems without MCC
Ancillary Services Used
Annual Statistics, 20XX

Source: Administrator's Annual Statistics 20XX.

there should not be less than four and usually not more than twelve bars or classes, and the frequency groups should not overlap.

Frequency Polygon

A **frequency polygon** is similar to a histogram in that it is a graph depicting the frequency of continuous data; however, a frequency polygon is in line form instead of bar form. The advantage of a frequency polygon is that several of them can be placed on the same graph to make comparisons. A frequency polygon uses the same axes as the histogram; that is, the x-axis displays the scale of the variable and the y-axis displays the frequency. A dot is placed at the midpoint of the class interval or frequency. A line drawn from one point to the next then connects the dots. Because the x-axis represents the entire frequency distribution, the line starts at zero cases and is drawn from the last frequency to the y-axis to end with zero. (See figure 11.11.)

Pictogram

A **pictogram** is an attractive alternative type of bar graph in that it uses pictures to show the frequency of the data. For example, if you want to show the top five cancer site deaths, you

Figure 11.5.   Pie graph showing nosocomial (hospital-acquired infections) by major service category

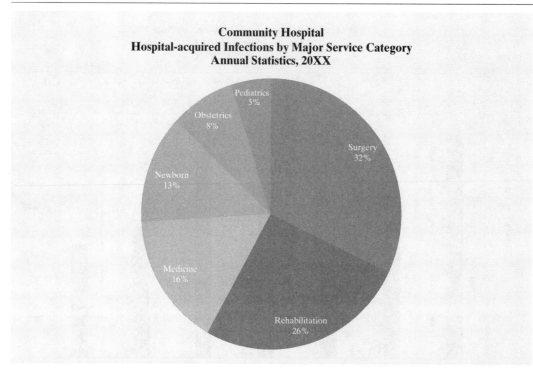

Figure 11.6.   Pie graph showing brain injury patients admitted from other facilities

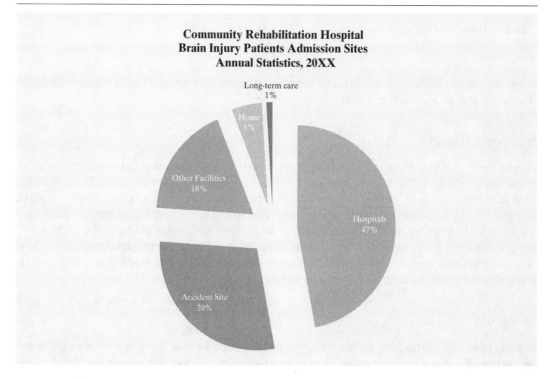

Figure 11.7. Example of a one-variable line graph

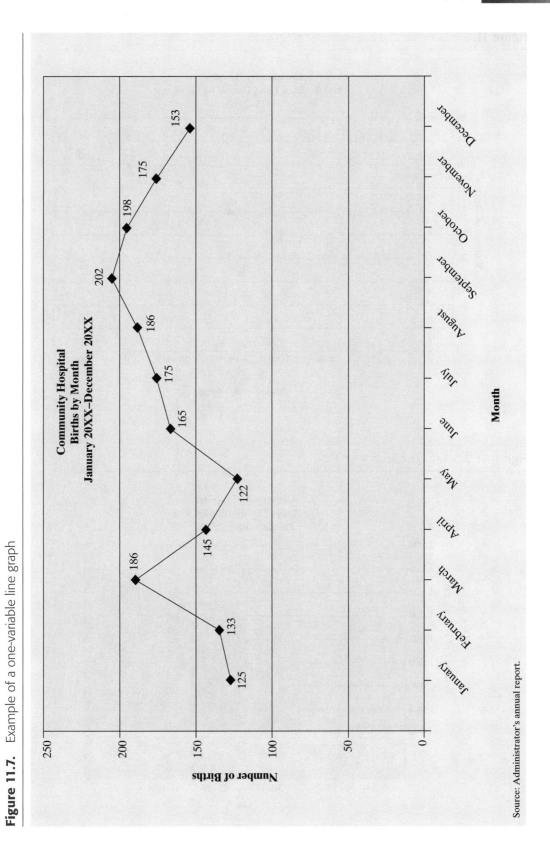

Figure 11.8.   Example of a two-variable line graph

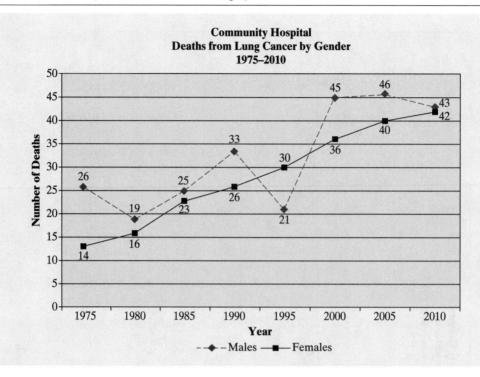

Figure 11.9.   Sample histogram #1

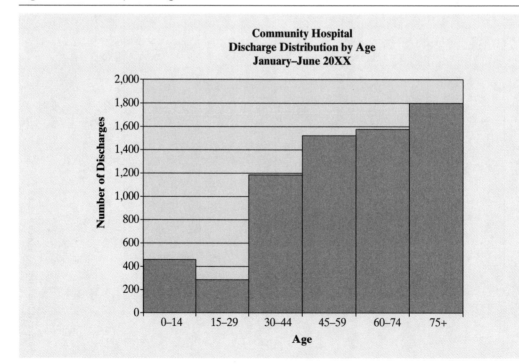

Figure 11.10. Sample histogram #2

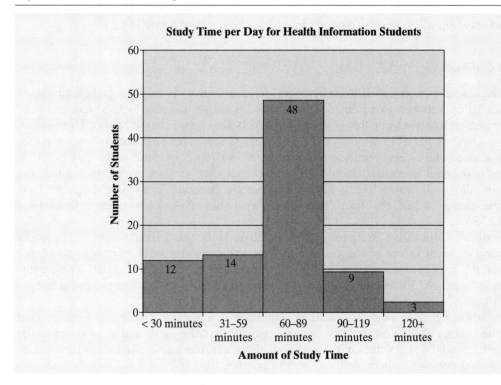

Figure 11.11. Frequency polygon

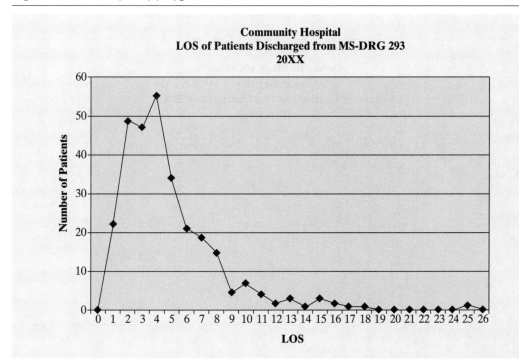

might use stick people. If you need to show exact numbers, a pictogram will probably not be a good choice for your presentation; however, they are very good at catching the attention of your audience and will give them a good sense of your data. (See figure 11.12.)

Scatter Diagram

A **scatter diagram** (also called a scattergram or scatter plot) is used to graphically show the relationship between two numerical variables. A scatter diagram is used to determine whether there is a correlation, that is, a relationship, between two characteristics. Correlation implies that as one variable changes, the other also changes. This does not always mean that there is a cause-and-effect relationship between two variables because there may be other variables that could cause the change. If the two characteristics are somehow related, the pattern of points will show a tight clustering in a certain direction. The closer the points look like a line in appearance, the more the two characteristics are likely to be correlated. (See figure 11.13.)

The slope of the values in figure 11.13 is positive. Notice that small values of the x-axis correspond to small values of the y-axis and large values of the x-axis correspond to large values of the y-axis; thus, a positive linear relationship is thought to exist. The scatter diagram in figure 11.13 shows a weak correlation because the scatter points are not clustered together tightly.

In contrast, figure 11.14 shows a scatter diagram with a negative linear relationship. That is, the small values of the x-axis correspond to large values of the y-axis and large values of the x-axis correspond to small values of the y-axis. Additionally, the scatter diagram in figure 11.14 shows a strong correlation because the cluster of points is tight.

Figure 11.15 illustrates a scatter diagram with no linear relationship because the scatter points are plotted randomly on the graph.

Figure 11.12.   Sample pictogram

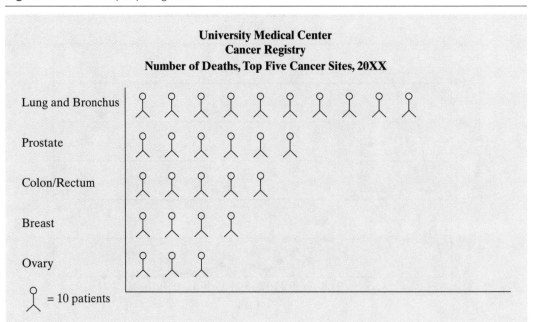

Figure 11.13. Sample scatter diagram showing a positive linear relationship

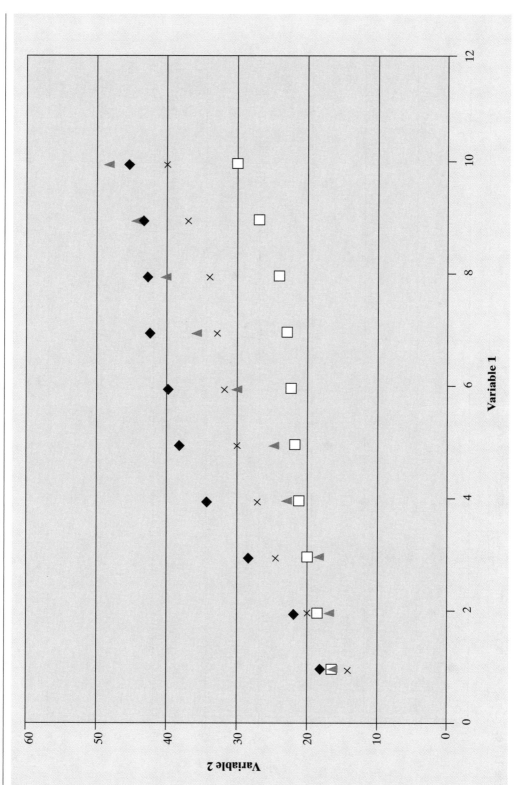

Figure 11.14. Sample scatter diagram showing a negative linear relationship

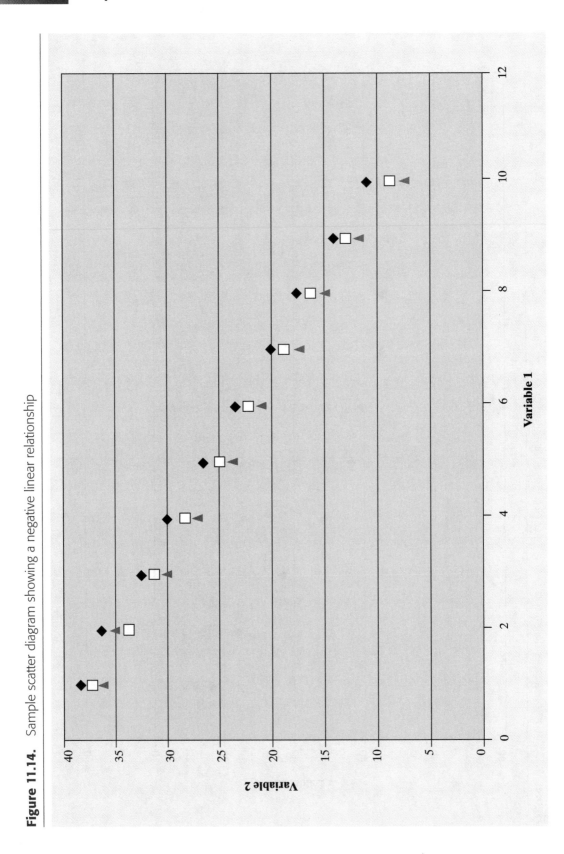

Figure 11.15. Sample scatter diagram showing no linear relationship

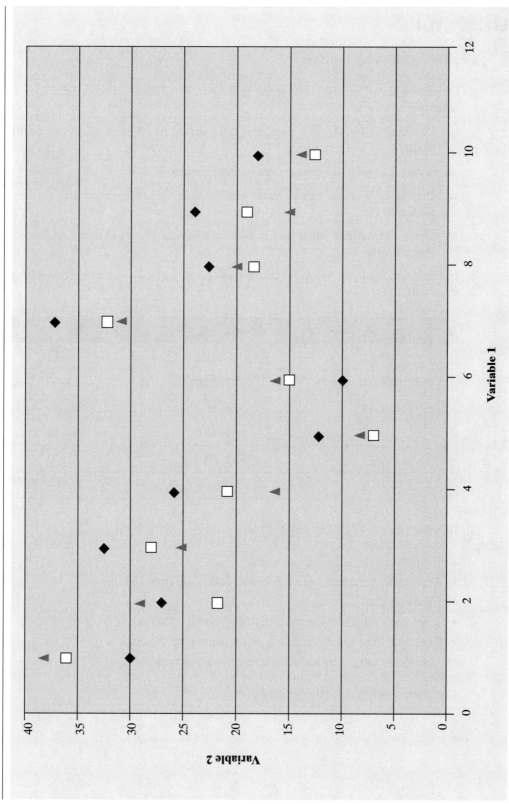

Exercise 11.4

Complete the following exercises.

1. Indicate whether a table or a graph is the preferred method of presentation in the following situations:

   a. Distribution by site, sex, race, and time period of all cancers in your healthcare facility

   b. Survival trends over time by sex for lung cancer

   c. Display of prostate cancer stage of disease for a presentation at a professional conference

   d. Detailed treatment distribution of breast cancer for a physician on the staff of your hospital

2. Indicate which of the following categories (A, B, and C) are mutually exclusive and clearly defined.

A	B	C
0–15	≤ 10.0	0–10
15–30	10.1–20.0	11–20
30–45	20.1–30.0	21–30
45–60	30.1–40.0	31–40
60+	40.1–50.0	41–50
	50.1+	51+

3. In September 20XX, Community Hospital discharged 150 patients.

   - 105 patients were discharged home
   - 6 patients were discharged home with follow-up home health
   - 5 patients died
   - 15 patients were transferred to a skilled nursing facility
   - 7 patients were transferred to another acute care facility
   - 12 patients were transferred to a rehabilitation hospital

   Complete a pie chart of this information.

4. Using the information in the table below, create a line graph of the data.

Community Hospital Number of Admissions to Cardiology Service January–June, 20XX	
Month	**Number of Admissions**
January	120
February	125
March	130
April	119
May	121
June	130

5. The cardiology team at Community Hospital would like to convince the hospital administration that a cardiac catheterization lab is needed because they are transferring patients from Community Hospital to University Hospital for their needed catheterizations. One of the cardiologists asks you to prepare a graph for a presentation to the admissions department of the number of transfers they have had over the past year. The data are listed below.

Community Hospital Cardiac Catheterization Transfers by Service January–December, 20XX			
Month	**Family Practice**	**Internal Medicine**	**Cardiology**
January	3	15	20
February	4	14	18
March	6	13	15
April	8	13	20
May	5	14	14
June	4	13	19
July	4	8	14
August	6	9	15
September	8	4	20
October	7	9	22
November	3	8	21
December	6	12	19

Exercise 11.5

Analyze the Administrator's Semiannual Reference Report that follows, then prepare the data displays indicated in questions 1 through 4. The data displays may be neatly hand drawn or created using a software program.

1. Create a histogram to display the distribution of total discharge days by age.

2. Create a bar graph to display the admission by day of week for Medicare patients in comparison to the admission by day of week for all patients.

3. Create a pie chart to display the percentage of patients discharged by major service category.

4. Create a table for length of stay distribution.

Administrator's Semiannual Reference Report
January–June 20XX

ALL PATIENTS, INCLUDING ONE-DAY STAYS (SEPARATE)

	ADMISSIONS					DISCHARGES			
	TOTAL PTS.	% OF PTS.	SURG. PTS.	AVG. PREOP	ONE-DAY STAYS	TOTAL PTS.	% OF PTS.	AVG. LOS	ONE-DAY STAYS
SUNDAY	1,187	17.9	774	1.7	146	809	12.1	8.1	46
MONDAY	755	11.3	426	2.8	124	576	8.7	6.2	144
TUESDAY	1,085	16.3	689	2.6	135	934	14.0	7.2	115
WEDNESDAY	1,035	15.5	622	3.5	141	934	14.0	7.7	147
THURSDAY	1,024	15.3	597	2.6	139	955	14.3	7.0	132
FRIDAY	808	12.1	359	3.9	145	965	14.5	7.7	141
SATURDAY	773	11.6	417	3.0	39	1,490	22.4	6.6	144

LENGTH OF STAY DISTRIBUTION				SUMMARY BY MAJOR SERVICE CATEGORY					
	TOTAL PTS.	% CASES			TOTAL PTS.	% OF PTS.	DIS DAYS	% DAYS	ALOS
SAME DAY	114	1.7		MEDICINE	2,005	30.0	21,052	30.6	10.5
1 DAY	755	11.3		SURGERY	1,401	21.0	7,845	11.4	5.6
2–4 DAYS	1,343	20.2		GYNECOLOGY	631	9.4	6,057	8.8	9.6
5–7 DAYS	1,555	23.3		OBSTETRICS	530	7.9	2,703	3.9	5.1
8–14 DAYS	1,469	22.0		NEWBORN	520	7.8	2,600	3.7	5.0
15–42 DAYS	1,217	18.3		PEDIATRICS	450	6.7	4,140	6.0	9.2
43+ DAYS	210	3.2		PSYCHIATRY	518	7.7	8,537	12.4	16.5
				OTHER	608	9.1	15,798	22.9	26.0

(continued on next page)

Administrator's Semiannual Reference Report
January–June 20XX

ADMISSION BY DAY OF THE WEEK BY PAYMENT STATUS

	SELF	BLUE CROSS	COMMERCIAL	GOV'T	WORK COMP	M-CAID	M-CARE	OTHER	Total
SUNDAY	31	413	188	0	2	41	273	2	950
MONDAY	19	300	103	0	11	46	280	1	760
TUESDAY	21	400	206	1	9	45	345	2	1,029
WEDNESDAY	20	503	240	2	22	35	223	3	1,048
THURSDAY	30	365	154	0	8	24	199	1	781
FRIDAY	28	40	179	0	0	42	294	0	583
SATURDAY	30	509	246	1	6	55	301	2	1,150
TOTAL PTS.	179	2,892	1,316	4	58	288	1,915	11	
% OF PTS.	2.6	43.4	19.7	0.6	0.8	4.3	28.7	0	
TOT DIS DAYS	1,109	26,895	16,818	36	609	2,670	20,491	104	
% OF DAYS	1.6	39.1	24.4	0	0.8	4	30	0	
AVG. LOS	6.2	9.3	12.8	9.0	10.5	9.3	11	9.5	

SUMMARY BY AGE

	TOTAL PTS.	% OF PTS.	TOT DIS DAYS	% DAYS	ALOS
0–14	429	6.4	1,749	2.5	4.1
15–18	229	3.4	817	1.2	3.6
19–34	1,144	17.2	9,746	14.2	8.5
35–49	1,488	22.3	14,647	21.3	9.8
50–64	1,570	23.6	18,101	26.3	11.5
65+	1,803	27.1	23,672	34.4	13.1
TOTAL	6,663		68,732		10.3

Exercise 11.6

University Hospital Cancer Registry records show the following incidence of cancer in female patients for the past year. Construct an appropriate graph of the data.

University Hospital Cancer Registry 10 Most Prevalent Cancer Sites—Female Patients 20XX	
Site	**Number of Cases**
Breast	122
Lung and bronchus	52
Colorectal	34
Uterus	25
Thyroid	21
Melanoma	15
Lymphoma	14
Kidney	12
Ovary	11
Pancreas	4

Exercise 11.7

University Hospital reported the following incidence of lung and bronchus cancer patients treated at the hospital during the past 10 years. Construct a line graph of the data.

University Hospital Cancer Registry Data Lung and Bronchus Cancer by Year and Gender		
Year	**Male**	**Female**
2006	172	48
2007	175	47
2008	169	49

(*continued on next page*)

University Hospital Cancer Registry Data Lung and Bronchus Cancer by Year and Gender		
Year	Male	Female
2009	165	50
2010	168	54
2011	121	93
2012	123	101
2013	130	118
2014	121	121
2015	112	123

Preparing Reports

Writing reports for your workplace is not the same as writing an article for a professional journal or preparing a report for an assignment in one of your classes, but the goal is the same. Communication is the goal, and it is achieved when you write your report in the style your audience prefers. Often your healthcare administration will let you know how reports are prepared and presented in your facility, or you could review previous reports that have been given to committees or your administration to use as a guide. Some reports are more formal than others. For example, for a committee meeting you may just provide some data in the form of graphs or tables to share with the members, whereas for a Cancer Conference, where information may be shared with the community, a more formal report will be in order.

Here are some general guidelines to follow:

- Include a title for the report.
- If your report is long, consider placing a paginated list of contents in the front of the report to make details easier to locate.
- If you are writing a formal report, include an introduction explaining the purpose of the report.
- The body of the report will include the narrative and any tables and graphs. These could be divided with titles.
  - Tables and graphs are great tools for presenting data. Tables show summarized and more detailed data, and graphs are useful for presenting relationships in visual form. The question of which to use depends on the audience.
  - Take a few minutes before you prepare a report to think about who will be reading or seeing your presentation. Will you be presenting information to your administrator about the need for new equipment in your department, will it be to a team who is deciding whether or not to investigate the need for a new

service in your facility, or will it be to a committee evaluating the quality of care provided in your hospital? Determine what you are trying to say to this person or group. Determine what details must be included; then decide what types of tables or graphs you want to provide.

○ Tables have several advantages over graphs:
  ▪ More information can be presented in a table.
  ▪ Exact values in tables can be helpful.
  ▪ Ordinarily, less work is involved in creating a table.
○ Graphs, on the other hand, also have advantages:
  ▪ Graphs are more attention-grabbing than tables.
  ▪ Graphs show trends more clearly.
  ▪ Graphs bring out facts that will stimulate thinking.
○ A narrative report will make the presentation more understandable and can explain what the values mean.
  ▪ Narrative reports can include historical information, for instance, what the data has shown over a specific period of time.
  ▪ The narrative can include factors that may influence the data such as seasonal changes in the patient population or reasons for significant increases or decreases in the data.
○ Make sure your data are correct because inaccurate data may lead to inaccurate decisions.
○ Be sure to include the sources of the data. (Bowden 2008)
• Write to the style of your workplace.
  ○ Be objective. Report all the pertinent information, both positive and negative points.
  ○ Use bias-free language. Avoid words such as "awesome" or "incredible."
  ○ Write in an impersonal style. Do not start your sentences with "I compared . . .", but rather, "A comparison showed . . ."
  ○ Be concise and strive for clarity.
  ○ Explain any abbreviations or acronyms.
• Proofread your document; brush up on your grammatical skills.
  ○ Read your report carefully to make sure the graphs and tables make sense and are easy to understand.
    ▪ You might even consider reading the report out loud to see how it sounds.
  ○ It is a good idea to ask another individual, another colleague or supervisor, to read your report to be certain it contains no mistakes and is logical.

Exercise 11.8

Prepare a report for your administration showing the results of your graphs from exercise 11.7. Add a cover page that includes the name of the hospital, the title of your report, a table of contents, tables of the data, and the graphs you prepared. Add a narrative report on the diagnosis of cancer of the bronchus and lung that describes the signs and symptoms, tests completed to reach the diagnosis, stages of the cancer, and types of cancer and treatment. Also, based on the data and graphs created in exercise 11.7, describe your facility's results over the last 10 years.

Chapter 11   Matching Quiz

Match the definition with the terms.

Definitions:

a. A graphic technique used to display frequency distributions of nominal or ordinal data that fall into categories; also called bar graph

b. Data that may be displayed by units of equal size and placed on a scale starting with zero and thus can be manipulated mathematically

c. An organized arrangement of data, usually in columns and rows

d. A graph that visually displays the linear relationships among factors

e. A type of data that represents observations that can be measured on an evenly distributed scale beginning at a point other than true zero

f. Four types of data (nominal, ordinal, interval, and ratio) that represent values or observations that can be sorted into a category; also called scales of measurement

g. A graphic technique used to illustrate the relationship between continuous measurements; consists of a line drawn to connect a series of points on an arithmetic scale and is often used to display time trends

h. A type of graph that shows data points collected over time and identifies emerging trends or patterns

i. A graphic technique in which the proportions of a category are displayed as portions of a circle

j. A graphic technique used to display the frequency distribution of continuous data (interval or ratio data) as either numbers or percentages in a series of bars

Terms:

1. _____ Histogram	**6.** _____ Table
2. _____ Interval data	**7.** _____ Pie chart
3. _____ Run chart	**8.** _____ Bar chart
4. _____ Ratio data	**9.** _____ Scatter diagram
5. _____ Line graph	**10.** _____ Categorical data

Chapter 11   Review

Complete the following exercises.

1. Which of the following graphs would be best to use to display the percentages of diagnoses seen at your mental health center?

   a. Frequency polygon

   b. Pie graph

   c. Bar graph

   d. Line graph

2. Physicians from the Community Physician's Clinic would like to demonstrate to the Community Hospital administration that additional exam rooms are needed to accommodate their patients. They ask the HIM manager to construct a graph showing the number of patients seen in the last year by the clinic physicians. The categories they wish to have displayed are Primary Care, 5,736; Medical Specialties, 2,473; Surgical Specialties, 2,022; and Hospital Outpatients, 984. Which type of graph would be appropriate?

   a. Line graph

   b. Bar graph

   c. Pie chart

   d. Scattergram

3. The administration at Community Physician's Hospital are interested in determining if they need to increase the number of physicians in order to see patients in a timely manner. The administrator asks the HIM manager to construct a graph that will show the following percentages about appointments in the following categories: patients who waited two to four weeks to see the physician, patients who waited one to two weeks to see a physician, patients who waited one week or less, and patients who were able to have an appointment on the day they called. Which would be the best graph to show this information?

   a. Line graph

   b. Bar graph

   c. Pie chart

   d. Scattergram

4. What type of numerical data contains only a finite number of results?

   a. Continuous

   b. Discrete

   c. Interval

   d. Ratio

5. When creating histograms, which is a true statement?

   a. Form classes of equal width.

   b. Always form frequency groups that do not overlap.

   c. Establish between four and 12 frequency groups.

   d. All of the above

6. What do the wedges or divisions in a pie graph represent?

   a. Frequency groups

   b. Various data

   c. Percentages

   d. Classes

7. The following graph shows:

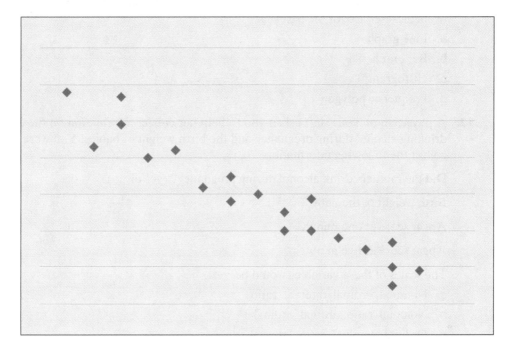

   a. Strong positive correlation

   b. Strong negative correlation

   c. Moderately positive correlation

   d. Moderately negative correlation

8. Which graph displays vertical bars to depict frequency distributions for continuous data?

   a. Histogram

   b. Line graph

   c. Pie graph

   d. Frequency distribution table

9. What is one of the simplest types of categorical data in which the values fall into unordered categories?

   a. Ordinal

   b. Nominal

   c. Ratio

   d. Interval

10. Which of the following graphs would be best for the cancer registrar to use to display the five-year survival rates of lung cancer patients in the years 20XX to 20XX at your hospital?

    a. Frequency polygon

    b. Bar graph

    c. Line graph

    d. Histogram

11. Which of the following graphs would be best to use to display the number of discharges by medical service for the past year?

    a. Line graph

    b. Bar graph

    c. Histogram

    d. Frequency polygon

12. A physician on your staff asked you to help her collect information on the effects of drinking alcohol during pregnancy and the birth weight of babies. You were asked to collect the following information.

    Did the mothers drink alcohol during pregnancy? (yes or no)

    Birth weight of the baby

    Apgar score at one minute

    Apgar score at five minutes

    The scales of these variables would be:

    a. Nominal, ordinal, interval, ratio

    b. Nominal, ratio, ordinal, ordinal

    c. Ordinal, nominal, ratio, interval

    d. Ratio, ordinal, interval, nominal

13. The family practice department at University Medical School offered the following information to its advisory board about placement of family practice graduates in your state for the past five years: Year 1 = 55 positions offered and 46 positions filled, Year 2 = 50 positions offered and 46 positions filled, Year 3 = 52 positions offered and 40 positions filled, Year 4 = 61 positions offered and 58 positions filled, and Year 5 = 64 positions offered and 62 positions filled. What type of graph would be most appropriate?

    a. Line graph

    b. Bar graph

    c. Pie chart

    d. Scattergram

14. When preparing a report for presentation, which of the following should be included?

    1. Title of the report

    2. Graphs will give more detail than tables

    3. Narrative will be helpful if included

    4. Content page must be included

a. 1, 2, and 3

b. 1 and 3

c. 2, 3, and 4

d. All of the above

15. In creating a frequency distribution table, which of the following statements is not a basic rule to follow?

   a. Choose classes that cover the smallest and largest values.

   b. Make certain that each item can go into only one class.

   c. As a general rule, use between 10 and 15 classes.

   d. Do not produce gaps between classes.

12

Basic Research Principles

Learning Objectives

At the conclusion of this chapter, you should be able to

- Compare and contrast the difference between quantitative and qualitative research
- Differentiate among the types of research, research methods, samples, data collection techniques, and data interpretation issues
- Determine the steps in the research process
- Explain the role of the Institutional Review Board (IRB) in research in healthcare facilities
- Apply ethical guidelines in the use of statistics

Key Terms

Alternative hypothesis
Applied research
Basic research
Causal research
Cluster sampling
Conclusive research
Convenience sampling
Correlational research
Data collection
Descriptive research
Ethnography
Evaluation research
Experimental research
Exploratory research
Fabrication
Falsification
Historical research

Hypothesis
Individually identifiable
   health information
Informed consent
Institutional Review Board
   (IRB)
Instrument
Judgment sampling
Literature review
Naturalistic inquiry
Null hypothesis
Observation
Observational research
Plagiarism
Primary research
Qualitative research
Quantitative research

Questionnaire
Quota sampling
Random sampling
Reliability
Research
Sample
Sample size
Secondary research
Snowball sampling
Stratified random sampling
Structured interview
Survey
Systematic random sampling
Unrestricted question
Validity

Research is an inquiry process aimed at discovering new information about a subject or revising old information. It includes investigation or experimentation aimed at the discovery of new facts, revision of accepted theories or law in light of these new facts, or practical application using the new facts. Health information research examines all aspects of health and can include studies on human subjects as well as public policy. The goal of health information research is to make discoveries that will benefit health information professionals.

Basic Research Principles

Research is the search toward the solution of problems. It answers questions that you or others may have and calls attention to theories that may be helpful in predicting future experiences.

Research is done in many fields and may be done in a variety of ways. Health research covers the wide gamut of laboratory research, clinical trials, and public health issues. This chapter covers the basic types of research and the steps in the research process, including data-collection techniques and the different types of samples.

Types of Research

There are generally two types of research: basic and applied. In **basic research**, the investigator is not concerned with the immediate applicability of his or her results but, rather, tries to look for understanding of natural processes. In **applied research**, the investigator has some kind of application in mind and wants to discover information about it that can be used to solve a problem or in some way contribute to society; it is more practical in nature.

Research Methodology

Research methodology is a set of procedures or strategies used by researchers to collect, analyze, and present data. At a higher and more general level, researchers in research methodology have described two overarching approaches to research: the qualitative approach and the quantitative approach.

Qualitative and Quantitative Research

Qualitative research describes events, persons, activities, processes, and so on without the use of numerical data. It is generally aimed at understanding the experiences and attitudes of patients, the community, or healthcare worker (McCusker and Gunaydin 2015).

An example of qualitative research would be interviews with health information practitioners to determine whether their past healthcare experiences affected their decision to enter the health information field or interviews with mothers of handicapped infants to determine how their lives were affected by the birth of their children. Qualitative research consists of interviews, observations, and written documents that may be used individually or in combination. "The richness of the data permits a fuller understanding of what is being studied than could be derived from experimental research methods" (Best and Kahn 2006, 251).

Quantitative research uses quantitative methods, or numbers, to describe a study, including some comparisons of the population and statistical analysis to describe the results. Quantitative research consists of observations, experiments, structured interviews, and **surveys**.

Table 12.1 illustrates some characteristics of quantitative and qualitative research.

Table 12.1. Characteristics of quantitative and qualitative research

Quantitative Research	Qualitative Research
Uses quantitative methods, including observations, structured interviews, experiments, and surveys	Describes observations without the use of numerical data, including interviews, observations, and written documents
Is objective	Is subjective
Sample is generally randomly selected	Sample is purposefully selected
Uses controlled measurements	Uses uncontrolled observations
Researcher is removed from the data; is an outside observer	Researcher is close to the data; has an inside perspective
Can be generalized and replicated	Is not generalized and may not be replicable
Is outcome oriented	Is process oriented

There is a trend toward combining the two methods, called mixed methods research. It is an approach in which researchers mix or combine quantitative and qualitative research techniques, methods, concepts, or language within one study and across related studies (Layman and Watzlaf 2009, 15). Mixed methods research holds strong potential for contributing to better understanding of problems and holds untapped potential that warrants further investigation (Pohl and Onwuegbuzie 2015).

One example of a technique that often uses both types of research methodologies is survey research. A single survey will often contain questions that result in both quantitative and qualitative data. For example, you might want to study the effects of a hospital's implementation of the electronic health record (EHR). Your survey could contain questions that require the interviewee to answer "On a scale of 1 to 5 with 1 being very good and 5 being very poor, how would you describe the implementation process of the new software for your facility's EHR." The same survey may very well contain additional questions such as, "In what ways would you change the process to better take into consideration the process used in your department?"

Exercise 12.1

Identify if the following are examples of quantitative or qualitative research.

   a. Qualitative research

   b. Quantitative research

   c. Mixed methods research

1. Researcher often has an inside perspective

2. Uses controlled measurements

3. Uses numbers to describe the results

    4. The sample is purposefully selected

    5. The study is process oriented

    6. Structured interviews are used

The Research Process

Although there are as many descriptions of the types of research as there are textbooks and articles about the subject, most agree that the research process involves the following six major steps:

1. Define the problem.
2. Review the literature.
3. Design the research.
4. Collect the data.
5. Analyze the data.
6. Draw conclusions.

Defining the Problem

Problem definition refers to forming a question regarding a topic you would like to study. The most important thing is to be clear about what you want to study. Often an analysis of historical data, also called secondary information, has gone into the problem definition.

Historical data analysis simply means looking at the past to see what has been done before; it prevents reinventing the wheel. In previous research, an investigator may have made recommendations for future studies. In addition, problems may be broken down into subcomponents or smaller problems. Figure 12.1 demonstrates an example of a problem and its possible subcomponents.

The definition also may define the scope of the study, that is, who or what will be included in the study. For example, a study that includes hospitals may be defined as including only those hospitals with fewer than 100 beds, a study that involves patients may include only those patients who are age 60 and over, or a study may include female patients only.

Figure 12.1.   Example of a research problem and its subcomponents

Problem/Question: Should a physician clinic in your community put an organized health information department into operation?

- Subcomponent 1. What are the health information services that could be provided?
- Subcomponent 2. What types of employees should be employed in this department?
- Subcomponent 3. What amount of space is needed for the department?
- Subcomponent 4. Where should the health information department be located?
- Subcomponent 5. What equipment does the department need to be operational?
- Subcomponent 6. What would be the total estimated cost of the project?

Reviewing the Literature

A **literature review** is an investigation of all the information about a topic. It is important to start any study with a review of literature on the research you want to conduct for three important reasons:

- To determine whether research has already been done on the question
- To determine whether any data sources can be used in the study
- To help make the hypothesis more specific

There are many sources of previous research. These may include journals, books, position papers, conference presentations, videos, interviews, and online databases, to name just a few.

Designing the Research and Collecting the Data

There are several types of research design, including the following:

- **Exploratory research** is often initially undertaken when a topic is not very clearly defined. The researcher has an idea that there may be a question that he would like answered and wants to find out more about that topic. This type of research allows the researcher to study a topic and gather information. It may generate a hypothesis. Exploratory research is generally informal and relies on literature review and informal discussions with others to find out more about a problem. Although exploratory research may not help answer the problem, it may provide insights into the problem. For example, a health information management (HIM) director may want to find out why claims are not being billed within the three-day requirement or why employees are coming to work late.

- **Historical research** involves an investigation and analysis of past events. This type of research also allows the researcher to apply previous researchers' experiences and conclusions in his or her professional practice. Researchers examine primary and secondary sources. Primary sources can include original documents, such as medical records, meeting minutes, certificates, newspaper and journal articles, eyewitness accounts, pictures, recordings, and research reports. Secondary data sources include data that come from a primary source such as indices, reports of a person who relates the testimony of an eyewitness, textbooks, and encyclopedias.

- **Conclusive research** is performed in order to reach some sort of conclusion or to help in decision making. This type of research may be done by using **primary research**, that is, data collected specifically for your study, or **secondary research**, that is, a literature review to see if previous studies can be used to answer your question. Secondary research may also include summaries of past works. There are two types of conclusive research:
    - **Descriptive research**, also called statistical research, provides data about the population you are studying, including the frequency that something occurs. These data might include studies on the status of the composition of the HIM workforce, employee morale in departments, coding accuracy, or the effects of EHR implementation. The most common collection techniques for descriptive research are case studies, observations, and surveys.

- ○ **Causal research** is conducted to try to answer questions about what causes certain things to occur. This type of research is difficult because there may always be an additional cause to consider. Causal research uses experimentation and simulation as its data-collection methods. An example of causal research may be to take the results of any descriptive research into the morale of the HIM department and further study if low morale causes an increase in the error rate of coding.

- **Correlational research** refers to studies that try to discover a relationship between variables. A variable is anything under study. In correlational research, the strength of the relationship is measured and there may be a positive or a negative relationship between variables. Correlational research determines only if there is a relationship between two or more variables; it does not determine the cause of those relationships. If a strong relationship is found, experimental research can be carried out to determine causality. (See chapter 11 for a more detailed discussion on correlation.) This type of research uses **questionnaires**, observations, and secondary data as its data-collection methods. Examples of correlational research might include studying whether there is a relationship between watching violence on television and behavior, whether graduating with a 4.0 grade point average from college affects the type of job a student gets after graduation, or whether there is a relationship between eating eggs and cholesterol levels.

- **Evaluation research** is a process used to determine what has happened during a given activity or in an institution. The purpose of evaluation research is to lead to a better understanding of whether a program is effective, whether a policy is working, or whether something that was agreed upon is the most cost-effective way of doing something. For example, evaluation research may be done each year to determine whether your school's health information program is meeting its goals.

- **Experimental and quasi-experimental research** entails manipulation of a situation in some way in order to test a hypothesis. In experimental research, certain variables are kept constant and an independent or experimental variable is manipulated. Researchers select both independent and dependent variables. Independent variables are the factors that researchers manipulate directly; dependent variables are the measured variables. Examples of experimental research include studies such as determining whether a certain medication is effective in treating Parkinsonism or studying whether the use of robotic technology in the operating suite is more beneficial to patients than the traditional surgical approach. Experimentation provides a method of hypothesis testing. Experimentation is the classic method of research where elements are manipulated and effects are observed. "It is the most sophisticated, exacting, and powerful method for discovering and developing an organized body of knowledge" (Best and Kahn 2006, 164). Quasi-experimental research is similar to experimental research but does not include randomization of participants. This research provides control of when and to whom the measurement is applied, but because there is not random assignment to experimental and control groups, the equivalence of the groups is not assured.

- **Observational research** requires researchers to observe, document, and analyze events and behaviors. This is part of qualitative research design. Qualitative researchers also use a technique referred to as triangulation or multiple data collection techniques. In this process data are verified through other data that were collected from other sources, other researchers, or different procedures.

Exercise 12.2

Identify the type of research in the following:

a. Exploratory research

b. Historical research

c. Descriptive research

d. Causal research

e. Correlational research

f. Evaluation research

g. Experimental research

1. _____ A health information manager would like more information about a new supervisory technique so he organizes a focus group of supervisors in the facility to generate ideas and clarify concepts.

2. _____ The wellness department director of your facility wants to test the effectiveness of an herbal supplement in the group of employees attending her weight management class. She divides the employees into two groups at random and each employee is given a pill to take every day, but the employees do not know what kind of pill they are taking; one is a sugar pill (the placebo) and one is the herbal supplement. The employees are evaluated after one month and no differences are found in the management of their weight, leading her to conclude that the herbal supplement was not effective.

3. _____ The behavioral health department at Community Hospital is interested in studying whether or not the smoking-cessation program they instituted for the employees is working.

4. _____ A researcher in your community is studying why there are differences in the number of lung cancer cases in your community versus the community 10 miles from your facility. The researcher surveyed residents in each community about their lifestyle choices. He found that citizens of your community smoke more than the other community.

5. _____ A researcher found that greater use of the Internet can decrease social support and lead to depression and loneliness.

6. _____ A researcher wants to study if eating too much sugar causes childhood diabetes.

7. _____ A health information researcher reviews the past 30 years of the *Journal of AHIMA* to identify health information managers' concerns in the workplace.

Statement of the Hypothesis

In formal research, a **hypothesis** is formed. A hypothesis is a statement of the predicted relationship among variables in measureable terms. It is a proposed solution or explanation the researcher has reached through the literature review, observation, theory, or models. More simply stated, it is the tentative answer to the question being studied.

The statement of the hypothesis is important because it allows the researcher to think about the variables and type of research design to use in the study. The research tests the hypothesis, proving it to be positive or negative (correct or incorrect). The fact that a hypothesis is rejected (that is, proven incorrect) does not necessarily mean that the research is poor but, rather, only that the results are different from what was expected. The formulation of the hypothesis in advance of the data-gathering process is necessary for an unbiased investigation.

There are two forms of the hypothesis:

- The **null hypothesis** states that there is no difference between the population means or proportions being compared or that there is no association between the two variables being compared. For example, in a clinical trial of a new medication, the null hypothesis is: The new medication is no better than the current medication. A detailed discussion of the null hypothesis is given in chapter 13.

- The **alternative hypothesis** is a statement of what the study is set up to establish. It states what the predicted association or difference between the variables is. For example, in the clinical trial of a new medication, the alternative hypothesis is: The new medication is better than the current medication.

Data-Collection Techniques

Data collection includes primary research, the data obtained from observations, and surveys and interviews. It also includes secondary research, which is the literature review or summaries of original studies. Regardless of the data-collection method used, the research must be valid and reliable.

- **Validity** is the degree to which scientific observations actually measure or record what they purport to measure. For example, if the researcher is using a written questionnaire to collect data, he or she will pretest it by giving it to someone who may have been included in the subject population in order to determine whether it is well written, clear, and inclusive of everything the researcher is looking for.

- **Reliability** is the repeatability of scientific observations. With reliability, the major question is: Can another researcher reproduce the study using a similar instrument and get similar results? A study may be reliable but not valid. That is, the study may be able to be replicated and yet not answer the research question.

The type of data-collection technique used depends on the type of research the investigator wishes to conduct. If the researcher wants to establish a causal relationship, he or she should conduct one of the experimental studies. However, if the researcher is breaking new ground in a poorly understood area of practice, he or she may want to consider an exploratory study in a qualitative design.

Some examples of data-collection methods include:

- *Surveys:* The survey method gathers data from a relatively large number of cases at a particular time. Surveys can include interviews and questionnaire surveys. In either case, the questions should be well thought out to ensure that they answer the questions of the research study. The questions can be restricted (structured) or closed ended when the investigator only wants certain answers. For example, "Yes" and "No" answers fall into this category. It is a good idea to provide for unanticipated responses. Providing an "Other" category permits respondents to indicate what might be their most important response, one the questionnaire builder had not anticipated. **Unrestricted or unstructured questions**, also referred to as open-ended questions, allow the participant to express a freer response in his or her own words. Open-ended questionnaires can be difficult to tabulate, and although they can be easier to write, it may be better to take additional time to write a closed-ended type of questionnaire because it is easier to interpret and tabulate. When standardized questions are used in the interview process, this is referred to as a **structured interview**. This will ensure that every participant in the study receives exactly the same questions in the same order. In this type of interview, the data is collected by an interviewer rather than a questionnaire. The interviewer reads the question exactly as it appears on the survey along with the answer choices. Open-ended questions may be included, and the interviewer must be able to capture the responses given exactly as they are given. The order of the questions is also important. Each participant must receive the questions in the same order. In this way there would be little impact of contextual effects, where the answers given to a survey question may depend on the previous question.

- *Observation:* Instead of asking questions, the investigator observes the participant.

  ○ In nonparticipant observation, the researcher is a neutral observer who does not interact with the participants.

  ○ In participant observation, the researcher may participate in the actions being observed but tries to maintain his or her objectivity.

  ○ Another type of observation is called **ethnography**, also called **naturalistic inquiry**. Using this method of observation, the researcher observes, listens to, and sometimes converses with the subjects in as free and natural an atmosphere as possible. The assumption is that the most important behavior of individuals in groups is a dynamic process of complex interactions and consists of more than one set of facts, statistics, or even discrete incidents. A position of neutrality, that is, the researcher observes, listens, and will occasionally talk with the participants, but never guides them to give certain answers, is important in this type of research. An example of naturalistic inquiry is a study conducted by Patzel (2001) wherein she conducted a study of women's use of resources in leaving abusive relationships.

- *Experimental study:* This type of data collection technique "provides a logical, systematic way to answer the question, 'If this is done under carefully controlled conditions, what will happen?'" (Best and Kahn 2006, 164). There are many types of experimental studies, and a complete discussion would be too lengthy and complex for this introductory section. Experimentation is a sophisticated technique for the collection of data and may not be appropriate for the beginning investigator.

Selection of an Instrument

The **instrument**, also called a tool, is a consistent way to collect data. Many different types of instruments are used in research studies, and whatever type is used should be one that fits the purpose of the research.

Researchers sometimes use instruments that have been published in databases and occasionally publish their own instrument with their research. However, researchers should not develop an instrument until they have established that one does not already exist. If you decide to develop your own instrument, develop the questions carefully and be sure to test them to ensure that you are gathering what you need to answer the question in your research problem.

It is a good idea to have someone review the questions to be sure that the questionnaire is easily read and understood and will give you the information you wish to collect. It would be too costly and time-consuming to have to repeat a survey because a question or two had been neglected or were not clearly worded.

Selection of Samples

Another consideration in data collection is the selection of subjects for the study. For example, a study on health information departments in the United States could try to include every HIM department in the nation, but it would likely prove impractical and could be costly and time-consuming. The next best thing is to use a **sample**. When chosen correctly, samples are considered to be representative of the population.

Generally, there are two types of sampling techniques: probability sampling and nonprobability sampling. Probability sampling uses some form of random selection. Probability sampling includes the following types:

- Simple **random sampling**: This sampling technique involves choosing individuals from the population in such a way that every individual has an equal chance of being selected.

- Statistics books include a table of random numbers that can be used in the selection of random samples. In order to draw a random sample, the researcher should begin by assigning a number to each subject in the population. This number depends on the number of subjects in the population. For example, if there are 105 subjects in the population, the first subject would be numbered 001, the second 002, and so on with the final subject being number 105. Similarly, if there are 2,582 subjects in the population, the first subject would be numbered 0001, the second 0002, and the last subject 2,582. The researcher must begin by selecting subjects at random using the table of random numbers. This can be done by moving across or down the table, as long as the correct number of digits is selected. If the population contains 1,000 subjects, each time the researcher selects a subject, he must select four digits. If he comes across a number not included in the number of subjects (for example, the researcher comes across 8,569 but only has 1,000 subjects), this number is simply discarded and he then moves on to the next number.

- In **systematic random sampling**, a systematic pattern is used with random sampling. For example, if you were choosing from a list of patients discharged during the past month, you might choose the first patient randomly and every fifth patient thereafter. In this sample, choice of the first patient determines the others.

- **Stratified random sampling**: To select a stratified random sample, divide the population into groups of similar individuals, called strata; choose a separate simple random sample (SRS) in each stratum; and then combine the SRSs to form the full sample. For example, you might want to make a selection based on gender, by patients with private insurance, or by separating hospitals by the number of beds in the facility.

- **Cluster sampling**: In this technique, the population is selected from groups, also known as clusters. For example, if the study includes HIM practitioners working in large cities, you first would choose the cities (the cluster) and then randomly choose the HIM practitioners from those cities. This is called two-stage cluster sampling. A difference between cluster and stratified sampling is that in cluster sampling the cluster is the sampling unit, whereas in stratified sampling, only specific elements of the strata are accepted as the sampling unit. Geographical sampling is a popular version of cluster sampling.

Almost all qualitative research methods rely on nonprobability sampling. Nonprobability sampling does not involve a random sampling of the population. Nonprobability sampling includes:

- **Judgment sampling**: In judgment sampling, the researcher relies on his or her own judgment to select subjects for a study. For example, in a study on health information departments in acute care hospitals that are using an EHR, the researcher might use his or her judgment to select a specific hospital size for the study from among large, small, and medium-sized hospitals that use EHRs. Interviewers who stop individuals on the street in order to ask their opinion on a topic is a population example of this type of sampling. The interviewer makes the judgment on whom to interview. This is sometimes referred to as purposive sampling.

- **Quota sampling**: In this type of sampling technique, the researcher first divides the population, as in stratified sampling, and then selects the number of subjects based on a specified proportion. In quota sampling, the selection of the sample is made by the researcher who has been given or decides on quotas to fill from the subgroup of the population. Continuing with the example of health information departments above, if 50 of the 100 hospitals in the state are using an EHR and 50 are not, the researcher may choose to base his or her study on 20 of the hospitals because that would be 20 percent of the total population of hospitals in the state. In simple terms, a quota sample involves getting participants when you can find them, keeping in mind that the participants will have certain common characteristics.

- **Convenience sampling**: In this sampling technique, selection is based on the availability of subjects who are "conveniently" available to participate in the study. Continuing with the example above, the researcher may decide to use only hospitals within a specific city or within a certain driving distance.

- **Snowball sampling**: Snowball sampling is a non-probability sampling technique that is used when characteristics needed to be possessed by participants are difficult to find (Dudovskiy 2011). For example, continuing with the example used above for HIM departments, if you wanted to study only those departments using a particular type of software and could not get that information from the vendor, you might have to rely on HIM professionals to refer you to others they know are using the same software. You would need to find the initial contact and then rely on the participant to direct you to subsequent participants.

Once the sample has been selected, the researcher will choose a delivery method for the instrument. This could include an electronic or web-based survey, a paper-based survey that is mailed to participants, individual face-to-face interviews, telephone interviews, or focus groups, where participants meet together at one location to discuss a topic using the interview method with an interviewer or moderator.

Exercise 12.3

Identify the type of sample in the following:

    a. Simple random sample

    b. Systematic random

    c. Stratified random

     d. Cluster

     e. Judgment

     f. Quota

     g. Convenience

     h. Snowball

1. _____ A health information professional is gathering information for a study from the coding professionals in her department.

2. _____ The marketing department of your facility will choose 50 patient satisfaction surveys from patients age 35 to 45.

3. _____ A researcher will study the incidence of cancer in your state. First he selects the city, then the hospitals, and finally the patients to study.

4. _____ A researcher would like to study nurse practitioners who treat diabetic children in your state. He finds the first nurse practitioner to interview then asks her to identify two others for him to interview. He intends to ask those two for two additional names and so on.

5. _____ Your college is conducting a study on study habits of students. The first thing they do is divide the student body into undergraduate and graduate students; then they select a random sample of each group to interview.

6. _____ You were asked by the health information committee to evaluate the discharge summaries on every tenth patient discharged last quarter.

7. _____ A health information researcher wants to report on the salary of professionals over the last year. She uses a database from the American Health Information Management Association in which every person has the same chance of being selected for the study.

8. _____ A health information researcher wants to study the effects of the Health Insurance Portability and Accountability Act (HIPAA) regulations on employees so she selects privacy officers with at least 5 years of experience to interview.

Sample Size

Usually there is a trade-off between the desirability of a large sample and the feasibility of a small one. The ideal **sample size** is one that is large enough to serve as an adequate representation of the population about which the researcher wishes to generalize and small enough to be selected economically in terms of subject availability, expense in both time and money, and complexity of data analysis. Here are tips about sample size:

- The larger the sample, the smaller the magnitude of sampling error.
- Survey studies ordinarily have a larger sample size than experimental studies.
- Questionnaires that are mailed can have a response rate as low as 20 percent depending on the content of the questionnaire (Kelly 2003) so a large initial sample is recommended.
- When planning to have subgroups from the study population, begin with a large group to make sure you have enough participants for the subgroups.

- Subject availability and costs are legitimate considerations in determining appropriate sample size (Best and Kahn 2006, 19–20).

Analyzing the Data

In this step of the research process, the investigator tries to determine what the data disclose. Data analysis takes a fair amount of time and should be undertaken carefully. Most researchers use a variety of techniques to describe the data. Two types of statistical applications are relevant to most quantitative research studies:

- Descriptive statistics describe the data. Measures of central tendency and measures of variation are included in descriptive statistics. These are discussed in detail in chapter 10.
- Inferential statistics allow the researcher to make inferences about the population characteristics (parameters) from the sample's characteristics. Analysis of variance (ANOVA) and t tests are examples of inferential statistics that are discussed in chapter 13.

Qualitative research relies on non-numerical observations, which include words, gestures, activities, time, space, images, artifacts, and perceptions (Layman and Watzlaf 2009, 255). Two methods of analysis for qualitative research include the following:

- Grounded theory is an approach for developing theory that is taken from data that has been systematically gathered and analyzed. This usually includes data that has been obtained from observation, interviews, and review of artifacts and texts (Cohen and Crabtree 2006). The researcher is continually moving in and out of the data. Using our example of HIM directors from above, the researcher may interview HIM directors and ask what has been their role in the development of the facility's EHR. After reviewing the data, the researcher may then decide to sample HIM directors with varying educational degrees to see if there are any differences. This constant moving in and out of the data is referred to as constant comparative method. This is only completed when there are no more ideas emerging from the data.
- Content analysis is the systematic and objective analysis of communication. Content analysis is used to examine a variety of communication in addition to written documentation including speech, body language, music, television shows, commercials, and movies. The purpose of content analysis is to study and predict behaviors (Layman and Watzlaf 2009, 257). In a study of role-modeling in the operating room, the researchers used content analysis and the identification of themes to systematically document the types of exemplary behaviors medical students saw when observing the operating room (OR) team during their anesthesia rotation in the OR. The researchers found that there were several themes such as teamwork, calmness, cooperativeness, teaching, and communication with patients. The researchers concluded that this type of exemplary behavior would contribute to their understanding of how professional behavior is viewed and potentially emulated by medical students (Curry et al. 2011).

Statistics Software Packages

There are many software packages on the market to help researchers analyze both their qualitative and quantitative data. A search on the Internet will return results showing many free software packages. These packages can help the researcher produce descriptive statistics along with charts or graphs. One such package is Epi-Info, which is free software from the Centers for

Disease Control and Prevention (CDC). It includes a program to create questionnaires along with allowing entry of data and analysis and creation of graphs and charts.

Another package available from the CDC is EZ-Text, which helps researchers enter data, create a codebook for the participant responses, manage and analyze qualitative databases, and export data into a variety of formats for analysis.

SPSS Statistical Package for Social Sciences (SPSS) is a statistical package that supports many industries. It offers a variety of analytical and graphic software. It also is used by many industries for its predictive analytics to help them make decisions. Other software packages include Tableau Data Visioning, which transforms spreadsheets and documents into professional graphic presentations, and R software, a free downloadable language and software package for statistical computing and graphics.

Drawing Conclusions

In the discussion of the conclusions, the researcher will try to answer whether or not the results supported the hypothesis or, if using the qualitative approach, identified the problem. The results from each hypothesis should be described. In the conclusion researchers also explain the significance, implications, and consequences of the findings of their study (Layman and Watzlaf 2009, 263). New knowledge about a particular issue is created. Researchers use this discussion to support their hypothesis or identified problem or explain how the findings do not support them and why. Any limitations discovered during data analysis are reported. For example, the study of health information departments mentioned earlier studied one city. That may be a limiting factor; that is, the conclusions may not apply to other geographical areas. In the presentation of the research findings, new hypotheses may be proposed if the data do not support the original hypothesis or if additional problems were identified, these are explained as well. Researchers usually include tables and graphs in this section of the research report to clarify and display the data. Researchers may also make recommendations for new research into areas where questions occurred or where data did not support the original hypothesis.

Data Interpretation Issues

It has been said that statistics can tell us anything we want them to or that it is easy to lie with statistics. Unfortunately, data can be misinterpreted in many ways. Sometimes misinterpretation is the result of mistakes made in calculation or presentation of the data. Other times techniques are used so that data are purposely misconstrued. HIM professionals have an ethical obligation to report data honestly and accurately. The Department of Health and Human Services (HHS) Office of Research Integrity (ORI) is responsible for developing policies, procedures, and regulations for detecting misconduct of research and overseeing projects from groups who receive federal money. Their Division of Investigative Oversight will monitor and investigate any reports of misconduct. Reports of misconduct and their resolutions are posted on their website. The ORI also offers a definition of research misconduct as including fabrication, falsification, and plagiarism. **Fabrication** means that the data or the reported results are made up. **Falsification** means that the research material, equipment, or processes were manipulated or the data were not accurately represented, they were changed or omitted from the report, or the results were not accurately reported. **Plagiarism** refers to taking another person's ideas or words without giving them credit. Misconduct does not include making an honest mistake or having differing opinions.

The American Statistics Association's Guidelines for Statistics Practice is a good resource to read before undertaking any research. It outlines the researcher's responsibility to the research, the subject, the research team, employers, the publications, and other researchers.

Misleading Presentation of Numbers

Statistics can be very powerful. Health information practitioners are generally the first individuals called upon to retrieve data for a facility; therefore, it is important for any "statistical communication" to be correct (Gelman and Nolan 2002).

The easiest way to fabricate data is to simply make up the numbers. As reported by the US Public Health Service, this is what happened in the case of Jon Sudbo. It was determined that he fabricated results in the reporting of information in a grant application and in its first-year progress report (ORI 2011). In another case investigated by the ORI, Dong Xiao, a cancer researcher, intentionally fabricated data in his findings, including graphs he created to describe a steroid that was being tested on prostate cancer growth (ORI 2015). It is misleading and dangerous for the public to trust the study results when data are untrue; it is also a waste of research funds.

Ignoring the Baseline

Another common error is comparing raw numbers without adjusting the baseline. For example, if Hospital A and Hospital B each had 40 deaths last month, do these data provide the best indication of the level of care given at Hospital A and Hospital B? A better comparison would be to look at the number of total discharges and deaths during the last month. If Hospital A had 200 total discharges and 40 deaths and Hospital B had 500 total discharges and 40 deaths, these additional data would change some inferences about each hospital. Knowing the case mix of each hospital (such as severity of cases and diagnoses) would provide additional data for a more accurate comparison.

Selection Bias

Statistical errors can also occur when a sample used in research does not represent the population. For example, if a report was generated on the length of stay of weekend admissions for the past year using as a sample patients admitted on Friday, Saturday, or Sunday and compared with a similar report from the previous year that used as a sample patients admitted on Saturday or Sunday, then the comparison would be biased. Comparison of the results in this example could be biased because the samples used did not represent the same days of the week. Some types of samples are inherently biased, such as convenience sampling in which subjects who are chosen are conveniently available or snowball sampling where the researcher must rely on a participant to refer another participant. The researcher should report the results but not imply that they reflect the whole population. In the case of Dong Xiao, the number of subjects (mice) was misrepresented. (He reported he studied the effects on 10 mice when there were only 4 in the experiment.)

Graphical Misrepresentations

Graphs can be manipulated to emphasize different points. For example, a bar graph can be designed so that the difference between bar heights is lessened. The smaller the increments on the y-axis, the more definition there is between the different bars. A pie chart can be manipulated to pull one wedge away from the rest of the chart. This would bring greater emphasis to that portion of the pie chart even though there may not be significant differences from the rest of the chart. It is also important to be careful with three-dimensional graphs as these may misrepresent data, causing the data to appear smaller or larger. In the case of Dong Xiao, a number of figures were also falsified to show that his results did have an effect on inhibiting cancer cells.

Sabotage

There are also cases of sabotage of a colleague's work. Vipul Bhrigu, a postdoctoral researcher, meticulously and systematically sabotaged the work of a graduate student in his lab by tampering with her experiments and poisoning her cell-culture media. The ORI judged this case as research misconduct, but this ruling has been challenged by at least one other researcher because it does not technically meet the definition of misconduct by the ORI (Rasmussen 2014, 412). Other cases of misbehavior in research have occurred. For example, in one survey that asked about the behavior of colleagues, "fabrication, falsification and modification had been observed, on average, by over 14% of respondents and other questionable practices by up to 72%." (Fanelli 2009). Moreover, he found that the researchers "admitted more frequently to have "modified" or "altered" research to "improve the outcome" than to have reported results they "knew to be untrue" (Fanelli 2009).

Importance of Data Validation

Computer-generated statistical reports are common in healthcare facilities. As discussed in chapter 9, when an HIM professional receives a statistical report, he or she should examine it carefully. The total number of admissions and discharges listed in a report should match coded records. The report should also be compared against the total number of discharges listed in the census data. If the totals do not match, it is important to determine the reasons for the discrepancies. Many reports give only whole numbers. The HIM professional may need to edit the report and its statistics to ensure consistency with usual reporting procedures, such as reporting numbers to the second decimal place. Doing so makes the information valuable to administration or medical staff.

Introduction to Institutional Review Boards

Healthcare organizations that conduct research on human subjects are required to have an **Institutional Review Board (IRB)**. The IRB is a committee primarily responsible for protecting the rights and welfare of research subjects. Professionals who serve on IRBs have extensive education and experience in clinical research. Most of these individuals have medical, doctoral, or other advanced degrees. IRB is a common term used in organizations; however, an institution may use whatever name it chooses. Some organizations refer to this group as an independent ethics committee, research ethics board, or human subjects committee.

The IRB functions as a kind of ethics committee that focuses on what is right or wrong and what is undesirable in order to protect the rights and welfare of anyone participating in the research study. Because human subjects may be involved, researchers are required to follow certain ethical principles that guide researcher behavior and morality. Research ethics provide

- A structure for analysis and decision making
- Support and reminders for researchers to protect human subjects
- Workable definitions of benefits and risks

Risk versus benefit is critical in weighing the advantages of biomedical research. A benefit may be specific to the individual subject or to others as a result of the research. Risks are considered minimal when the probability and magnitude of harm or discomfort anticipated in the proposed research are not greater than those encountered in daily life.

IRBs are responsible for reviewing the research procedures before the study is started and may require periodic reviews during the study. They may approve, modify, or deny requests for research in their facility. If a research project is denied by the IRB, they must notify the researcher and give him or her an opportunity to respond to the denial. Any research on humans must be done carefully to ensure that subjects are not abused in any way. Referring to the earlier example of a study consisting of interviews with mothers of handicapped infants, even though there would not be any physical pain to the mothers, questions asked in the study theoretically could cause the mothers emotional pain. The researcher must obtain permission from the IRB before any research study is started and prepare a plan for the research. This means that the researcher must have thought through the research carefully, prepared any questionnaires, and decided how to select a sample and how to collect data in order to prepare the documentation necessary for the IRB, including informed consent forms for the subjects to read and sign. The IRB should continually review research until it is completed.

In most cases, biomedical research requires that subjects give an informed consent. **Informed consent** is a person's voluntary agreement to participate in research or to undergo a diagnostic, therapeutic, or preventive procedure. It is based on adequate knowledge and an understanding of relevant information provided by the investigators. In giving informed consent, subjects do not waive any of their legal rights nor do they release the investigator, sponsor, or institution from liability for negligence. Federal regulations require that certain information be provided to each human subject, including

- A statement that the study involves research, the purpose of the research, the expected time frame of their participation, a description of the procedures to be followed, and the identification of procedures that are experimental
- A description of reasonably foreseeable risks or discomforts
- A description of the benefits to the subject or others who may reasonably benefit from the research
- A disclosure of any appropriate alternative procedures or courses of treatment that might be advantageous to the subject
- A statement describing the extent to which confidentiality of records identifying the subject will be maintained
- For research involving more than minimal risk, an explanation of whether any compensation or medical treatments are available if injury occurs, and if so, what they consist of or where further information may be obtained
- An explanation of whom to contact for answers to pertinent questions about the research and whom to contact in the event of a research-related injury
- A statement that participation is voluntary, that refusal to participate will involve no penalty or loss of benefits to which the subject may be entitled, and that the subject may discontinue participation at any time without penalty or loss of benefits to which the subject may be entitled (HHS 1998)

Federal regulations also require that informed consent be in a language that is understandable to the subject. The consent form must be translated into that language. Subjects who are not literate in their language must have an interpreter present to explain the study and to translate questions and answers between subject and investigator. A model consent form appears in figure 12.2.

Privacy Considerations in Clinical and Biomedical Research

In response to a congressional mandate in HIPAA, the HHS issued regulations titled Standards for Privacy of Individually Identifiable Health Information. Known as the Privacy Rule, it protects medical records and other **individually identifiable health information,** from being used or disclosed in any form. Individually identifiable refers to whether or not someone could tell or in some way could determine to whom the information refers. The rule became effective on April 14, 2001, and organizations covered by the rule (covered entities) were expected to be in compliance by April 14, 2003.

Figure 12.2. Template for informed consent for research involving human subjects

---

Consent to Investigational Treatment or Procedure

I, _____ , hereby authorize or direct _____ or associates of his/her choosing to perform the following treatment or procedure (describe in general terms), upon _____ (myself).

The experimental (research) portion of the treatment or procedure is:

1. Purpose of the procedure or treatment
2. Possible appropriate alternative procedure or treatment (not to participate in the study is always an option)
3. Discomforts and risks reasonably to be expected
4. Possible benefits for subjects/society
5. Anticipated duration of subject's participation (including number of visits)

I hereby acknowledge that _____ has provided information about the procedure described above, about my rights as a subject, and he/she answered all questions to my satisfaction. I understand that I may contact him/her at phone number _____ should I have additional questions. He/she has explained the risks described above, and I understand them; he/she has also offered to explain all possible risks or complications.

I understand that, where appropriate, the US Food and Drug Administration may inspect records pertaining to this study. I understand further that records obtained during my participation in this study that may contain my name or other personal identifiers may be made available to the sponsor of this study. Beyond this, I understand that my participation will remain confidential.

I understand that I am free to withdraw my consent and participation in this project at any time after notifying the project director without prejudicing future care. No guarantee has been given to me concerning this treatment or procedure.

I understand that in signing this form, beyond giving consent, I am not waiving any legal rights that I might have and I am not releasing the investigator, the sponsor, or institution or its agents from any legal liability for damages that they might otherwise have.

In the event of injury resulting from participation in this study, I also understand that immediate medical treatment is available at _____ and that the costs of such treatment will be at my expense; financial compensation beyond that required by law is not available. Questions about this should be directed to the Office of Research Risks _____ .

I have read and fully understand the consent form. I sign it freely and voluntarily. A copy has been given to me.

The Privacy Rule establishes a category of protected health information (PHI), which may be used or disclosed only in certain circumstances or under certain conditions. PHI is a subset of what is called individually identifiable health information. It includes what healthcare professionals typically regard as a patient's PHI, such as information in the patient's medical records as well as billing information for services rendered. PHI also includes identifiable health information about subjects of clinical research. Patient information considered "protected" is listed on the HHS website (HHS 2016).

Health information is any information, oral or recorded in any form, that "(1) Is created or received by a health care provider, health plan, public health authority, employer, life insurer, school or university, or health care clearinghouse; and (2) Relates to the past, present, or future physical or mental health or condition of an individual; the provision of health care to an individual; or the past, present, or future payment for the provision of health care to an individual" (45 CFR 160.103).

The Privacy Rule defines the means by which human research subjects are informed of how their personal medical information will be used or disclosed. It also outlines their right to access the information. Further, it protects the privacy of individually identifiable information while ensuring that researchers continue to have access to the medical information they need to conduct their research. Investigators are permitted to use and disclose PHI for research with individual authorization or without individual authorization under limited circumstances.

A valid Privacy Rule authorization is an individual's signed permission allowing a covered entity to use or disclose the patient's PHI for the purpose(s) and to the recipient(s) stated in the authorization. When an authorization is obtained for biomedical research purposes, the Privacy Rule requires that it pertain only to a specific research study, not to future unspecified projects. The core elements of the Privacy Rule authorization are

- A description of the PHI to be used or disclosed, identifying the information in a specific and meaningful manner
- The names or other specific identification of the person or persons authorized to make the requested use or disclosure
- The names or other specific identification of the person or persons to whom the covered entity may make the requested use or disclosure
- A description of each purpose of the requested use or disclosure
- An authorization expiration date or expiration event that relates to the individual or to the purpose of the use or disclosure
- The signature of the individual and the date. If the individual's legally authorized representative signs the authorization, a description of his or her authority to act for the individual also must be provided

In addition, the authorization must include statements indicating

- That the individual has the right to revoke the authorization at any time and must be provided with the procedure for doing so
- Whether treatment, payment, enrollment, or eligibility of benefits can be contingent upon authorization, including research-related treatment and consequences of refusing to sign the authorization, if applicable
- Any potential risk that the PHI will be redisclosed by the recipient and no longer protected by the Privacy Rule

Finally, the authorization must be written in plain language, and a copy must be provided to the individual. A model HIPAA consent form appears in figure 12.3; optional elements that may be included in the HIPAA consent form are listed in figure 12.4.

Some facilities may also have a research protocol monitoring committee that reviews any research before and during the study to ensure that there are no adverse effects on the participants. It may even recommend closure of research that is not meeting safety standards, does not have scientific merit, or is not meeting the goals of the research.

Figure 12.3. Model HIPAA consent: Required elements

Authorization to Use or Disclose (Release) Health Information That Identifies You for a Research Study

If you sign this document, you give permission to __(name of healthcare providers)__ at _____(name of covered entity)_____ to use or disclose (release) your health information that identifies you for the research study described here:

(provide a description of the research study, such as title and purpose)

The health information that we may use or disclose (release) for this research includes:

The health information listed above may be used by and/or disclosed (released) to:

_____(name of covered entity)_____ is required by law to protect your health information. By signing this document, you authorize ____(name of covered entity)____ to use and/or disclose (release) your information for this research. Those persons who receive your health information may not be required by federal privacy laws (such as the Privacy Rule) to protect it and may share your information with others without your permission, if permitted by laws governing them.

Please note that (include the appropriate statement):

- You do not have to sign this authorization, but if you do not, you may not receive research-related treatment.

  (when the research involves treatment and is conducted by the covered entity or when the covered entity provides healthcare solely for the purpose of creating protected health information to disclose to a researcher)

- (Name of covered entity) may not condition (withhold or refuse) treating you based upon whether you sign this authorization.

  (when the research does not involve research-related treatment by the covered entity or when the covered entity is not providing healthcare solely for the purpose of creating protected health information to disclose to a researcher)

Please note that (include the appropriate statement):

- You may change your mind and revoke (take back) this authorization at any time, except to the extent that (name of covered entity) has already acted based on this authorization. To revoke this authorization, you must write to (name of covered entity and contact information).

  (where the research study is conducted by an entity other than the covered entity)

- You may change your mind and revoke (take back) this authorization at any time. Even if you revoke this authorization, (name of persons at the covered entity involved in the research) may still use or disclose health information they already have obtained about you as necessary to maintain the integrity or reliability of the current research. To revoke this authorization, you must write to (name of covered entity and contact information).

This authorization does not have an expiration date.

Source: HHS 2004.

Figure 12.4. Model HIPAA consent: Optional elements

**Authorization to Use or Disclose (Release) Health Information
That Identifies You for a Research Study**

- Your health information will be used or disclosed when required by law.

- Your health information may be shared with a public health authority that is authorized by law to collect or receive such information for the purpose of preventing or controlling disease, injury, or disability, and conducting public health surveillance, investigations, or interventions.

- No publication or public presentation about the research described above will reveal your identity without another authorization from you.

- All information that does or can identify you is removed from your health information; the remaining information will no longer be subject to this authorization and may be used or disclosed for other purposes.

- **When the research for which the use or disclosure is made involves treatment and is conducted by a covered entity:** To maintain the integrity of this research study, you generally will not have access to your personal health information related to this research until the study is complete. At the conclusion of the research and at your request, you generally will have access to your health information that (name of covered entity) maintains in a designated record set that includes medical information or billing records used in whole or in part by your doctors or other healthcare providers at (name of covered entity) to make decisions about individuals. Access to your health information in a designated record set is described in the Notice of Privacy Practices provided to you by (name of covered entity). If it is necessary for your care, your health information will be provided to you or your physician.

- If you revoke this authorization, you may no longer be allowed to participate in the research described in this authorization.

Source: HHS 2004.

Ethical Guidelines in Statistics

The HIM professional has an obligation to follow ethical guidelines in statistical practice. Statistics play an important part in clinical and healthcare administrative decision making. Therefore, statistical data collection, calculation, display, and interpretation must be appropriate and accurate. To help ensure data quality, HIM professionals should follow the edicts of the IRB at their facilities and follow accepted ethical practice. When using statistics, HIM professionals must assure that they understand the capabilities and limitations of statistics. They must also use appropriate statistical methods and techniques for the question under study.

The American Statistical Association (ASA) has developed Ethical Guidelines for Statistical Practice. They advocate for integrity in the professional work of researchers, particularly when private interests may inappropriately influence the reporting of statistics. Their guidelines in part read that statisticians should

- Present their findings and interpretations honestly and objectively
- Avoid untrue, deceptive, or undocumented statements
- Disclose any financial or other interests that may affect, or appear to affect, their professional statements (ASA 1999)

Hopefully, one's research will raise new questions about what should be studied and suggest needs for future research. The researcher should always include conclusions about whether or not the problem is better understood or perhaps even resolved by the study.

Health information researchers provide other HIM professionals with knowledge and methods to answer questions and to decipher problems in the work setting. Researchers should be commended for their hard work because they must be very patient and unhurried. Research requires expertise and practice and is rarely spectacular work. However, it has contributed not only to a better place to practice health information management but also to a better place to live and a greater understanding of the world around us.

Those students who would like to be involved in research and who need to develop skills in research should follow these steps:

1. Take at least one course in statistics and research methodologies.
2. Begin to read research studies in professional journals to see how others have performed their research.
3. Agree to work with a skilled health information researcher on a study to gain experience. You can find this information by contacting the author of a research study that you enjoyed reading. It is highly likely he or she will be performing another research study.
4. Learn how to present data effectively both in written form and verbally.

Statistics is the servant, not the master, of logic; it is a means rather than an end of research. "Unless basic assumptions are valid, unless the right data are carefully gathered, recorded, and tabulated; and unless the analysis and interpretations are logical, statistics can make no contribution to the search for truth" (Best and Kahn 2006, 397).

Exercise 12.4

Put the steps of the research process in order.

Order	Description
	Analyze the data
	Design the research
	Define the problem
	Draw conclusions
	Review the literature
	Collect the data

Chapter 12   Matching Quiz

Match the definition with the terms.

Definitions:

a. The process of selecting subjects for a sample from each cluster within a population

b. A type of research instrument with which the members of the population being studied are asked questions and respond orally

c. A systematic investigation of all the knowledge available about a topic from sources such as books, journal articles, theses, and dissertations

d. The appropriation of another person's ideas, processes, results, or words without giving appropriate credit

e. An administrative body that provides oversight for the research studies conducted within a healthcare institution

f. A statement that describes a research question in measurable terms

g. Making up data or results and recording or reporting them

h. A sample in which every element in the population has an equal chance of being selected

i. The use of subjects who are nearby or at hand

j. A technique where the population is first segmented into mutually exclusive subgroups, and then judgment is used to select the subjects or units from each segment based on a specified proportion

Terms:

1. _____ Cluster sampling

2. _____ Fabrication

3. _____ Hypothesis

4. _____ Institutional Review Board

5. _____ Convenience sampling

6. _____ Literature review

7. _____ Plagiarism

8. _____ Random sample

9. _____ Quota sampling

10. _____ Survey

Chapter 12   Review

Complete the following exercises.

1. The degree to which scientific observations actually measure or record what they purport to measure is referred to as _____.
   a. Integrity
   b. Validity
   c. Reliability
   d. Theory

2. The type of research that uses methods or numbers, including comparisons of the population and statistical analysis, to describe results is called _____.
   a. Qualitative research
   b. Quantitative research
   c. Hypothetical research
   d. Theoretical research

3. This type of sample consists of individuals from the population chosen in such a way that every individual has an equal chance of being selected.
   a. Cluster sample
   b. Quota sample
   c. Simple random sample
   d. Judgment sample

4. A statement of the predicted relationship of what the researcher is studying is called a(n) _____.
   a. Educated guess
   b. Essay
   c. Theory
   d. Hypothesis

5. Data can be misinterpreted in which of the following ways?
   a. Fabrication of data
   b. Graphical misrepresentations
   c. Selection bias
   d. All of the above

6. The portion of the research in which the researcher explains the significance and findings of the study is called _____.
   a. Analyzing the data
   b. Drawing conclusions
   c. Sample selection
   d. Selecting the instrument

7. Which type of research entails manipulation of a situation in some way in order to test a hypothesis?
   a. Correlational research
   b. Experimental research
   c. Evaluation research
   d. Hypothetical research

8. Which of the following is the repeatability of scientific observations?
   a. Reliability
   b. Validity
   c. Theory
   d. Integrity

9. Which data-collection method gathers data from a relatively large number of cases at a particular time?

   a. Survey

   b. Observation

   c. Essay

   d. Experimental study

10. In which type of sample does the researcher rely on his or her opinion to select the subjects?

    a. Simple random sample

    b. Judgment sample

    c. Cluster sample

    d. Quota sample

11. A tool used by the researcher to collect data is referred to as the _____.

    a. Survey

    b. Instrument

    c. Research mechanism

    d. Apparatus

12. The type of research describing events, persons, and so on without the use of numerical data is called:

    a. Qualitative research

    b. Quantitative research

    c. Theoretical research

    d. Hypothetical research

13. A committee within an organization whose primary responsibility is to protect the rights and welfare of research subjects is referred to as _____.

    a. Research committee

    b. Health information committee

    c. Institutional review board

    d. Therapeutics committee

14. What are generally the two types of research?

    a. Quantitative and qualitative

    b. Basic and applied

    c. Scientific and hypothetical

    d. Theory and hypothesis

15. A method of observation in which the researcher observes and often speaks with the subjects in as free and natural an atmosphere as possible is called _____.

    a. Freedom of inquiry

    b. Conclusive inquiry

    c. Ethnography

    d. Controlled research

Inferential Statistics in Healthcare

Learning Objectives

At the conclusion of this chapter, you should be able to

- Explain inferential statistics
- Compare and contrast descriptive and inferential statistics
- Interpret the standard error of the mean and confidence intervals
- Identify and describe the null hypothesis
- Understand the importance of *t* tests and the chi-square
- Interpret ANOVA

Key Terms

Analysis of variance (ANOVA)	Descriptive statistics	*t* test
	Inferential statistics	Type I error
Chi-square	Null hypothesis	Type II error
Confidence interval	Standard error of the mean	

In health information management (HIM) practice, descriptive statistics, covered in chapter 10, are most often used in an HIM department. Terms such as mortality and morbidity are examples of descriptive statistics. Healthcare researchers, in contrast, are interested in understanding the characteristics of and reaching conclusions about a population from a sample, which is called inferential statistics. We will see the use of this type of statistics in health information research as well. For example, studies about readmission risk or the electronic health record use and data analytics, which will be covered in chapter 14, often include inferential statistics. This chapter introduces key concepts and calculations in inferential statistics with the goal of providing a general understanding for health information management practitioners.

Inferential Statistics

In chapter 10 we learned that **descriptive statistics** describe a population and are used to describe data in ways that are manageable and easily understood. **Inferential statistics** allow us to generalize from a sample to a population with a certain amount of confidence regarding our findings. Without inferential statistics, it would be very difficult, short of conducting a census, to describe the characteristics of a population. The ability to interpret inferential statistics requires a pre-existing understanding of descriptive statistical measures and computations.

Errors in sampling procedures are inevitable; even with random sampling, there is no guarantee that the sample drawn will be representative of the population. For this reason, inferential statistics are limited to certain amounts of confidence.

This chapter discusses the interpretation of common inferential statistical measures, including standard error of the mean, confidence intervals, the null hypothesis, t tests, analysis of variance (ANOVA), and chi-square.

It is not the intention of this chapter to replace your general statistics course requirement. This chapter merely provides a review of concepts you have learned in that course with exercises from a healthcare perspective. An exhaustive explanation of these concepts, including mathematical computation, is beyond the scope of this book.

Standard Error of the Mean and Confidence Intervals

When trying to determine the characteristics of a population, the mean or average from one sample may not be sufficient because of random sampling error. A more accurate representation could be found by taking many large samples, calculating the mean for each sample, and then finding the standard deviation of all the sample means. This value is called the **standard error of the mean**, abbreviated SE_m, and comes from the standard deviation of many sample means. The graphical representation of all the sample means is a normal distribution when the sample size is reasonably large.

Finding the SE_m in the manner described above can be tedious, and it may not be realistic to find the SE_m of the sample means. For this reason, statisticians have found a formula for approximating the SE_m from only one random sample ($SE_m = sd/sqrt(n)$). (A discussion of the theory leading to this formula is not covered in this book.) When the SE_m has been computed, it is generally reported in one of two ways.

1. The data may be displayed in research reports as follows:

$$\bar{x} = 150, sd = 10, n = 75, SE_m = 1.15$$

Where:
$$\bar{x} = \text{mean}$$
$$sd = \text{standard deviation}$$
$$n = \text{number of observations}$$
$$SE_m = \text{standard error of the mean}$$

Based on the characteristics of normal distributions and treating the SE_m as a margin of error, by adding the SE_m (1.15) to and subtracting it from the sample mean (150), it can be said that we are 68 percent sure that the interval 148.85 to 151.15 contains the population mean. This is called a **confidence interval** (abbreviated CI).

$$150 - 1.15 = 148.85$$
$$150 + 1.15 = 151.15$$

Similarly, it can be said that we are 95 percent sure that the interval 147.70 to 152.30 contains the population mean.

$$150 - (2 \times 1.15) = 147.70$$
$$150 + (2 \times 1.15) = 152.30$$

2. The data may be displayed in a research report as follows:

$$\bar{x} = 60, sd = 4, n = 16, SE_m = 1$$
$$68\% \text{ CI} = 59 \text{ to } 61$$
$$95\% \text{ CI} = 58 \text{ to } 62$$
$$99.7\% \text{ CI} = 57 \text{ to } 63$$

In this example, the confidence intervals have already been computed.

In a normal distribution, confidence intervals are computed by adding one standard error of the mean to and subtracting one from the mean, then adding two standard errors of the mean to and subtracting two from the mean, and so on. The percentages above come from a normal distribution (see Chapter 10 for more information about normal distribution):

- 68 percent of all scores in a normal distribution fall within + or − 1 standard deviation away from the mean
- 95 percent of all scores in a normal distribution fall within + or − 2 standard deviations away from the mean
- 99.7 percent of all scores in a normal distribution fall within + or − 3 standard deviations away from the mean

A confidence interval is the range of scores in which we are estimating the population mean to be. In the example above, the CIs let us know, with a certain amount of confidence, where the mean will lie.

It is important to note that the larger the sample size, the more confidence there is in the mean and the smaller the chance for sampling errors, meaning a smaller SE_m. Further, the more homogenous a population (less variation), the smaller the SE_m. In fact, if a population were all the same (no variation) the SE_m would be zero.

Exercise 13.1

Given the information below, find the 68%, 95%, and 99.7% confidence intervals. Round to one decimal place.

$$\bar{x} = 14, sd = 2, n = 30, SE_m = 0.4$$

68% CI = _____

95% CI = _____

99.7% CI = _____

The Null Hypothesis

The **null hypothesis** states that the difference between two population means is zero. This statement is generally made based on two sample means. For example, let's suppose we obtain a sample of the heights of 15-year-old girls at high school A and a second sample of the heights of 15-year-old girls at high school B. These are the means:

High school A: $\bar{x} = 5.7$ ft.
High school B: $\bar{x} = 5.6$ ft.

From these results, it would appear that 15-year-old girls at high school A are taller than 15-year-old girls at high school B. However, this may not be true; in fact, the difference may be due to errors in sampling and the mean of the heights of girls at high school A (population mean) may equal the heights of girls at high school B (population mean). This is a statement of a null hypothesis.

The null hypothesis can be expressed as follows:

$$H_0: \mu_1 - \mu_2 = 0$$

H_0 represents the null hypothesis.
μ_1 represents the population mean for group 1.
μ_2 represents the population mean for group 2.

When conducting research, most researchers are searching for differences in population means and are therefore not looking to confirm the null hypothesis. In fact, most research is carried out to reject the null hypothesis. Therefore, researchers may develop an alternative hypothesis to test against the null. The alternative hypothesis can be expressed in one of three ways:

$$H_1 = \mu_1 > \mu_2$$

H_1 represents the alternative hypothesis.
μ_1 represents the population mean for group 1, hypothesized to be larger than group 2.
μ_2 represents the population mean for group 2, hypothesized to be smaller than group 1.

or

$$H_1 = \mu_1 < \mu_2$$

H_1 represents the alternative hypothesis.
μ_1 represents the population mean for group 1, hypothesized to be smaller than group 2.
μ_2 represents the population mean for group 2, hypothesized to be larger than group 1.

or

$$H_1 = \mu_1 \neq \mu_2$$

H_1 represents the alternative hypothesis.

μ_1 represents the population mean for group 1, hypothesized to be different from group 2 without sufficient information to determine which group is larger.

μ_2 represents the population mean for group 2, hypothesized to be different from group 1 without sufficient information to determine which group is larger.

The first alternative hypothesis states that group 1 is larger than group 2; this would be the same as the samples would imply, that 15-year-old girls from high school A are taller than 15-year-old girls from high school B. The second alternative hypothesis states that group 1 is smaller than group 2; this would indicate the samples do not represent the population, and that 15-year-old girls from high school A are not taller than 15-year-old girls from high school B. The third alternative hypothesis states that group 1 and group 2 are different, but there is not enough information to determine which population of girls has the higher mean height.

Because there is always a chance that the null hypothesis is true, testing it will lead to a probability (p) that it is true. The smaller the p value (probability that the null hypothesis is true), the more evidence that we should reject the null hypothesis. As a rule of thumb accepted by most statisticians in hypothesis testing, if the probability that the null hypothesis is true is 5 percent or less, the null hypothesis is rejected.

In hypothesis testing, rejecting the null hypothesis with this level of confidence is, in effect, describing the relationship between the means as statistically significant. This is generally the manner in which the null hypothesis is discussed in academic journals.

Probabilities of the null hypothesis are expressed as follows:

$p < 5\%$ The probability that the null hypothesis is true is less than 5 percent.

$p < 1\%$ The probability that the null hypothesis is true is less than 1 percent.

$p < 0.1\%$ The probability that the null hypothesis is true is less than 0.1 percent.

Where: p = the probability that the null hypothesis is true given the values present in the sample. Remember, we are generalizing from a sample to make conclusions about the population.

These different probabilities represent different statistical significance levels; the lower the percentage that the null hypothesis is true, the more significant the finding. Thus, a $p \leq 0.1\%$ is more significant a finding than a $p \leq 5\%$.

Exercise 13.2

Given the following probabilities that the null hypothesis is true, determine whether to reject the null hypothesis or fail to reject the null hypothesis:

1. $p < 5.8\%$ _____

2. $p < 0.7\%$ _____

3. $p < 0.15\%$ _____

4. $p < 2.6\%$ _____

5. Which probability above is the most statistically significant?

Dealing with levels of uncertainty in hypothesis testing creates two types of errors: Type I errors and Type II errors. A **Type I error** occurs when the null hypothesis is rejected, yet it is actually true. A **Type II error** occurs when the null hypothesis is not rejected, yet it is false. Following are examples of both types of errors.

Type I Error

According to the National Cancer Institute, a woman's chance of being diagnosed with breast cancer from age 50 through age 59 is 2.38 percent (2012). With this knowledge, going to see a doctor because of a lump on her breast presents a risk that the doctor will diagnose the patient with breast cancer even if she does not have breast cancer. Consider the following null hypothesis: there is no difference between women diagnosed with breast cancer and women not diagnosed with breast cancer. Rejecting the null hypothesis in this instance would be assuming that the doctor will not diagnose her with breast cancer as there is a difference between the two populations (women diagnosed with breast cancer and women not diagnosed with breast cancer). However, if she is diagnosed with breast cancer, this would be an example of a Type I error. Simply said, the patient could receive a positive test result when, in fact, she does not have breast cancer.

Type II Error

A Type I error is controlled by the researcher setting the acceptable error rate. A Type II error is driven by the sample size and the particular test used. Suppose a drug company has developed a new drug for a serious disease and the new drug is effective. If, however, the null hypothesis is not rejected because the drug company selected a level of significance that is too high, the results of the study will have to be described as insignificant and the drug may not receive government approval (Pyrczak 2010, 83). This is an example of a Type II error.

When describing the null hypothesis, it is never "accepted." Rather, we say "reject the null hypothesis" or "fail to reject the null hypothesis."

Exercise 13.3

Use the following information to provide an example of a Type I and Type II Error.

A pharmaceutical company tests a promising new medicine designed to lower cholesterol when taken daily. The pharmaceutical company conducts a study to determine the effectiveness of the medication against a placebo. Consider the null hypothesis: there is no difference between the effectiveness of the new medication and the placebo in lowering cholesterol.

      Type I Error: _____

      Type II Error: _____

The *t* Test

A *t* test is an example of a test of the null hypothesis to determine if a set of results is statistically significant. As mentioned previously, for the results to be considered statistically significant, the probability that the null hypothesis is true should be 5 percent or less. The results of a *t* test can be written several ways. Consider the following example.

Example:

Group	$\bar{x}$	Standard Deviation (sd)	n
A	5.3	1.6	10
B	6.6	1.0	10

With this group of data, the results of the *t* test (computed using computer software or a calculator) can be written as follows:

The null hypothesis: There is no difference between the groups.

$$H_0: \mu_1 - \mu_2 = 0 \text{ (the difference between the means is zero)}$$

1. Statistically significant ($t = 2.18$, $df = 18$, $p < 0.05$)

2. Statistically significant at the 0.05 level ($t = 2.18$, $df = 18$)

3. Reject H_0 at the 0.05 level ($t = 2.18$, $df = 18$)

Where: t = the value produced by the *t* test

df = The degrees of freedom are found by taking $n - 1$ for the number of groups. In the sample above, there are two groups, therefore:

$df = (n_1 - 1) + (n_2 - 1)$
$df = (10 - 1) + (10 - 1) = 18$
$df = 18$

Statements 1 through 3 above all reject the null hypothesis and say that there is a statistically significant difference between the population means of Group A and Group B ($5.3 - 6.6 = -1.3$).

However, the sample data may not support the conclusion that there is a statistically significant difference between the means. Consider the following example.

Example:

Group	$\bar{x}$	Standard Deviation (sd)	n
A	25	3	8
B	24	3	8

$$H_0: \mu_1 - \mu_2 = 0 \text{ (the difference between the means is zero)}$$

1. Not statistically significant ($t = 0.67$, $df = 14$, $p > 0.05$)

2. H_0 is not rejected at the 0.05 level ($t = 0.67$, $df = 14$)

These statements do not reject the null hypothesis and say that the difference between the sample means is not statistically significant ($25 - 24 = 1$). The null hypothesis is not rejected because the probability of the null hypothesis actually occurring is greater than 5 percent; for this reason, the difference between the means is not statistically significant.

Example:

Group	$\bar{x}$	Standard Deviation (sd)	n
A	18	2.5	7
B	17	8	7

The null hypothesis: There is no difference between the groups.

H_0: $\mu_1 - \mu_2 = 0$ (the difference between the means is zero)

($t = 0.32$, $df = 12$, $p > 0.05$) Do not reject the null hypothesis.

Exercise 13.4

Given the information in the example above, would you reject the null hypothesis or not? How would you state your findings?

It is important to note that understanding the computation involved in testing the null hypothesis is reserved for an advanced statistics course and is not part of the daily activities of a healthcare practitioner. How to interpret the results of these tests, however, is important. For this reason, the next two sections on ANOVA and chi-square are briefly introduced.

ANOVA

Although t tests are used to test the difference between two means, an **analysis of variance (ANOVA)** test is used to test the differences among more than two means. Sometimes ANOVA is referred to as an F test. In the special case when only two means are tested, the F test will yield a p value that is the same as a t test for testing the difference between two population means.

In the following example, the means from four samples are listed. Using ANOVA will test to determine if any of six differences among the means is statistically significant.

	LOS Group 1: Patients with Private Insurance	LOS Group 2: Patients with Medicare/Medicaid
Males	$\bar{x} = 10$	$\bar{x} = 23$
Females	$\bar{x} = 15$	$\bar{x} = 17$

Males with Private Insurance (Group A): $\bar{x} = 10$
Males with Medicare/Medicaid (Group B): $\bar{x} = 23$
Females with Private Insurance (Group C): $\bar{x} = 15$
Females with Medicare/Medicaid (Group D): $\bar{x} = 17$

Differences tested by ANOVA:

1. Between A and B

2. Between A and C

3. Between A and D

4. Between B and C

5. Between B and D

6. Between C and D

This is the power of ANOVA, the ability to test many differences among means at once. If the results from an ANOVA are statistically significant (reject the null hypothesis that at least one of the pairs of means is different), the researcher's next step is to figure out what differences are significant. However, if the results are not statistically significant (the null hypothesis is not rejected), the work is done.

Chi-Square

Chi-square (represented by the symbol χ^2) is a test of significance that deals with nominal data and frequencies, specifically data where the standard deviation and mean are not meaningful descriptions. Note that calculation is possible, just not meaningful. Using computer software to conduct a chi-square test is simple and quickly yields results. Consider the following example.

Example: Employees at a large healthcare facility were randomly asked whether they smoked and whether they had parents who smoked. The results of the 150 employees sampled were:

	Parents Who Smoke	Parents Who Do Not Smoke
Employee smokes	45	25
Employee does not smoke	30	50

These data in this table suggest that those employees with parents who did not smoke were likelier not to smoke (50 versus 25) than were those employees with parents who smoked (30 versus 45). From this sample alone, there appears to be a relationship between smoking and having parents who smoke. However, there is a possibility that the null hypothesis, that the relationship does not exist in this population, is true. A chi-square test can determine whether the relationship is statistically significant. A chi-square test using the values above yielded these results:

$$\chi^2 = 10.71, df = 1, p < 0.01$$

Based on the results, there is a less than 1 percent chance that the null hypothesis is true. Said another way, the results are statistically significant; there is a relationship between employees who do not smoke having parents who do not smoke.

Notice below that the degrees of freedom are determined differently for chi-square. The degrees of freedom are found by taking $(r-1) \times (c-1)$ for the number of categories where r = the number of rows and c = the number of columns.

$$df = (r-1)(c-1)$$
$$df = (2-1)(2-1) = (1)(1) = 1$$
$$df = 1$$

Chapter 13   Matching Quiz

Match the definition with the terms.

Definitions:

a. Test used to assess the differences among more than two means

b. A test of significance, represented by χ^2, that deals with nominal data and frequencies, specifically data where the standard deviation and mean are not meaningful descriptions

c. A healthcare statistic that is calculated from the standard error of the mean, it is an estimate of the true limits within which the true population mean lies; the range of values that may reasonably contain the true population mean

d. Statistics that describe populations

e. Statistics that are used to make inferences from a smaller group of data to a large one

f. A hypothesis that states there is no association between the independent and dependent variables in a research study

g. A value that is found by taking many large samples, calculating the mean for each sample, and then finding the standard deviation of all the sample means

h. A test of the null hypothesis to determine if a set of results is statistically significant

i. Occurs when the null hypothesis is rejected, yet it is actually true

j. Occurs when the null hypothesis is not rejected, yet it is false

Terms:

1. _____ Type II error
2. _____ Null hypothesis
3. _____ Confidence interval
4. _____ Descriptive statistics
5. _____ Type I error
6. _____ Analysis of variance
7. _____ *t*-test
8. _____ Chi-square
9. _____ Inferential statistics
10. _____ Standard error of the mean

Chapter 13   Review

1. Define inferential statistics.

2. Explain the difference between descriptive and inferential statistics.

3. Identify which choices would be considered descriptive statistics and which would be considered inferential statistics.

   Of 500 randomly selected people in New York City, 210 people had O+ blood.

   a. "42 percent of the people in New York City have O+ blood." Is the statement descriptive statistics or inferential statistics?

   b. "58 percent of the people of New York City do not have type O+ blood." Is the statement descriptive statistics or inferential statistics?

   c. "42 percent of all people living in New York State have type O+ blood." Is the statement descriptive statistics or inferential statistics?

4. Identify which choices would be considered descriptive statistics and which would be considered inferential statistics.

   On the last three Friday evenings, City Hospital diagnosed a number of heroin overdoses. There were four on January 14, 20XX, two on January 21, 20XX, and six on January 28, 20XX.

   a. "City Hospital averaged four heroin overdoses in their ER for the last three Friday evenings."

   b. "City Hospital never has more than six heroin overdoes on Friday evenings."

   c. "Friday nights are the busiest time for heroin overdoses at City Hospital."

5. The standard error of the mean comes from the standard deviation of many population means.

   a. True

   b. False

6. Create a null hypothesis for the following research question: What are the differences between emergency room shifts on medication errors?

7. Create a null hypothesis for the following research question: On a clinical trial of a new drug, what will be the effects over a currently used drug?

8. Reword the following research hypothesis to a null hypothesis: Smoking during pregnancy increases the risk of a child being born prematurely.

9. Reword the following research hypothesis to a null hypothesis: Regular exercise in older adults decreases blood pressure levels.

10. Based on the results below, how would you describe the relationship between heart attack patients being treated with aspirin and whether or not they lived?

	Male Heart Attack Patients Treated with Aspirin	Male Heart Attack Patients Not Treated with Aspirin
Male patients who lived	15	4
Male patients who did not live	2	8

$$\chi^2 = 9.39, \, df = 1, \, p \leq 0.01$$

11. Using the following information, determine if the differences between the means are significant.

    Medical Terminology Class

    Group A = Number of word elements remembered by students using flash cards

    Group B = Number of word elements remembered by students not using flash cards

Group	$\bar{x}$	Standard Deviation (*sd*)	*n*
A	75	2.0	10
B	50	3.5	10

    The null hypothesis: There is no difference between the groups.

    $$H_0: \mu_1 - \mu_2 = 0 \text{ (the difference between the means is zero)}$$

    $$(t = 19.61, df = 18, p < 0.01)$$

12. Given the following p values, which would be considered more significant?
    a. $p \leq 0.3$
    b. $p \leq 0.02$
    c. $p \leq 0.25$

13. Given the following null hypothesis, give an example of a Type I error.

    H_0: There is no difference between the number of males or females who go to their primary care physician for an annual exam.

14. Given the following null hypothesis, give an example of a Type II error.

    H_0: There is no difference in the level of understanding of this chapter between students who have previously taken a statistics course and students who have not previously taken a statistics course.

15. Given the following information, determine the 68 percent, 95 percent, and 99.7 percent confidence intervals. Round to two decimal places.

    $$\bar{x} = 4.33, SE_m = 3$$

CHAPTER 14 | Data Analytics

Learning Objectives

At the conclusion of this chapter, you should be able to

- Compare and contrast among the three types of data analytics
- Determine how data analytics is used in making healthcare decisions

Key Terms

Big Data
Clinical data warehouse
Dashboard
Data analysis
Data analytics

Data mining
Descriptive analytics
Evidence-based medicine
Health data analyst
Health informatics

Information governance
Predictive analytics
Predictive modeling
Prescriptive analytics
Real time analytics

With the advent of electronic health records (EHRs) a new field of information science has emerged that is concerned with the management of health data—**health informatics**. This field combines information technology with healthcare and develops ways to control stored health information. Because of the proliferation of data and the need to make it meaningful, the next challenge for healthcare is the move toward data analytics. This area will make it possible for data analysts to use the data from the EHRs along with data from other systems, such as research results, to provide better care for patients and monitor the cost of that care more closely.

Introduction to Data Analytics

Healthcare is a business that relies on tremendous amounts of decision-making both in the clinical and administrative aspects of healthcare. EHRs have expanded the amount of data available to physicians and administrators. **Big data** is a term used for the massive amounts of information that can be interpreted by analytics to provide an overview of trends or patterns. The primary purpose of any healthcare data should be to help healthcare practitioners provide the best care available to patients. A trend in healthcare is to move toward **evidence-based medicine**, which involves systematically reviewing clinical data and making treatment decisions based on the best available information (Kayyoll et al. 2013). This would be tedious and most impossible for a physician to complete manually.

Healthcare administrators also use data to make sound business decisions regarding financial aspects of the facility. **Data analysis** is defined as the task of transforming, summarizing, or modeling data to allow the user to make meaningful conclusions. For example, data analytics can help healthcare administrators identify fraud in their billing claims. Data analytics can link various components, including provider and equipment supplier names, aliases, and demographic data, to detect unusual or hidden relationships.

Health data analysts are responsible for taking health data and transforming it into information that is easily understood. The American Health Information Management Association (AHIMA) offers a credential called certified health data analyst (CHDA). Practitioners who earn this credential have the knowledge to acquire, manage, analyze, interpret, and transform data into accurate, consistent, and timely information, while balancing the "big picture" strategic vision with day-to-day details (AHIMA 2015). Individuals with this credential are prepared for the role of data analyst or content analyst. A data analyst works with policies and procedures on how data will be acquired and studies the data to translate it into information that administrators can use to make business decisions, while a content analyst is responsible for supporting the development and design of clinical information systems by working with clinicians to determine what they need to make good clinical decisions. Another role could be an informaticist who is responsible for tracking outcomes for analysis and billing.

Data analytics is the science of examining raw data with the purpose of drawing conclusions about that information. Analytics can be descriptive, predictive, or prescriptive.

- **Descriptive analytics** is just the summarization of data.
- **Predictive analytics** is a branch of data mining concerned with the prediction of future probabilities and trends, also called forecasting.
- **Prescriptive analytics** is related to descriptive and predictive analytics but it tries to automatically process new data to improve the accuracy of predictions and provide better decision options. (SearchCIO 2012)

Types of Healthcare Data

Healthcare data are divided into two broad categories of quantitative and qualitative data. Quantitative data are numeric while qualitative data describe observations. Quantitative data can be numerically counted. They deal with measurements. Quantitative data are categorized into the categories of interval and ratio. As covered in chapter 11, interval data are numeric, in which we know the order and the differences between the values. Ratio data have a defined unit of measure, and the intervals between successive values are equal.

Qualitative data are divided into the nominal scale and ordinal scale. As discussed in chapter 11, in nominal data, observations are organized into categories in which there is no recognition of order and ordinal data are types of data where the values are in ordered categories and the order of the numbers is meaningful, but not the numbers themselves.

Data are also categorized in terms of internal and external data. Internal data sources are those which are obtained from inside an organization. In healthcare this includes health records, registries, surveys taken of patient satisfaction or other performance improvement studies, annual or other reports, committee minutes.

External data sources refers to data collected outside an organization. For example, a census, reports from the Centers for Medicare and Medicaid Services (CMS) or the Centers for Disease Control (CDC), economic databases, journals, even social media have links to outside data. Healthcare organizations use both internal and external data to help them in decision-making.

Data analytics relies on both descriptive and inferential statistics. Remember from chapter 10 that descriptive statistics describes a population. The typical value may be described by using the mean, median, or mode. The spread of the data may be described using range, variance, and standard deviation. Inferential statistics, as covered in chapter 13, allow us to generalize from a sample to a population with a certain amount of confidence regarding our findings. Inferential statistics are used to test hypotheses or make decisions about the population. These statistics have a probability of making an error. In the previous chapter, this was referred to as a Type I or Type II error. Inferential statistics also offers a confidence level, that is, the probability that the value of a parameter falls within a specified range of values. For example, a confidence level of 95 percent means that there is a probability of at least 95 percent that the result is reliable.

Most studies conducted by a health data analyst require a type of sample. These were covered in detail in chapter 12. The most common type of probability sample used is the random sample. These include simple, stratified, systematic and cluster sampling. The sample size is determined by the amount of precision desired for the study. There are a number of software tools available to help analysts calculate the size as discussed in chapter 12, Statistical Package for the Social Sciences (SPSS) and Statistical Analysis System (SAS) are common. Another program that is often used is called RAT-STATS. It is free to download from the Office of Inspector General's Office of Audit Services. This statistical software program helps facilities perform billing reviews by generating random numbers to random samples, evaluate sample results, and estimate a sample size.

Types of Data Analytics

Healthcare facilities use data analytics to help them make business and clinical decisions. However, new technologies will allow data to be used immediately. This immediate use of data will permit facilities to stay competitive and flexible.

Descriptive Analytics

Descriptive analytics describes raw data. This type of analytics is useful because it helps us see what was done in the past. We can learn from our past behaviors and begin to look at how we can effect some change in the future. Most of the statistics we use fall into this category. We use this type of analytics when we want to understand at an aggregate level what is happening with our patients in our healthcare facilities.

Predictive Analytics

Predictive analytics are about understanding the future keeping in mind that nothing can predict the future with 100 percent certainty. This type of analytics takes the information the healthcare facility has in its EHRs and data warehouses and tries to make the best guess based on patterns. Facilities use this type of analytics when they want to look into the future. Called forecasting, this type of analytics helps determine the probability that something will happen.

Data Mining

Data mining is the process of extracting and analyzing large volumes of data from a database for the purpose of identifying hidden and sometimes subtle relationships or patterns and using those relationships to predict behaviors. Data mining uses both graphical techniques and descriptive statistics to identify trends and patterns in data (White 2013, 7).

For example, data mining can be used to determine which type of patients are using the most resources or abusing resources or to help healthcare facilities make management decisions and help physicians make good clinical decisions for patients.

Data mining has successfully helped healthcare organizations fight healthcare fraud. The National Healthcare Anti-Fraud Association (NHCAA) estimated that fraudulent payments for healthcare services accounts for about 3 percent of the total health expenditures in 2007. They place the range of fraud to be from $70 billion to over $200 billion (Lamont 2009, 1). Fraud in healthcare includes a variety of activities, such as charging for services that were never performed, assigning codes that would receive a higher reimbursement, or creating nonexistent patients. Data mining can detect patterns that do not match what would typically be seen in certain claims—higher than average charges, tests and services that are not usually performed, treatments that do not match the diagnosis, and demographics to identify patients that lead the facility to suspect identity theft.

Clinical Data Warehouse

A **clinical data warehouse** is a collection of data that reflects all aspects of hospital operations and that is used for reporting and analysis. Rather than backing up data, a warehouse lets users find subject-oriented information on demand (Byer 2011). Warehouses are found in many departments in the healthcare facility including the pharmacy, registration, accounting services, and the laboratory. Combining these data into a warehouse allows for many users of the data. The clinical data warehouse can make patient care more efficient and quality outcomes easier to assess. They can also use the warehouse for gathering data for grant-funded research studies. Because of the volume of data available in the health record along with articles in medical journals, researchers will be able to identify associations, trends, and patterns in the data more easily.

Predictive Modeling

Predictive modeling is a process used in predictive analysis to identify patterns that can be used to determine the odds of a particular outcome based on the observed data. That is, statistics from the past are reviewed to determine what is likely to happen in the future. Predictive modeling is used by many companies that want to predict future trends. For example, insurance companies use predictive modeling, or analysis, to determine how insurance policies will be priced. They "investigate thousands of predictors—including such things as what other policies an insured [individual] has, whether they pay their bills on time, and various characteristics of the area in which the risk is located" (Insurance Journal 2012). The auto insurance industry is also able to use telematics—the computer and electronic technology involved in our cars—to record driving behavior data from its customers (Insurance Journal 2012). In the case of healthcare, predictive modeling statistical techniques are used to determine the likelihood of certain events occurring together (White 2011).

Predictive modeling can help healthcare organizations reduce costs and improve patient care. For example, many health insurance companies use predictive modeling techniques to identify claims that are suspicious in order to have them reviewed for accuracy. CMS is moving toward predictive modeling to detect improper Medicare claims. Predictive modeling flags suspicious claims and requires them to be reviewed individually. In an effort to improve patient care and prevent one million heart attacks and strokes by 2017, the Department of Health and Human Services (HHS) has launched its Million Hearts: Cardiovascular Disease Risk Reduction Model (Letourneau 2015).

Predictive modeling goes beyond just collecting data. At Advocate Health Care, a large health system based in Illinois, a predictive analytics project identifies which patients might be readmitted within 30 days after discharge. Another project they have undertaken includes an initiative to identify patients who are likely candidates for interventions to prevent disease, better manage their health conditions outside the hospital, and prevent future hospitalizations, all of which could save insurers and the system money (Evans 2014).

Real-time Analytics

Unlike retrospective analytical tools, such as predictive modeling, **real-time analytics** refers to data that can be accessed as they come into a computer system. Real-time analytics, also referred to as streaming analytics, implies instantaneous results; however, the data may not be immediately available, but rather within a few minutes. The most valuable data in this category are those that are collected and analyzed during the customer interaction, not the review afterward. The analysis that counts is not the results of the last three months, or even the last three days, but the last 30 seconds—probably less (Babcock 2015). The University of Texas Southwestern Medical Center in Dallas is analyzing data from their EHRs to study readmissions of congestive heart failure patients. The EHR analytics model used in the study draws on 29 clinical, social, and behavioral factors within 24 hours of a patient's admission for heart failure, making it possible to match the intensity of the readmission intervention to the patient's risk of readmission on any given day. This real-time program allows physicians to focus on the patients with the highest risk of readmission and has been successful in reducing the number of hospital returns (Bresnick 2013).

Prescriptive Analytics

Prescriptive analytics is a relatively new field of analytics that allows users to prescribe a number of different possible actions. This type of analytics predicts what will happen, but also provides recommendations that will take advantage of the predictions. By providing information about the possible future, this allows facilities to look at the predicted outcomes and come to a decision. Because this is relatively new, most companies are not yet using them in their daily course of business (Halo 2014).

Using Data Analytics for Decision-Making

Healthcare organizations are beginning to rely on data analytics to learn about their patient populations. The more information they have, the more they can make informed decisions.

Data analytics can help healthcare providers in clinical decision support. For example, data analytics can be used to help physicians search through past cases to make an informed decision on one particular patient. Having all patient information, such as lab and x-ray results, medications, and physician orders, on one electronic dashboard (or e-dashboard) can improve how physicians view the data and make decisions about their patients. A **dashboard** is a visual display of the most important information that a physician would need to see about his patients. These can usually be customized by facility or an individual. Data analytics can also help facilities with coordinating a patient's care, that is, monitoring when patients are transferred to other physicians or services. Healthcare providers can use data analytics to help illness from recurring by looking for patterns in the data that are linked to an illness.

Data analytics can also help healthcare executives in a variety of ways. For example, employees can monitor hospital inventory so they will know when to order materials rather than keep a large inventory on hand. Organizations can also compare their facilities with others and then establish benchmarks to improve care. Something as simple as determining wait times in clinics can have a financial impact on the organization. When a facility falls short of its benchmarks, it can apply educational programs to teach employees how to improve processes.

Data is one of the most useful tools available to a health information professional. An HIM professional's educational background and experience makes him or her particularly adept at dealing with data analytics. AHIMA's *Healthcare Data Analysis Toolkit* lists a number of skills needed in order to be successful as a data analyst:

- Has basic understanding of coding systems (CPT/HCPCS, DRG, ICD-10-CM, ICD-10-PCS, National Drug Code [NDC])
- Demonstrates strong verbal and written communication skills
- Demonstrates excellent organizational and time-management skills
- Exhibits keen attention to detail and problem-solving skills
- Knows Microsoft Office, especially Excel and Access (Bronnert et al. 2011)

Health information professionals are in a unique position because they understand coding systems in which all diseases are categorized and can communicate with the many departments of the healthcare facility, including the administrative and clinical sides of healthcare. Their educational programs require computer skills. We are one of the few allied health fields that requires a statistics course in their educational requirements.

Big data is growing exponentially. If someone can think of a way to track healthcare it will be done. For example, some companies have developed ways to track patients with their smart phones or other medical devices to determine how patients are behaving. One example is from Propeller Health, a company that developed a GPS-enabled software that keeps track of patients with chronic respiratory diseases. It keeps track of medications and inhaler use and can be used with rescue and controller medications for tracking symptoms. The sensor on the inhaler wirelessly connects to the patient's smart phone to record data, which can be shared with the patient's physician.

Reminders that can be sent to patients with chronic diseases to remind them to take their medications or make an appointment to have lab tests completed are all part of big data in healthcare. There will be many more opportunities to help patients in the future. The potential for cutting healthcare costs also is possible. It is estimated that $300 billion to $450 billion in reduced healthcare spending could be conservative, as many insights and innovations are still ahead (Kayyoll et al. 2013). Facilities and individuals willing to put in the time and energy to learn more about data analytics will reap the rewards.

In Medicine 2064, Dr. Daniel Kraft explains his vision of healthcare, in which patients work together with their physicians in participatory medicine to create specialized medications specifically for them. He states we are on the technological cusp now with the big data we are collecting. It will not be necessary to wait for a patient to get sick to provide treatment; physicians will be able to know how to prevent disease before it happens (Kraft 2014).

Information Governance

As EHRs continue to evolve, and as data analytics continue to develop more information, healthcare facilities will need to organize and manage this information. An initiative that is gaining momentum in this area is **information governance (IG)**. IG is defined as an organization-wide framework for managing information throughout its lifecycle and supporting the organization's strategy, operations, and regulatory, legal, and environmental requirements. IG applies to all information kept in a facility. IG includes policies, procedures, and processes developed in a healthcare facility that support the facility's efforts to gain value from and understand their information in order to meet the organization's goals as well as protect itself against legal action. It includes more than traditional health information management practices but also information security, compliance, quality management, and risk management. IG ensures the trustworthiness of information.

Chapter 14 Matching Quiz

Match the definition with the terms.

Definitions:

a. The visual display, on a single screen, of the most important information that a physician would need to see about his patients
b. Massive amounts of information that can be interpreted by analytics to provide an overview of trends or patterns
c. The process of extracting and analyzing large volumes of data from a database
d. The task of transforming, summarizing, or modeling data to allow the user to make meaningful conclusions
e. Branch of data mining concerned with the prediction of future probabilities and trends
f. A collection of data that reflects all aspects of hospital operations that is used for reporting and analysis
g. Allows users to prescribe a number of different possible actions
h. The summarization of data
i. Data that can be accessed as it comes into a computer system
j. The science of examining raw data with the purpose of drawing conclusions about that information

Terms:

1. _____ Data analytics	6. _____ Real-time analytics
2. _____ Big data	7. _____ Predictive analysis
3. _____ Clinical data warehouse	8. _____ Data mining
4. _____ Descriptive analytics	9. _____ Data analysis
5. _____ Prescriptive analytics	10. _____ Dashboard

Chapter 14 Review

1. Your administrator has asked you to generate a report that gives the number of hypertension patients last year. This is an example of _____.
   a. Descriptive analytics
   b. Predictive analytics
   c. Prescriptive analytics
   d. Real-time analytics

2. The medical director has asked for a report that will tell him the probability of one of his patients with hypertension will result in a cerebrovascular accident. This is an example of _____.
   a. Descriptive analytics
   b. Predictive analytics
   c. Prescriptive analytics
   d. Real-time analytics

3. The medical director would also like to know if he should try a new medication to prevent one of his hypertensive patients from having a CVA. This is an example of _____.
   a. Descriptive analytics
   b. Predictive analytics
   c. Prescriptive analytics
   d. Real-time analytics

4. Community Hospital is using a system that will help them detect when intracranial pressure becomes high in patients with a recent CVA that will quickly send an alert to the physician. This is an example of _____.
   a. Descriptive analytics
   b. Predictive analytics
   c. Prescriptive analytics
   d. Real-time analytics

5. A managed care organization is using a system that examines the past healthcare behaviors of their patients to determine their future costs for their healthcare. This is an example of _____.

   a. Descriptive analytics

   b. Predictive modeling

   c. Prescriptive analytics

   d. Real-time analytics

6. The term that describes the use of most current scientific research to treat patients is referred to as _____.

   a. Big data

   b. Evidence-based medicine

   c. Predictive analytics

   d. Real-time analytics

7. One of the pediatricians at Community Physician's Clinic worked with a software vendor to get a display of the patients she currently has in the hospital on her smart phone that lets her know current information, such as lab results, vital signs, and medications given. This is called a _____.

   a. Big data

   b. Descriptive analytics screen

   c. Dashboard

   d. Descriptive tablet

8. Which of the following types of data do not have a natural order?

   a. Nominal

   b. Ordinal

   c. Ratio

   d. Interval

9. One of the questions on the patient satisfaction survey that is sent to the patient after discharge asks for the number of times the nurses checked the patient's vital signs in a day. This is an example of which type of data?

   a. Nominal

   b. Interval

   c. Qualitative

   d. Quantitative

10. A statewide database is used by your performance improvement department each month to compare other facilities' readmission rates to your facility's rates. This is an example of _____.

    a. Internal data

    b. External data

    c. Ratio data

    d. Nominal data

11. Which of the following are used to test hypotheses or make decisions about the population?

    a. Descriptive statistics

    b. Descriptive analytics

    c. Inferential statistics

    d. External data

12. The process of extracting and analyzing large volumes of data from a database for the purpose of identifying hidden and sometimes subtle relationships or patterns and using those relationships to predict behaviors is called _____.

    a. Data mining

    b. Data warehouse

    c. Data searching

    d. Big data

13. Your facility is looking at new software that will improve the outcomes of patients by giving recommendations on how to treat the patient in various disease categories. This is an example of _____.

    a. Descriptive analytics

    b. Inferential statistics

    c. Predictive analytics

    d. Prescriptive analytics

14. The business office at Community Hospital is looking at software that can help them with decreasing their fraud and abuse cases. The software claims to be able to flag those patients that would most likely be involved in fraud by examining many databases at the same time and finding those patients with demographic discrepancies. This is an example of _____.

    a. Descriptive analytics

    b. Predictive analytics

    c. Inferential statistics

    d. Descriptive statistics

15. The physicians and pharmacy at Community Hospital have access to controlled substance history information immediately at the patient's bedside which now allows the physician to make better decisions about prescribing medications for the patient. This is an example of _____.

    a. Descriptive analytics

    b. Real-time analytics

    c. Prescriptive analytics

    d. Inferential statistics

References

45 CFR 160.103: General Administrative Requirements Definitions Subpart A. 2013. http://www.ecfr.gov/cgi-bin/text-idx?node=se45.1.160_1103&rgn=div8.

American Health Information Management Association. 2015. Certified health data analyst (CDHA). www.ahima.org/certification/cdha.

American Statistical Association. 1999. Ethical guidelines for statistical practice. http://www.amstat.org/about/ethicalguidelines.cfm.

Babcock, C. 2015 (June 23). Big data moves toward real-time analysis. http://www.informationweek.com/big-data/software-platforms/big-data-moves-toward-real-time-analysis/a/d-id/1320952.

Best, J. and J. Kahn. 2006. *Research in Education*, 7th ed. Boston: Pearson Education, Inc.

Bowden, J. 2008. *Writing a Report: How to Prepare, Write and Present Really Effective Reports*. Oxford, UK: How to Books Ltd.

Bresnick, J. 2013 (August 2). Real-time EHR data analytics helps reduce readmissions by 5%. *EHR Intelligence.* https://ehrintelligence.com/news/real-time-ehr-data-analytics-helps-reduce-readmissions-by-5/.

Bronnert, J., J. Clark, L. Hyde, J. Solberg, S. White, and M. Wolin 2011. *Health Data Analysis Toolkit*. Chicago: AHIMA.

Byer, C. 2011 (October 25). Using health care data analytics to improve information management. *Tech Target*. http://searchhealthit.techtarget.com/tutorial/Using-health-care-data-analytics-to-improve-information-management.

Centers for Disease Control and Prevention. 2016a. CDC Wonder. Underlying causes of death, 2010. http://wonder.cdc.gov/controller/datarequest/D76.

Centers for Disease Control and Prevention. 2016b. National Healthcare Safety Network (NHSN) overview. http://www.cdc.gov/nhsn/pdfs/pscmanual/pcsmanual_current.pdf.

Centers for Disease Control and Prevention (CDC). 2016c. National Healthcare Safety Network: Surgical site infection (SSI) event. http://www.cdc.gov/nhsn/PDFs/pscManual/9pscSSIcurrent.pdf.

Centers for Disease Control and Prevention (CDC). 2015a. Deaths and mortality: FastStats. http://www.cdc.gov/nchs/fastats/deaths.htm.

Centers for Disease Control and Prevention (CDC). 2015b. National Healthcare Safety Network. http://www.cdc.gov/nhsn/index.html.

Centers for Disease Control and Prevention. 2013. Deaths and mortality: Final data for 2013. http://www.cdc.gov/nchs/data/nvsr/nvsr64/nvsr64_02.pdf.

Centers for Disease Control and Prevention. 2012. Consumption of cigarettes and combustible tobacco—United States, 2000–2011. *MMWR* 61(30):565–569. http://www.cdc.gov/mmwr/preview /mmwrhtml/mm6130a1.htm.

Cohen D, Crabtree B. 2006 (July). Qualitative research guidelines project. Robert Wood Foundation. http://www.qualres.org/HomeGrou-3589.html.

Curry, S., C. Cortland, and M. Graham. 2011. Role-modelling in the operating room: Medical student observations of exemplary behavior. *Medical Education* 45(9):946–957.

Department of Health and Human Services (HHS). 2016. Guidance regarding methods for de-identification of protected health information in accordance with the Health Insurance Portability and Accountability Act (HIPAA) Privacy Rule. Accessed March 3, 2016. http://www.hhs.gov/hipaa /for-professionals/privacy/special-topics/de-identification/index.html.

Department of Health and Human Services (HHS). 2014. The health consequences of smoking—50 years of progress: A report of the Surgeon General, 2014: 677. http://www.surgeongeneral.gov/library /reports/50-years-of-progress/full-report.pdf.

Department of Health and Human Services (HHS). 2004. HIPAA authorization for research: NIH Publication Number 04-5529. https://privacyruleandresearch.nih.gov/pdf/authorization.pdf.

Dudovskiy, J. 2011. Research Methods. http://research-methodology.net/.

Evans, M. 2014 (July 12). Data collection could stump next phase of predictive analytics. *Modern Healthcare.* http://www.modernhealthcare.com/article/20140712/MAGAZINE/307129969.

Fanelli, D. 2009. How many scientists fabricate and falsify research? A systematic review and meta-analysis of survey data. *PLoS ONE* 4(5):e5738. doi: 10.1371/journal.pone.0005738. http://journals.plos. org/plosone/article?id=10.1371/journal.pone.0005738.

Folkerts, B. Coordinator, HIM Program, Hutchinson Community College. 2016 (January 19). E-mail exchange to author.

Gelman, A. and D. Nolan. 2002. *Teaching Statistics: A Bag of Tricks.* New York: Oxford University Press. http://stat.columbia.edu/~gelman/bag-of-tricks/chap10.pdf.

Halo Business Intelligence. 2014. Descriptive, predictive, and prescriptive analytics explained: the two-minute guide to understanding and selecting the right analytics. https://halobi.com/2014/10/descriptive-predictive-and-prescriptive-analytics-explained/.

Huffman, E. K. 1994. *Health Information Management.* Berwyn, IL: Physician's Record Company.

Institute of Information Science and Technology (IIST). 2015. Deciles, quartiles and percentiles. Accessed October 15. http://www-ist.massey.ac.nz/dstirlin/CAST/CAST/Scentre/centre5.html.

Insurance Journal. 2012 (June 18). How predictive modeling has revolutionized insurance. http://www.insurancejournal.com/news/national/2012/06/18/251957.htm.

Jacobsen, K. 2012. *Introduction to health research methods: A Practical guide.* Sudbury, MA: Jones and Bartlett.

Kalra, A., R. Fisher, and P. Axelrod. 2010. Decreased length of stay and cumulative hospitalized days despite increased patient admissions and readmissions in an area of urban poverty. *Journal of General Internal Medicine* 25(9):930–935. http://www.ncbi.nlm.nih.gov/pmc/articles/PMC2917661/.

Kayyoll, B., D. Knott, and S. VanKulken. 2013 The big-data revolution in US healthcare: Accelerating value and innovation. http://www.mckinsey.com/insights/health_systems_and_services/the_big-data _revolution_in_us_health_care.

Kelly, K., B. Clark, V. Brown, and J. Sitzia. 2003. Good practice in the conduct and reporting of survey research. *International Journal for Quality in Health Care* 15(3):261–266. http://intqhc.oxfordjournals.org /content/15/3/261.

Kraft, D. 2014 (September 16). Alger YouTube video: Medicine 2064. https://www.youtube.com /watch?v=iOgt85cPU8Q&feature=youtu.be.

Lamont, J. 2009 (June). KM challenges fraud. *KM World* 18:6. http://www.kmworld.com/Articles /Editorial/Features/KM-challenges-fraud-53982.aspx.

Layman, E. and V. Watzlaf. 2009. *Health Informatics Research Methods: Principles and Practice*. Chicago: AHIMA.

Letourneau, R. 2015 (October 2). "How CMS aims to prevent 1M heart attacks, strokes." *HealthLeaders Media*. http://healthleadersmedia.com/content/QUA-321274/How-CMS-Aims-to-Prevent-1M-Heart -Attacks-Strokes.html.

Martin, J.A., B.E. Hamilton, S.J. Ventura, M.J.K. Osterman, E. Wilson, and T.J. Mathews. 2012. Births: Final data for 2010. National vital statistics reports; vol 61, no 1. Hyattsville, MD: National Center for Health Statistics.

McCusker, K. and S. Gunaydin. 2015. Research using qualitative, quantitative or mixed methods and choice based on the research. *Perfusion* 30(7):537–542.

Miller, P.J. and F.L. Waterstraat. 2004. Apples to apples: Using autobenchmarking to measure productivity. *Journal of AHIMA* 75(1):44–49.

National Center for Health Statistics. 2015. About the National Vital Statistics System. http://www.cdc .gov/nchs/nvss/about_nvss.htm#evital_update.

National Center for Health Statistics. 2011 (August). The changing profile of autopsied deaths in the United States, 1972–2007. NCHS Data Brief 67. http://www.cdc.gov/nchs/data/databriefs/db67.pdf.

National Cancer Institute. 2012 (September 24). Breast cancer risk in American women. http://www.cancer.gov/types/breast/risk-fact-sheet.

National Conference of State Legislatures (NCSL). 2015 (September). Certificate of need: State health laws and programs. http://www.ncsl.org/research/health/con-certificate-of-need-state-laws.aspx.

The Office of Research Integrity. 2015 (January 22). Case summary: Xiao, Dong. http://ori.hhs.gov /content/case-summary-xiao-dong.

The Office of Research Integrity. 2011 (April 19). Case summary: Sudbo, Jon. http://ori.hhs.gov/content /case-summary-sudbo-jon.

Onwuegbuzie, A. and C. Poth. 2015. Afterword. *International Journal of Qualitative Methods* 14(2):122–125.

Optum. 2012 (February 3). An inpatient prospective payment system refresher: MS-DRGs. *Advance Healthcare Network for Health Information Management Professionals*. http://health-information. advanceweb.com/Web-Extras/CCS-Prep/An-Inpatient-Prospective-Payment-System-Refresher-MS -DRGs-2.aspx.

Patzel, B. 2001. Women's use of resources in leaving abusive relationships: A naturalistic inquiry. *Issues in Mental Health Nursing* 22(8): 729–747.

Pendergrass, J. 2015. Interviewed by L. Horton. Personal interview. October 8. Hutchinson Regional Medical Center, Hutchinson, Kansas.

Poth, C. and A. Onwuegbuzie. 2015. Editors' introduction. *International Journal of Qualitative Methods* 14(2):1–4.

Prabhat, J. 2012. Counting the dead is one of the world's best investments to reduce premature mortality. *Hypothesis* 2012, 10(1): e3, doi:10.5779/hypothesis.v10i1.254.

Pronovost, P., D. Angus, T. Dorman, K. Robinson, T. Dremsizov, and T. Young. 2002. Physician staffing patterns and clinical outcomes in critically ill patients. *JAMA* 288(17): 2151–2162.

Pyrczak, F. 2010. *Making Sense of Statistics: A Conceptual Overview.* Los Angeles: Pyrczak Publishing.

Rasmussen, L. 2014. The case of Vipul Bhrigu and the federal definition of research misconduct. *Science and Engineering Ethics* 20(2):411–421.

Sauers, P. 2016a. Interviewed by L. Horton. Personal interview. January 19. Ellsworth County Medical Center, Hutchinson, Kansas.

Sauers, P. 2016b (January 13). E-mail exchange to L. Horton.

SearchCIO. 2012. Predictive analytics. http://searchcio.techtarget.com/definition/Prescriptive-analytics.

Shambaugh, E., J.L. Young, C. Zippin, D. Lum, C. Akers, and M.A. Weiss. 1994. SEER Program Self-Instructional Manual for Cancer Registrars—Book 7: Statistics and Epidemiology for Cancer Registries. Publication No. 94-3766. Washington, DC: US Department of Health and Human Services.

Slavenburg, R. 2016 (January 14). E-mail exchange to L Horton.

US Census Bureau. 2013. American Fact Finder. American estimate of the resident population: April 1, 2010 to July 1, 2013. 2013 population estimates." http://factfinder.census.gov/faces/tableservices/jsf/pages/productview.xhtml?src=bkmk.

Voth, K. 2015 (October 6). Interviewed by L. Horton. Personal interview. Hutchinson Clinic, Hutchinson, Kansas.

WebMD. 2014 (September 9). Types of anesthesia. http://www.webmd.com/pain-management/tc/anesthesia-topic-overview.

White, S. 2013. *A Practical Approach to Analyzing Healthcare Data.* Chicago: AHIMA.

White, S. 2011 (Sept.). Predictive modeling 101. *Journal of AHIMA* 82(9):46–47.

World Health Organization. 2016. About WHO. http://www.who.int/about/what-we-do/en/.

APPENDIX A | Formulas

Formulae Listed Alphabetically by Name

Adjusted Hospital Autopsy Rate (p. 128) [Chapter 7]

$$\frac{Total\ hospital\ autopsies \times 100}{Total\ number\ of\ deaths\ of\ hospital\ patients\ whose\ bodies\ are\ available\ for\ autopsy}$$

Anesthesia Death Rate (p. 100) [Chapter 6]

$$\frac{Total\ deaths\ caused\ by\ anesthetic\ agents \times 100}{Total\ number\ of\ anesthetics\ administered}$$

Average (p. 25) [Chapter 2]

$$\frac{Sum\ of\ all\ the\ values}{Number\ of\ all\ the\ values\ involved} = \bar{X}$$

Average Daily Inpatient Census (p. 45) [Chapter 3]

$$\frac{Total\ inpatient\ service\ days\ for\ a\ period\ (excluding\ newborns)}{Total\ number\ of\ days\ in\ the\ period}$$

Average Daily Inpatient Census for a Patient Care Unit (p. 47) [Chapter 3]

$$\frac{Total\ inpatient\ service\ days\ for\ the\ unit\ for\ the\ period}{Total\ number\ of\ days\ in\ the\ period}$$

Average Daily Newborn Census (p. 46) [Chapter 3]

$$\frac{Total\ newborn\ inpatient\ service\ days\ for\ a\ period}{Total\ number\ of\ days\ in\ the\ period}$$

Average Length of Stay (p. 78) [Chapter 5]

$$\frac{Total\ length\ of\ stay\ (discharge\ days)}{Total\ discharges\ (including\ deaths)}$$

Average Newborn Length of Stay (p. 79) [Chapter 5]

$$\frac{Total\ newborn\ discharge\ days}{Total\ newborn\ discharges\ (including\ deaths)}$$

Bed Occupancy Ratio (p. 56) [Chapter 4]

$$\frac{Total\ inpatient\ service\ days\ in\ a\ period \times 100}{Total\ bed\ count\ days\ in\ the\ period\ (Bed\ count \times Number\ of\ days\ in\ the\ period)}$$

Bed Turnover Rate, Direct Formula (p. 64) [Chapter 4]

$$\frac{Number\ of\ discharges\ (including\ deaths)\ for\ a\ period}{Average\ bed\ count\ during\ the\ period}$$

Bed Turnover Rate, Indirect Formula (p. 64) [Chapter 4]

$$\frac{Occupancy\ rate \times Number\ of\ days\ in\ a\ period}{Average\ length\ of\ stay}$$

Cancer Mortality Rate (p. 112) [Chapter 6]

$$\frac{Number\ of\ cancer\ deaths\ during\ a\ period \times 100,000}{Total\ number\ in\ population\ at\ risk}$$

Case Fatality Rate (p. 93) [Chapter 6]

$$\frac{Number\ of\ people\ who\ die\ of\ a\ disease\ in\ a\ specified\ period \times 100}{Number\ of\ people\ who\ have\ the\ disease}$$

Case-Mix (p. 204) [Chapter 9]

$$\frac{Sum\ of\ the\ weights\ of\ MS\text{-}DRGs\ (Medicare\ severity\ diagnosis\text{-}related\ groups)\ for\ patients\ discharged\ during\ a\ given\ period}{Total\ number\ of\ patients\ discharged}$$

Cesarean Section Rate (p. 156) [Chapter 8]

$$\frac{Total\ number\ of\ C\text{-}sections\ performed\ in\ a\ period \times 100}{Total\ number\ of\ deliveries\ in\ the\ period\ (including\ C\text{-}sections)}$$

Complication Rate (p. 154) [Chapter 8]

$$\frac{Total\ number\ of\ complications\ for\ a\ period \times 100}{Total\ number\ of\ discharges\ (including\ deaths)\ in\ the\ same\ period}$$

Consultation Rate (p. 158) [Chapter 8]

$$\frac{Total\ number\ of\ patients\ receiving\ a\ consultation \times 100}{Total\ number\ of\ patients\ discharged}$$

Fetal Autopsy Rate (p. 133) [Chapter 7]

$$\frac{Autopsies\ performed\ on\ intermediate\ and\ late\ fetal\ deaths\ for\ a\ period \times 100}{Total\ intermediate\ and\ late\ fetal\ deaths\ for\ the\ same\ period}$$

Fetal Death Rate (p. 109) [Chapter 6]

$$\frac{Total\ number\ of\ intermediate\ and/or\ late\ fetal\ deaths\ for\ a\ period \times 100}{Total\ number\ of\ live\ births + Intermediate\ and\ late\ fetal\ deaths\ for\ the\ period}$$

Gross Autopsy Rate (p. 122) [Chapter 7]

$$\frac{Total\ autopsies\ on\ inpatient\ deaths\ for\ a\ period \times 100}{Total\ inpatient\ deaths\ for\ the\ period}$$

Gross (Hospital) Death Rate (p. 93) [Chapter 6]

$$\frac{Number\ of\ inpatient\ deaths\ (including\ NB)\ in\ a\ period \times 100}{Number\ of\ discharges\ (including\ A\&C\ and\ NB\ deaths)\ in\ the\ same\ period}$$

Infection Rate (p. 147) [Chapter 8]

$$\frac{Total\ number\ of\ infections \times 100}{Total\ number\ of\ discharges\ (including\ deaths)\ for\ the\ period}$$

Labor Productivity (p. 185) [Chapter 9]

$$Completed\ work = Total\ work\ output - Defective\ work$$

$$Labor\ productivity = \frac{Completed\ work}{Hours\ worked\ to\ produce\ total\ work\ output}$$

Maternal Death Rate (p. 103) [Chapter 6]

$$\frac{Number\ of\ direct\ maternal\ deaths\ for\ a\ period \times 100}{Number\ of\ obstetrical\ discharges\ (including\ deaths)\ for\ the\ period}$$

Mean (p. 221) [Chapter 10]

$$\frac{Total\ sum\ of\ all\ the\ values}{Number\ of\ the\ values\ involved} = \bar{X}$$

or

$$\frac{\Sigma\ scores}{N} = \frac{Sum\ of\ all\ scores}{Total\ number\ of\ scores}$$

Net Autopsy Rate (p. 124) [Chapter 7]

$$\frac{Total\ autopsies\ on\ inpatient\ deaths\ for\ a\ period \times 100}{Total\ inpatient\ deaths - Unautopsied\ coroners'\ or\ medical\ examiners'\ cases}$$

Net Death Rate (p. 96) [Chapter 6]

$$\frac{Total\ number\ of\ inpatient\ deaths\ (including\ NB)\ minus\ deaths < 48\ hours\ for\ a\ given\ period \times 100}{Total\ number\ of\ discharges\ (including\ NB\ deaths)\ minus\ deaths < 48\ hours\ from\ the\ same\ period}$$

Newborn Autopsy Rate (p. 132) [Chapter 7]

$$\frac{Newborn\ autopsies\ for\ a\ period \times 100}{Total\ newborn\ deaths\ for\ the\ period}$$

Newborn Bassinet Occupancy Ratio (p. 61) [Chapter 4]

$$\frac{Total\ newborn\ inpatient\ service\ days\ for\ a\ period \times 100}{Total\ newborn\ bassinet\ count \times Number\ of\ days\ in\ the\ period}$$

Newborn Mortality Rate (p. 107) [Chapter 6]

$$\frac{Total\ number\ of\ newborn\ deaths\ for\ a\ period \times 100}{Total\ number\ of\ newborn\ discharges\ (including\ deaths)\ for\ the\ period}$$

Nosocomial Infection Rate (p. 147) [Chapter 8]

$$\frac{Total\ number\ of\ nosocomial\ infections\ for\ a\ period \times 100}{Total\ number\ of\ discharges, including\ deaths,\ for\ the\ same\ period}$$

Other Rates (p. 161) [Chapter 8]

$$\frac{Number\ of\ times\ something\ happened \times 100}{Number\ of\ times\ something\ could\ have\ happened}$$

Payback Period (p. 195) [Chapter 9]

$$\frac{Total\ cost\ of\ project}{Annual\ incremental\ cash\ flow}$$

Postoperative Death Rate (p. 97) [Chapter 6]

$$\frac{Total\ number\ of\ deaths\ (within\ 10\ days\ after\ surgery) \times 100}{Total\ number\ of\ patients\ who\ were\ operated\ on\ for\ the\ period}$$

Postoperative Infection Rate (p. 150) [Chapter 8]

$$\frac{Total\ number\ of\ infections\ in\ clean\ surgical\ cases\ for\ a\ period \times 100}{Total\ number\ of\ surgical\ operations\ for\ the\ period}$$

Rate (p. 24) [Chapter 2]

$$Rate = \frac{Part}{Base},\ or\ R = \frac{P}{B}$$

Return on Investment (p. 195) [Chapter 9]

$$\frac{Average\ annual\ incremental\ cash\ flow}{Total\ cost\ of\ the\ project}$$

Staffing Level (p. 186) [Chapter 9]

$$\frac{Patient\ encounters}{Productivity} = Number\ of\ FTEs\ needed$$

Standard Deviation (p. 231) [Chapter 10]

$$SD = \sqrt{\frac{\Sigma(X - \bar{X})^2}{(N-1)}}$$

Unit Labor Costs (p. 174) [Chapter 9]

$$\frac{Total\ (sum)\ coding\ professional\ annual\ compensation}{Total\ (sum)\ coding\ professional\ annual\ productivity}$$

Variance (p. 229) [Chapter 10]

$$s^2 = \frac{(X_1 - \bar{X})^2 + (X_2 - \bar{X})^2 + (X_3 - \bar{X})^2 \; and \; so \; on}{N - 1}$$

Vital Statistics Infant Mortality Rate (p. 107) [Chapter 6]

$$\frac{Number \; of \; infant \; deaths \, (neonatal \; and \; postneonatal) \, during \; a \; period \times 1,000}{Number \; of \; live \; births \; during \; the \; period}$$

Vital Statistics Maternal Mortality Rate (p. 103) [Chapter 6]

$$\frac{Number \; of \; deaths \; attributed \; to \; maternal \; conditions \; during \; a \; period \times 100,000}{Number \; of \; births \; during \; the \; period}$$

Vital Statistics Neonatal Mortality Rate (p. 107) [Chapter 6]

$$\frac{Number \; of \; neonatal \; deaths \; during \; a \; period \times 1,000}{Number \; of \; live \; births \; during \; the \; period}$$

World Health Organization formula for Maternal Mortality Ratio (p. 106) [Chapter 6]

$$\frac{Number \; of \; maternal \; deaths \times 100,000}{Number \; of \; live \; births}$$

Formulas Listed by Chapter in Which They Appear

Chapter 2

Average (p. 25)
Rate (p. 24)

Chapter 3

Average Daily Inpatient Census (p. 45)
Average Daily Inpatient Census for a Patient Care Unit (p. 47)
Average Daily Newborn Census (p. 46)

Chapter 4

Bed Occupancy Ratio (p. 56)
Bed Turnover Rate, Direct Formula (p. 64)
Bed Turnover Rate, Indirect Formula (p. 64)
Newborn Bassinet Occupancy Ratio (p. 61)

Chapter 5

Average Length of Stay (p. 78)
Average Newborn Length of Stay (p. 79)

Chapter 6

Anesthesia Death Rate (p. 100)
Cancer Mortality Rate (p. 112)
Case Fatality Rate (p. 93)
Fetal Death Rate (p. 109)
Gross (Hospital) Death Rate (p. 93)
Maternal Death Rate (p. 103)
Net Death Rate (p. 96)
Newborn Mortality Rate (p. 107)
Postoperative Death Rate (p. 97)
Vital Statistics Infant Mortality Rate (p. 107)
Vital Statistics Maternal Mortality Rate (p. 103)
Vital Statistics Neonatal Mortality Rate (p. 107)
World Health Organization formula for Maternal Mortality Ratio (p. 106)

Chapter 7

Adjusted Hospital Autopsy Rate (p. 128)
Fetal Autopsy Rate (p. 133)
Gross Autopsy Rate (p. 122)
Net Autopsy Rate (p. 124)
Newborn Autopsy Rate (p. 132)

Chapter 8

Cesarean Section Rate (p. 156)
Complication Rate (p. 154)
Consultation Rate (p. 158)
Infection Rate (p. 147)
Nosocomial Infection Rate (p. 147)
Other Rates (p. 161)
Postoperative Infection Rate (p. 150)

Chapter 9

Case-Mix (p. 204)
Labor Productivity (p. 185)
Payback Period (p. 195)
Return on Investment (p. 195)
Staffing Level (p. 186)
Unit Labor Costs (p. 174)

Chapter 10

Mean (p. 221)
Standard Deviation (p. 231)
Variance (p. 229)

APPENDIX

B | Glossary of Healthcare Services and Statistical Terms

Accuracy: A characteristic of data that are free from significant error, up to date, and representative of relevant facts

Adjusted hospital autopsy rate: The proportion of hospital autopsies performed following the deaths of patients whose bodies are available for autopsy

Admission date: In the home health prospective payment system, the date of first service; in the acute care prospective payment system, the year, month, and day of inpatient admission, beginning with a hospital's formal acceptance of a patient who is to receive healthcare services while receiving room, board, and continuous nursing services

Aggregate data: Data extracted from individual health records and combined to form de-identified information about groups of patients that can be compared and analyzed

Agency for Healthcare Research and Quality: An agency within the Department of Health and Human Services whose mission is to produce evidence to make healthcare safer, higher quality, more accessible, equitable, and affordable, and to work within the US Department of Health and Human Services and with other partners to make sure that the evidence is understood and used

Alternative hypothesis: A hypothesis that states that there is an association between independent and dependent variables

Ambulatory care: Preventive or corrective healthcare services provided on a nonresident basis in a provider's office, clinic setting, or hospital outpatient setting

Analysis of variance (ANOVA): Test used to assess the differences among more than two means

Ancillary service visit: The appearance of an outpatient in a unit of a hospital or outpatient facility to receive services, tests, or procedures that ordinarily are not counted as encounters for healthcare services

Ancillary services: Tests and procedures ordered by a physician to provide information for use in patient diagnosis or treatment

Anesthesia: Loss of feeling or awareness, as when an anesthetic is administered before surgery

Anesthesia death rate: The ratio of deaths caused by anesthetic agents to the number of anesthetics administered during a specified period of time

Applied research: A type of research that focuses on the use of scientific theories to improve actual practice as in medical research applied to the treatment of patients

Arithmetic mean length of stay (AMLOS):   The average length of stay for all patients

Autopsy: The postmortem examination of the organs and tissues of a body to determine the cause of death or pathological conditions

Autopsy rate: The proportion or percentage of deaths in a healthcare organization that are followed by the performance of an autopsy

Available for hospital autopsy: A situation in which the required conditions have been met to allow an autopsy to be performed on a hospital patient who has died

Average: The value obtained by dividing the sum of a set of numbers by the number of values

Average daily inpatient census: The mean number of hospital inpatients present in the hospital each day for a given period of time

Average duration of hospitalization: *See* **average length of stay**

Average length of stay (ALOS):   The mean length of stay for hospital inpatients discharged during a given period of time

Bar chart: A graphic technique used to display frequency distributions of nominal or ordinal data that fall into categories; also called bar graph

Bar graph: *See* **bar chart**

Basic research: A type of research that focuses on the development and refinement of theories

Bed capacity: The number of beds that a facility has been designed and constructed to house

Bed complement: *See* **bed count**

Bed count: The number of inpatient beds set up and staffed for use on a given day; also called bed complement

Bed count day: A unit of measure that denotes the presence of one inpatient bed (either occupied or vacant) set up and staffed for use in one 24-hour period

Bed occupancy ratio: The proportion of beds occupied, defined as the ratio of inpatient service days to bed count days during a specified period of time

Bed size: The total number of inpatient beds for which a facility is equipped and staffed to provide patient care services

Bed turnover rate: The average number of times a bed changes occupants during a given period of time

Big data: Massive amounts of information that can be interpreted by analytics to provide an overview of trends or patterns

Boarder: An individual such as a parent, caregiver, or other family member who receives lodging at a healthcare facility but is not a patient

Boarder baby: A newborn who remains in the nursery following discharge because the mother is still hospitalized, or a premature infant who no longer needs intensive care but remains for observation

Budget: A plan that converts the organization's goals and objectives into targets for revenue and spending

Calculation of inpatient service days: The measurement of the services received by all inpatients in one 24-hour period

Calculation of transfers: A medical care unit that shows transfers on and off the unit as subdivisions of patients admitted to and discharged from the unit

Cancer mortality rate: The proportion of patients who die from cancer

Cancer registrar: An individual who is responsible for capturing a complete summary of the history, diagnosis, treatment and disease status for every cancer patient

Cancer registry: A collection of information about the occurrence of cancer, the types of cancers that occur and their locations within the body, the extent of cancer at the time of diagnosis (disease stage), and the kinds of treatment that patients receive

Capital budget: The allocation of resources for long-term investments and projects

Case fatality rate: The total number of deaths due to a specific illness during a given time period divided by the total number of cases during the same period

Case-mix: A method of grouping patients according to a predefined set of characteristics

Case-mix index: The average relative weight of all cases treated at a given facility or by a given physician, which reflects the resource intensity or clinical severity of a specific group in relation to the other groups in the classification system

Categorical data: Four types of data (nominal, ordinal, interval, and ratio) that represent values or observations that can be sorted into a category; also called scales of measurement

Causal research: A type of conclusive research that tries to answer questions about what causes certain things to occur

Cause-specific death rate: The total number of deaths due to a specific illness during a given time period divided by the estimated population for the same time period

Census: The number of inpatients present in a healthcare facility at any given time

Census day: *See* **inpatient service day**

Census statistics: Statistics that examine the number of patients being treated at specific times, the lengths of their stay, and the number of times a bed changes occupants

Census survey: A survey that collects data from all the members of a population

Centers for Disease Control and Prevention (CDC):   A group of federal agencies that oversees health promotion and disease control and prevention activities in the United States

Centers for Medicare and Medicaid Services (CMS): The division of the Department of Health and Human Services that is responsible for developing healthcare policy in the United States and for administering the Medicare program and the federal portion of the Medicaid program; called the Health Care Financing Administration (HCFA) prior to 2001

Certificate of need: A state-directed program that requires healthcare facilities to submit detailed plans and justifications for the purchase of new equipment, new buildings, or new service offerings that cost in excess of a certain amount

Cesarean section: A surgical operation for delivering a child by cutting through the wall of the mother's abdomen

Cesarean section rate: The ratio of all Cesarean sections to the total number of deliveries, including Cesarean sections, during a specified period of time

Chi-square: A test of significance, represented by χ^2, that deals with nominal data and frequencies, specifically data where the standard deviation and mean are not meaningful descriptions

Chronic: Of long duration

Clean surgical case: A surgical case in which no infection existed prior to surgery

Clinical autopsy: An autopsy in which permission is granted by the next of kin

Clinical data warehouse: A collection of data that reflects all aspects of hospital operations that is used for reporting and analysis

Clinic outpatient: A patient who is admitted to a clinical service of a clinic or hospital for diagnosis or treatment on an ambulatory basis

Clinical research: A specialized area of research that primarily investigates the efficacy of preventive, diagnostic, and therapeutic procedures; also called medical research

Cluster sampling: The process of selecting subjects for a sample from each cluster within a population (for example, a family, school, or community)

Community-acquired infection: An infectious disease contracted as the result of exposure before or after a patient's period of hospitalization

Complete master census: A total census for a facility showing the names and locations of patients present in the hospital at a particular point in time

Complication: A medical condition that arises during an inpatient hospitalization (for example, a postoperative wound infection)

Complication rate: The total number of hospital inpatients with a complication for a given period divided by the total number of discharges and deaths for the same period

Conclusive research: A type of research performed in order to come to some sort of conclusion or help in decision making; includes descriptive research and causal research

Concomitant: Accessory; taking place at the same time

Confidence interval: A healthcare statistic that is calculated from the standard error of the mean, it is an estimate of the true limits within which the true population mean lies; the range of values that may reasonably contain the true population mean

Consultation: The response by one healthcare professional to another healthcare professional's request to provide recommendations and/or opinions regarding the care of a particular patient or resident

Consultation rate: The total number of hospital inpatients receiving consultations for a given period divided by the total number of discharges and deaths for the same period

Continuous data: Data that represent measurable quantities but are not restricted to certain specified values

Control group: A comparison study group whose members do not undergo the treatment under study

Convenience sample: The "convenient" use of subjects who are nearby or at hand, also known as accidental samples or haphazard samples

Convenience sampling: A sampling technique where the selection of units from the population is based on easy availability and/or accessibility

Coroner: A public officer whose principal duty is to inquire via an inquest into the cause of any death that there is reason to suppose is not due to natural causes

Coroner's case: A death that appears to be suspicious and requires action from the coroner to determine the cause of death

Correlational research: A design of research that determines the existence and degree of relationships among factors

Cost–benefit analysis: A process that uses quantitative techniques to evaluate and measure the benefit of providing products or services compared to the cost of providing them

Crude birth rate: The number of live births divided by the population at risk

Crude death rate: The total number of deaths in a given population for a given period of time divided by the estimated population for the same period of time

Daily census: The number of inpatients present at the census-taking time each day, plus any inpatients who were both admitted after the previous census-taking time and discharged before the next census-taking time

Daily inpatient census: The number of inpatients present at census-taking time each day, plus any inpatients who were both admitted and discharged after the census-taking time the previous day

Dashboard: A visual display of the most important information needed to achieve one or more objectives; consolidated and arranged on a single screen so the information can be monitored at a glance

Data: The dates, numbers, images, symbols, letters, and words that represent basic facts and observations about people, processes, measurements, and conditions

Data accuracy: The extent to which data are free of identifiable errors

Data analysis: The task of transforming, summarizing, or modeling data to allow the user to make meaningful conclusions

Data analytics: The science of examining raw data with the purpose of drawing conclusions about that information

Data collection: The process by which data are gathered

Data mining: The process of extracting and analyzing large volumes of data from a database for the purpose of identifying hidden and sometimes subtle relationships or patterns and using those relationships to predict behaviors

Data warehouse: A repository of historical data organized for reporting and analysis. It facilitates data access by having data from many sources in one place, linked together, and easily searchable

Date of encounter (outpatient and physician services):   The year, month, and day of a visit or other healthcare encounter

Date of procedure (inpatient):   The year, month, and day of each significant procedure

Date of service (DOS):   The date a test, procedure, or service was rendered

Days of stay: *See* **length of stay**

Dead on arrival (DOA):   The condition of a patient who arrives at a healthcare facility with no signs of life and who was pronounced dead by a physician

Death rate: The proportion of inpatient hospitalizations that end in death

Decile: The tenth equal part of a distribution

Decimal: Numbered or proceeding by tens; based on the number 10; expressed in or utilizing a decimal system, especially with a decimal point

Delivery: The process of delivering a liveborn infant or dead fetus (and placenta) by manual, instrumental, or surgical means

Denominator: The part of a fraction below the line signifying division that functions as the divisor of the numerator and, in fractions with 1 as the numerator, indicates into how many parts the unit is divided

Dependent variable: A measurable variable in a research study that depends on an independent variable

Descriptive analytics: The summarization of data

Descriptive research: A type of conclusive research that determines and reports the current status of topics and subjects

Descriptive statistics: Statistics that describe populations

Discharge date: The year, month, and day that an inpatient was formally released from the hospital and room, board, and continuous nursing services were terminated

Discharge days: *See* **length of stay** and **total length of stay**

Discharge diagnosis list: A complete set of discharge diagnoses applicable to a single patient episode, such as an inpatient hospitalization

Discharge transfer: The transfer of an inpatient to another healthcare institution at the time of discharge

Discrete data: Data that represent separate and distinct values or observations; that is, data that contain only finite numbers and have only specified values

Disposition: For outpatients, the healthcare practitioner's description of the patient's status at discharge (no follow-up planned, follow-up planned or scheduled, referred elsewhere, expired), for inpatients, a core health data element that identifies the circumstances under which the patient left the hospital (discharged alive, discharged to home or self-care, discharged and transferred to another short-term general hospital for inpatient care, discharged and transferred to a skilled nursing facility, discharged and transferred to an intermediate care facility, discharged and transferred to another type of institution for inpatient care or referred for outpatient services to another institution, discharged and transferred to home under care of an organized home health services organization, discharged and transferred to home under care of a home intravenous therapy provider, left against medical advice or discontinued care, expired, status not stated)

Duration of inpatient hospitalization: *See* **length of stay**

Early fetal death: The death of a product of human conception that is fewer than 20 weeks of gestation and 500 grams or less in weight before its complete expulsion or extraction from the mother

Electronic health record (EHR):   A computerized record of health information and associated processes; also called computer-based patient record

Electronic medical record (EMR):   A form of computer-based health record in which information is stored in whole files instead of by individual data elements

Electronic signature: Any representation of a signature in digital form, including an image of a handwritten signature; also, the authentication of a computer entry in a health record made by the individual making the entry

Emergency patient: A patient who is admitted to the emergency services department of a hospital for the diagnosis and treatment of a condition that requires immediate medical, dental, or allied health services in order to sustain life or to prevent critical consequences

Emergency services department: The department of a hospital responsible for the provision of medical and surgical care to patients arriving at the hospital in need of immediate care. The emergency department is also called the emergency room or ER

Encounter: The direct personal contact between a patient and a physician or other person authorized by state licensure law and, if applicable, by medical staff bylaws to order or furnish healthcare services for the diagnosis or treatment of the patient

Episode of care: A period of relatively continuous medical care performed by healthcare professionals in relation to a particular clinical problem or situation

Ethnography: A method of observational research that investigates culture in naturalistic settings using both qualitative and quantitative approaches

Evaluation research: A design of research that examines the effectiveness of policies, programs, or organizations

Evidence-based medicine: The judicious use of the best current available scientific research in making decisions about the care of patients

Exacerbation: To make more violent, bitter, or severe

Experimental research: A research design used to establish cause and effect; also, a controlled investigation in which subjects are assigned randomly to groups that experience carefully controlled interventions that are manipulated by the experimenter according to a strict protocol; also called experimental study

Exploratory research: A research design used because a problem has not been clearly defined or its scope is unclear

Fabrication: Making up data or results and recording or reporting them

Falsification: Manipulating research materials, equipment, or processes, or changing or omitting data or results such that the research is not accurately represented in the research record

Fetal autopsy rate: The number of autopsies performed on intermediate and late fetal deaths for a given time period divided by the total number of intermediate and late fetal deaths for the same time period

Fetal death: The death of a product of human conception before its complete expulsion or extraction from the mother regardless of the duration of the pregnancy; also called stillborn

Fetal death rate: A proportion that compares the number of intermediate and/or late fetal deaths to the total number of live births and intermediate or late fetal deaths during the same period of time

Fiscal year: Any consecutive 12-month period an organization uses as its accounting period

Forensic autopsy: An autopsy in which a legal representative has ordered an autopsy to be performed

Fraction: One or more parts of a whole

Frequency distribution: A table or graph that displays the number of times (frequency) a particular observation occurs

Frequency distribution table: A table consisting of a set of classes or categories along with the numerical counts that correspond to nominal and ordinal data

Frequency polygon: A type of line graph that represents a frequency distribution

Full-time equivalent employees (FTEs): The total number of workers, including part-time, in an area as the equivalent of full-time positions

Gender: The biological sex of the patient as recorded at the start of care

Graph: A graphic tool used to show numerical data in a pictorial representation

Gross autopsy rate: The number of inpatient autopsies conducted during a given time period divided by the total number of inpatient deaths for the same time period

Gross death rate: The number of inpatient deaths that occurred during a given time period divided by the total number of inpatient discharges, including deaths, for the same time period

Health data analysts: Individuals responsible for taking health data and transforming it into information that is easily understood

Histogram: A graphic technique used to display the frequency distribution of continuous data (interval or ratio data) as either numbers or percentages in a series of bars

Historical research: A research design used to investigate past events

Home health (HH): An umbrella term that refers to the medical and nonmedical services provided to patients and their families in their places of residence; also called home care

Home health agency (HHA): A program or organization that provides a blend of home-based medical and social services to homebound patients and their families for the purpose of promoting, maintaining, or restoring health or of minimizing the effects of illness, injury, or disability

Home healthcare: Home healthcare is healthcare that is provided by a home health agency and occurs within one's home

Home healthcare patient: A patient who receives care within their own home provided by a home health agency

Hospice: An interdisciplinary program of palliative care and supportive services that addresses the physical, spiritual, social, and economic needs of terminally ill patients and their families

Hospice care: The medical care provided to persons with life expectancies of six months or less who elect to forgo standard treatment of their illness and to receive only palliative care

Hospital: A healthcare entity that has an organized medical staff and permanent facilities that include inpatient beds and continuous medical and nursing services and that provides diagnostic and therapeutic services for patients, as well as overnight accommodations and nutritional services

Hospital ambulatory care: All hospital-directed preventive, therapeutic, and rehabilitative services provided by physicians and their surrogates to patients who are not hospital inpatients

Hospital autopsy: A postmortem (after-death) examination performed on the body of a person who has at some time been a hospital patient by a hospital pathologist or a physician of the medical staff who has been delegated the responsibility

Hospital autopsy rate: The total number of autopsies performed by a hospital pathologist for a given time period divided by the number of deaths of hospital patients (inpatients and outpatients) whose bodies were available for autopsy for the same time period

Hospital death rate: The number of inpatient deaths for a given period of time divided by the total number of live discharges and deaths for the same time period

Hospital inpatient: A patient who is provided with room, board, and continuous general nursing services in an area of an acute care facility where patients generally stay at least overnight

Hospital inpatient autopsy: A postmortem (after-death) examination performed on the body of a patient who died during an inpatient hospitalization by a hospital pathologist or a physician of the medical staff who has been delegated the responsibility

Hospital inpatient beds: Accommodations with supporting services (such as food, laundry, and housekeeping) for hospital inpatients, excluding those for the newborn nursery, but including incubators and bassinets in nurseries for premature or sick newborn infants

Hospital live birth: In an inpatient facility, the complete expulsion or extraction of a product of human conception from the mother, regardless of the duration of pregnancy, which, after such expulsion or extraction, breathes or shows any other evidence of life, such as beating of the heart, pulsation of the umbilical cord, or definite movement of voluntary muscles

Hospital newborn bassinet: Accommodations including incubators and isolettes in the newborn nursery with supporting services (such as food, laundry, and housekeeping) for hospital newborn inpatients

Hospital newborn inpatient: A patient born in the hospital at the beginning of the current inpatient hospitalization

Hospital outpatient: A hospital patient who receives services in one or more of a hospital's facilities when he or she is not currently an inpatient or a home care patient

Hospital outpatient care unit: An organized unit of a hospital that provides facilities and medical services exclusively or primarily to patients who are generally ambulatory and who do not currently require or are not currently receiving services as an inpatient of the hospital

Hospital-acquired infection: *See* **nosocomial infection**

Hospitalization: The period during an individual's life when he or she is a patient in a single hospital without interruption except by possible intervening leaves of absence

Hybrid health record: A combination of paper and electronic records

Hypothesis: A statement that describes a research question in measurable terms

Iatrogenic: Induced inadvertently by a physician or surgeon or by medical treatment or diagnostic procedures

Incidence rate: A computation that compares the number of new cases of a specific disease for a given time period to the population at risk for the disease during the same time period

Individually identifiable health information: According to HIPAA privacy provisions, that information which specifically identifies the patient to whom the information relates, such as age, gender, date of birth, and address

Induced termination of pregnancy: The purposeful interruption of an intrauterine pregnancy that was not intended to produce a liveborn infant and that did not result in a live birth

Infant death: The death of a liveborn infant at any time from the moment of birth to the end of the first year of life (364 days, 23 hours, 59 minutes from the moment of birth)

Infant mortality rate: The number of deaths of individuals under one year of age during a given time period divided by the number of live births reported for the same time period

Infection rate: The ratio of all infections to the number of discharges, including deaths

Inferential statistics: Statistics that are used to make inferences from a smaller group of data to a large one

Information: Data that have been deliberately selected, processed, and organized to be useful

Information governance: An organization-wide framework for managing information throughout its lifecycle and supporting the organization's strategy, operations, and regulatory, legal, and environmental requirements

Inpatient: *See* **hospital inpatient**

Inpatient admission: An acute care facility's formal acceptance of a patient who is to be provided with room, board, and continuous nursing service in an area of the facility where patients generally stay at least overnight

Inpatient bed count: *See* **bed count**

Inpatient bed occupancy rate: The total number of inpatient service days for a given time period divided by the total number of inpatient bed count days for the same time period; also called percentage of occupancy

Inpatient census: *See* **census**

Inpatient days of stay: *See* **length of stay**

Inpatient discharge: The termination of hospitalization through the formal release of an inpatient from a hospital

Inpatient service day: A unit of measure equivalent to the services received by one inpatient during one 24-hour period

Institutional death rate: *See* **net death rate**

Institutional Review Board (IRB):   An administrative body that provides oversight for the research studies conducted within a healthcare institution

Instrument: A standardized and uniform way to collect data

Intermediate fetal death: The death of a product of human conception before its complete expulsion or extraction from the mother that has completed 20 weeks of gestation (but less than 28 weeks) and weighs 501 to 1,000 grams

Internal validity: An attribute of a study's design that contributes to the accuracy of its findings

Interval data: A type of data that represents observations that can be measured on an evenly distributed scale beginning at a point other than true zero

Interview guide: A list of written questions to be asked during an interview

Intrahospital transfer: A change in medical care unit, medical staff unit, or responsible physician during hospitalization

Intranet: A private network that works like the Internet but can only be accessed by certain individuals, such as employees of a company

Intrarater reliability: A measure of a research instrument's reliability in which the same person repeating the test will get reasonably similar findings

Judgment sampling: A sampling technique where the researcher relies on his or her own judgment to select the subjects

Knowledge: The information, understanding, and experience that give individuals the power to make informed decisions

Late fetal death: The death of a product of human conception that is 28 weeks or more of gestation and weighs 1,001 grams or more before its complete expulsion or extraction from the mother

Leave of absence: The authorized absence of an inpatient from a hospital or other facility for a specified period of time occurring after admission and prior to discharge

Leave of absence day: A day occurring after the admission and prior to the discharge of a hospital inpatient when the patient is not present at the census-taking hour because he or she is on leave of absence from the healthcare facility

Length of stay (LOS):   The total number of patient days for an inpatient episode, calculated by subtracting the date of admission from the date of discharge

Line graph: A graphic technique used to illustrate the relationship between continuous measurements; consists of a line drawn to connect a series of points on an arithmetic scale and is often used to display time trends

Literature review: A systematic investigation of all the knowledge available about a topic from sources such as books, journal articles, theses, and dissertations

Low-birth-weight neonate: Any newborn baby, regardless of gestational age, whose weight at birth is less than 2,500 grams

Managed care: A generic term for reimbursement and delivery systems that integrate the financing and provision of healthcare services by means of entering contractual agreements with selected providers to furnish comprehensive healthcare services and developing explicit criteria for the selection of healthcare providers, formal programs of ongoing quality improvement and utilization review, and significant financial incentives for members to use providers associated with the plan

Managed care organization (MCO):   A type of healthcare organization that delivers medical care and manages all aspects of the care or the payment for care by limiting providers of care, discounting payment to providers of care, or limiting access to care

Maternal death: The death of any woman, from any cause, related to or aggravated by pregnancy or its management (regardless of duration or site of pregnancy), but not from accidental or incidental causes

Maternal death rate: For a hospital, the total number of maternal deaths directly related to pregnancy for a given time period divided by the total number of obstetrical discharges for the same time period; for a community, the total number of deaths attributed to maternal conditions during a given time period in a specific geographic area divided by the total number of live births for the same time period in the same area

Mean: A measure of central tendency that is determined by calculating the arithmetic average of the observations in a frequency distribution

Measure: A term referring to the quantifiable data about a function or process

Measurement: The systematic process of data collection, repeated over time or at a single point in time

Measures of central tendency: The typical or average numbers that are descriptive of the entire collection of data for a specific population

Median: A measure of central tendency that shows the midpoint of a frequency distribution when the observations have been arranged in order from lowest to highest

Medical examiner: *See* **coroner**

Medical services: The activities relating to medical care performed by physicians, nurses, and other healthcare professional and technical personnel under the direction of a physician

Medicare-severity diagnosis related groups (MS-DRG):   Payment groups designed for the Medicare population that recognize severity of illness, resource use, and patient complexity. Patients who have similar clinical characteristics and similar costs are assigned to an MS-DRG, which is linked to a fixed payment amount based on the average cost of patients in the group. Patients can be assigned to an MS-DRG based on diagnosis, surgical procedures, age, and other administrative information

Method: A way of performing an action or task; also, a strategy used by a researcher to collect, analyze, and present data

Military time: Time measured in hours numbered to 24 (as 0100 or 2300) from one midnight to the next

Mode: A measure of central tendency that consists of the most frequent observation in a frequency distribution

Morbidity: A term referring to the state of being diseased (including illness, injury, or deviation from normal health); the number of sick persons or cases of disease in relationship to a specific population

Morgue: The place where the bodies of persons who have died are kept until identified and claimed by relatives or released for burial

Mortality: A term referring to the incidence of death in a specific population; also, the loss of subjects during the course of a clinical research study, or attrition

Mortality rate: A rate that measures the risk of death for the cause under study in a defined population during a given time period

Multivariate: In reference to research studies, a term meaning that many variables were involved

Naturalistic observation: A type of nonparticipant observation in which researchers observe certain behaviors and events as they occur naturally

Necropsy: *See* **autopsy**

Neonatal death: The death of a liveborn infant within the first 27 days, 23 hours, and 59 minutes following the moment of birth

Neonatal mortality rate: The number of deaths of infants under 28 days of age during a given time period divided by the total number of births for the same time period

Neonatal period: The period of an infant's life from the hour of birth through the first 27 days, 23 hours, and 59 minutes of life

Net autopsy rate: The ratio of inpatient autopsies compared to inpatient deaths calculated by dividing the total number of inpatient autopsies performed by the hospital pathologist for a given time period by the total number of inpatient deaths minus unautopsied coroners' or medical examiners' cases for the same time period

Net death rate: The total number of inpatient deaths minus the number of deaths that occurred less than 48 hours after admission for a given time period divided by the total number of inpatient discharges minus the number of deaths that occurred less than 48 hours after admission for the same time period

Newborn (NB):   An inpatient who was born in a hospital at the beginning of the current inpatient hospitalization

Newborn autopsy rate: The number of autopsies performed on newborns who died during a given time period divided by the total number of newborns who died during the same time period

Newborn bassinet count: The number of available hospital newborn bassinets, both occupied and vacant, on any given day

Newborn bassinet count day: A unit of measure that denotes the presence of one newborn bassinet, either occupied or vacant, set up and staffed for use in one 24-hour period

Newborn death: The death of a liveborn infant born in the hospital who later dies during the same admission

Newborn death rate: The number of newborns who died divided by the total number of newborns, both alive and dead; also called newborn mortality rate

Newborn mortality rate: The number of newborns who died divided by the total number of newborns, both alive and dead

Nominal data: A type of data that represents values or observations that can be labeled or named and where the values fall into unordered categories; also called dichotomous data

Normal distribution of data: A continuous frequency distribution characterized by a bell-shaped curve; that is, the mean, median, and mode are equal and most of the measurements are near the center of the frequency

Nosocomial infection: An infection acquired by a patient while receiving care or services in a healthcare organization; also called hospital-acquired infection

Nosocomial infection rate: The number of hospital-acquired infections for a given time period divided by the total number of inpatient discharges for the same time period

Null hypothesis: A hypothesis that states there is no association between the independent and dependent variables in a research study

Numerator: The part of a fraction that is above the line and signifies the number of parts of the denominator taken

Numerical data: Data that include discrete data and continuous data

Nursing facility: A comprehensive term for long-term care facilities that provide nursing care and related services on a 24-hour basis for residents requiring medical, nursing, or rehabilitative care

Observation: Service in which providers observe and monitor a patient to decide whether the patient needs to be admitted to inpatient care or can be discharged to home or outpatient area, usually charged by the hour

Observation patient: A patient who presents with a medical condition with a significant degree of instability and disability and who needs to be monitored, evaluated, and assessed to determine whether he or she should be admitted for inpatient care or discharged for care in another setting

Occasion of service: A specified, identifiable service that involves the care of a patient but is not an encounter (for example, a lab test ordered during an encounter)

Occupancy percent/ratio: *See* **bed occupancy ratio**

Operation: *See* **surgical operation**

Operational budget: A type of budget that allocates and controls resources to meet an organization's goals and objectives for the fiscal year

Ordinal data: A type of data that represents values or observations that can be ranked or ordered

Outlier: An extreme statistical value that falls outside the normal range

Outpatient: A patient who receives ambulatory care services in a hospital-based clinic or department

Patient: A living or deceased individual who is receiving or has received healthcare services

Patient care unit (PCU):   An organizational entity of a healthcare facility organized both physically and functionally to provide care

Patient day: *See* **inpatient service day**

Payback period: A financial method used to evaluate the value of a capital expenditure by calculating the time frame that must pass before inflow of cash from a project equals or exceeds outflow of cash

Percentage: A value computed on the basis of the whole divided into 100 parts

Percent/percentage of occupancy: *See* **inpatient bed occupancy rate**

Perinatal death: An all-inclusive term that refers to both stillborn infants and neonatal deaths

Pictogram: A graphic technique in which pictures are used in the display of data

Pie chart: A graphic technique in which the proportions of a category are displayed as portions of a circle (like pieces of a pie)

Pie graph: *See* **pie chart**

Plagiarism: The appropriation of another person's ideas, processes, results, or words without giving appropriate credit

Population: The universe of data under investigation from which a sample is taken

Postmortem examination: *See* **autopsy**

Postneonatal death: The death of a liveborn infant from 28 days to the end of the first year of life (364 days, 23 hours, and 59 minutes from the moment of birth)

Postneonatal mortality rate: The number of deaths of persons aged 28 days up to, but not including, one year during a given time period divided by the number of live births for the same time period

Postoperative death rate: The ratio of deaths within 10 days after surgery to the total number of operations performed during a specified period of time

Postoperative infection rate: The number of infections that occur in clean surgical cases for a given time period divided by the total number of operations within the same time period

Postpartum: Occurring after childbirth

Postterm neonate: Any neonate whose birth occurs from the beginning of the first day of the 43rd week (295th day) following onset of the last menstrual period

Predictive analytics: A branch of data mining concerned with the prediction of future probabilities and trends; also called forecasting

Predictive modeling: A process used to identify patterns that can be used to predict the odds of a particular outcome based on the observed data

Pre-existing condition: Any injury, disease, or physical condition occurring prior to an arbitrary date

Prepartum: Occurring prior to childbirth

Prescriptive analytics: Data analytics technique that tries to determine the best solution or outcome among various choices

Preterm infant: An infant with a birth weight between 1,000 and 2,499 grams and/or a gestation between 28 and 37 completed weeks

Preterm neonate: Any neonate whose birth occurs through the end of the last day of the 38th week (266th day) following onset of the last menstrual period

Primary data source: Record developed by healthcare professionals in the process of providing patient care

Primary research: Data collected specifically for a study

Procedure: *See* **surgical procedure**

Productivity: A unit of performance defined by management in quantitative standards

Profiling: A measurement of the quality, utilization, and cost of medical resources provided by physicians, or groups of physicians, that is made by employers, third-party payers, government entities, and other purchasers of healthcare

Proportion: The relation of one part to another or to the whole with respect to magnitude, quantity, or degree

Puerperal: The period immediately following childbirth

Qualitative research: A philosophy of research that assumes that multiple contextual truths exist and bias is always present; also called naturalism

Quantitative research: A philosophy of research that assumes that there is a single truth across time and place and that researchers are able to adopt a neutral, unbiased stance and establish causation; also called positivism

Quartile: The fourth equal part of a distribution

Questionnaire: A type of survey in which the members of the population are questioned through the use of electronic or paper forms

Quota sampling: A sampling technique where the population is first segmented into mutually exclusive subgroups, just as in stratified sampling, and then judgment is used to select the subjects or units from each segment based on a specified proportion

Quotient: The number resulting from the division of one number by another

Random sample: A sample in which every element in the population has an equal chance of being selected

Random sampling: An unbiased selection of subjects that includes methods such as simple random sampling, stratified random sampling, systematic sampling, and cluster sampling

Randomization: The assignment of subjects to experimental or control groups based on chance

Range: Distance or extent between possible extremes

Ranked data: A type of ordinal data where the observations are first arranged from highest to lowest according to magnitude and then assigned numbers that correspond to each observation's place in the sequence

Rate: A measure used to compare an event over time; a comparison of the number of times an event did happen (numerator) with the number of times an event could have happened (denominator)

Ratio: A calculation found by dividing one quantity by another; also, a general term that can include a number of specific measures such as proportion, percentage, and rate

Ratio data: Data that may be displayed by units of equal size and placed on a scale starting with zero and thus can be manipulated mathematically (for example, 0, 5, 10, 15, 20)

Real-time analytics: Data that can be accessed is it comes into a computer system

Recap: Abbreviation of *recapitulation*

Recapitulation: A concise summary of data

Recurrence: To occur again after an interval

Release of information: The process of disclosing patient information from the medical record to another party. Federal, state and local regulations exist to govern the release of a patient's medical record information

Relevance: How applicable information is to some matter

Reliability: A measure of consistency of data items based on their reproducibility and an estimation of their error of measurement

Research: Investigation or experimentation aimed at the discovery and interpretation of facts, revision of accepted theories or laws in the light of new facts, or practical application of such new or revised theories or laws; the collecting of information about a particular subject

Research data: Data used for the purpose of answering a proposed question or testing a hypothesis

Return on investment (ROI): The financial analysis of the extent of value a major purchase will provide

Rounding: The process of approximating a number

Run chart: A type of graph that shows data points collected over time and identifies emerging trends or patterns

Sample: A set of units selected for study that represents a population

Sample size: The number of subjects needed in a study to represent a population

Sample size calculation: The qualitative and quantitative procedures to determine an appropriate sample size

Sample survey: A type of survey that collects data from representative members of a population

Scales of measurement: *See* **categorical data**

Scatter diagram: A graph that visually displays the linear relationships among factors

Secondary data source: Data derived from the primary patient record, such as an index or database

Secondary record: A record derived from the primary record and containing selected data elements

Secondary research: Data collected from a literature review

Skewness: The horizontal stretching of a frequency distribution to one side or the other so that one tail is longer than the other

Snowball sampling: A method of sampling in which existing study subjects recruit future subjects from their among their acquaintances, hence the recruits grow in snowball fashion

Spreadsheet: Worksheet into which text, numbers, and formulas are entered to assist with calculations

Standard error of the mean: A value that is found by taking many large samples, calculating the mean for each sample, and then finding the standard deviation of all the sample means

Standard deviation: A measure of variability that describes the deviation from the mean of a frequency distribution in the original units of measurement; the square root of the variance

Statistics: A branch of mathematics concerned with collecting, organizing, summarizing, and analyzing data

Stillbirth: The birth of a fetus, regardless of gestational age, that shows no evidence of life (such as heartbeats or respirations) after complete expulsion or extraction from the mother during childbirth

Stratified random sampling: The process of selecting the same percentages of subjects for a study sample as they exist in the subgroups (strata) of the population

Structured interview: An interview format that uses a set of standardized questions that are asked of all applicants

Surgical death rate: *See* **postoperative death rate**

Surgical operation: One or more surgical procedures performed at one time for one patient via a common approach or for a common purpose

Surgical procedure: Any single, separate, systematic process upon or within the body that can be complete in itself; is normally performed by a physician, dentist, or other licensed practitioner; can be performed with or without instruments; and is performed to restore disunited or deficient parts, remove diseased or injured tissues, extract foreign matter, assist in obstetrical delivery, or aid in diagnosis

Survey: A type of research instrument with which the members of the population being studied are asked questions and respond orally

Swing bed hospital: A hospital participating in Medicare that has approval to provide post-hospital skilled care; the hospital can use its beds, as needed, for either acute care or skilled nursing care

Systematic random sampling: The process of selecting a sample of subjects for a study by drawing every nth unit on a list

***t* test:**   A test of the null hypothesis to determine if a set of results is statistically significant.

Table: An organized arrangement of data, usually in columns and rows

Term neonate: Any neonate whose birth occurs from the beginning of the first day of the 39th week (267th day) through the end of the last day of the 42nd week (294th day) following onset of the last menstrual period

Total bed count days: The sum of inpatient bed count days for each of the days during a specified period of time

Total discharge days: *See* **total length of stay**

Total inpatient service days: The sum of all inpatient service days for each of the days during a specified period of time

Total length of stay: The sum of the days of stay of any group of inpatients discharged during a specific period of time; also called discharge days

Transfer: The movement of a patient from one treatment service or location to another; *see also* **intrahospital transfer**

Tumor registry: See **Cancer registry**

Type I error: Occurs when the null hypothesis is rejected, yet it is actually true

Type II error: Occurs when the null hypothesis is not rejected, yet it is false

Unit labor cost: Cost determined by dividing the total annual compensation by total annual productivity

Unrestricted question: A type of question that allows free-form responses; also called open-ended question

Utilization management: A program that evaluates the healthcare facility's efficiency in providing necessary care to patients in the most effective manner

Validity: The extent to which data correspond to the actual state of affairs or that an instrument measures what it purports to measure; also, a term referring to a test's ability to accurately and consistently measure what it purports to measure

Variability: The difference between each score and every other score in a frequency distribution

Variable: A characteristic or property that may take on different values

Variance: A disagreement between two parts; the square of the standard deviation

Variance analysis: An assessment of a department's financial transactions to identify differences between the budget amount and the actual amount of a line item

Visit: A single encounter with a healthcare professional that includes all the services supplied during the encounter

Vital statistics: Data related to births, deaths, marriages, and fetal deaths

Well newborn: A newborn born at term, under sterile conditions, with no diseases, conditions, disorders, syndromes, injuries, malformations, or defects diagnosed, and no operations other than routine circumcision performed

Whole number: Any of the set of nonnegative integers

World Health Organization (WHO):   The United Nations specialized agency created to ensure the attainment by all peoples of the highest possible levels of health and responsible for a number of international classifications, including *The International Statistical Classification of Diseases & Related Health Problems* (ICD-10) and *The International Classification of Functioning, Disability & Health* (ICF)

APPENDIX

C

Answers to Odd-Numbered Chapter Exercises

Chapter 1

Exercise 1.1

Type of Healthcare Information	Type of Data Source
1. Productivity reports pulled from patient visit report	Secondary
2. Tumor registry	Secondary
3. State vital statistics	Primary
4. Hospital census	Primary
5. Hospital disease index	Secondary
6. Patient health record	Primary
7. Health insurance data pulled from national census	Secondary

Chapter 2

Exercise 2.1

1. $\dfrac{20}{40}$

   Answer: $\dfrac{2}{4} = \dfrac{1}{2}$

   Cross out one zero from numerator and denominator, then divide each by common factor (2)

2. $\dfrac{4}{6}$

   Answer: $\dfrac{2}{3}$

   Divide the numerator and denominator by common factor (2)

3. $\dfrac{12}{54}$

   Answer: $\dfrac{2}{9}$

   Divide the numerator and denominator by common factor (6)

4. $\dfrac{8}{12}$

   Answer: $\dfrac{2}{3}$

   Divide the numerator and denominator by common factor (4)

5. $\dfrac{16}{28}$

   Answer: $\dfrac{4}{7}$

   Divide the numerator and denominator by common factor (4)

Exercise 2.3

1. 42

   Answer: 40
   42 is closer to 40 than 50, so round to 40.

2. 338

   Answer: 340
   338 is closer to 340 than 330, so round to 440.

3. 217

   Answer: 220
   217 is closer to 220 than 210, so round to 220.

4. 6,989

   Answer: 6,990
   6,989 is closer to 6,990 than 6,980, so round to 6,990.

5. 8,532

   Answer: 8,530
   8,532 is closer to 8,530 than 8,540, so round to 8,530.

6. 156

   Answer: 200
   156 is closer to 200 than 100, so round to 200.

7. 321

   Answer: 300
   321 is closer to 300 than 400, so round to 300.

8. 3,807

    Answer: 3,800
    3,807 is closer to 3,800 than 3,900, so round to 3,800.

9. 4,357

    Answer: 4,400
    4,357 is closer to 4,400 than 4,300, so round to 4,400.

10. 8,175

    Answer: 8,200
    8,175 is closer to 8,200 than 8,100, so round to 8,200.

11. 38.1

    Answer: 38
    38.1 is closer to 38 than 39 so round to 38. The 1 in the tenths position is less than 5, so do not round up.

12. 55.6

    Answer: 56
    55.6 is closer to 56 than 55 so round to 56. The 6 in the tenths position is more than 5, so round up.

13. 14.7

    Answer: 15
    14.7 is closer to 15 than 14 so round to 15. The 7 in the tenths position is more than 5, so round up.

14. 625.2

    Answer: 625
    625.2 is closer to 625 than 626 so round to 625. The 2 in the tenths position is less than 5, so do not round up.

15. 100.5

    Answer: 101
    100.5 is halfway between 100 and 101, so round to 101.

16. 19.76

    Answer: 19.8
    19.76 is closer to 19.8 than 19.7, so round to 19.8. The 6 in the hundredths position is more than 5, so round up.

17. 34.62

    Answer: 34.6
    34.62 is closer to 34.6 than 34.7, so round to 34.6. The 2 in the hundredths position is less than 5, so do not round up.

18. 172.87

Answer: 172.9

172.87 is closer to 172.8 than 172.8 so round to 172.9. The 7 in the hundredths position is more than 5 so round up.

19. 99.98

Answer: 100.0

99.98 is closer to 100.0 than 99.9, so round to 100.0. The 8 in the hundredths position is more than 5, so round up. Notice here that the 9 in the tenths position will be rounded to a 10—the 0 will go in the tenths position, then the 1 is added to 99 to get 100.

20. 125.96

Answer: 126.0

125.96 is closer to 126.0 than 125.9, so round to 126.0. The 6 in the hundredths position is more than 5, so round up.

21. 8.36801

Answer: 8.37

8.36801 is closer to 8.37 than 8.36, so round to 8.37. The 8 in the thousandths position is more than 5, so round up.

22. 14.5264

Answer: 14.53

14.5264 is closer to 14.53 than 14.52, so round to 14.53. The 6 in the thousandths position is more than 5, so round up.

23. 0.87642

Answer: 0.88

0.87642 is closer to 0.88 than 0.87 so round to 0.88. The 6 in the thousandths position is more than 5 so round up. Also, remember when requested to round to decimal places and your answer is less than a whole number, add the "0" to the left of the decimal point.

24. 27.99999

Answer: 28.00

27.99999 is closer to 28.00 than 27.99, so round to 28.00. The 9 in the thousandths position is more than 5 so round up. Notice here that the 9 in the tenths position will be rounded to a 10—the 0 will go in the tenths position, then the 1 is added to 27 to get 28.

25. 15.90176

Answer: 15.90

15.90176 is closer to 15.90 than 15.91, so round to 15.90. The 1 in the thousandths position is less than 5, so round down.

Exercise 2.5

	Fraction	Decimal	Percentage
Sickle cell	$\dfrac{20}{40}$ $\dfrac{10}{20}$ $\mathbf{\dfrac{1}{2}}$	$\dfrac{1}{2} = 0.50$ 1 divided by 2	$0.5 \times 100 = 50\%$
Hemophilia	$\dfrac{12}{40}$ $\dfrac{6}{20}$ $\mathbf{\dfrac{3}{10}}$	$\dfrac{3}{10} = 0.30$ 3 divided by 10	$0.3 \times 100 = 30\%$
Ewing's	$\dfrac{6}{40}$ $\dfrac{3}{20}$ $\mathbf{\dfrac{3}{20}}$	$\dfrac{3}{20} = 0.15$ 3 divided by 20	$0.15 \times 100 = 15\%$
Wilms'	$\dfrac{2}{40}$ $\dfrac{1}{20}$ $\mathbf{\dfrac{1}{20}}$	$\dfrac{1}{20} = 0.05$ 1 divided by 20	$0.05 \times 100 = 5\%$

Exercise 2.7

1. $\dfrac{12}{(12+225)} = 0.05$

2. $\dfrac{6}{(6+44)} = 0.12$

3. $\dfrac{458}{(458+192)} = 0.70$

4. $\dfrac{182}{(182+88)} = 0.67$

5. $\dfrac{14}{(14+21)} = 0.40$

Chapter 3

Exercise 3.1

1. Yes. *The counts could have differed. Any number of admissions, discharges, or transfers could have occurred between 12 midnight and 1 a.m. on either day.*

2. No. *The total hospital census would be inconsistent. Every PCU in the hospital should follow the same administrative procedure.*

3. No. *The patient cannot be in two places at the same time. If both units are counting heads only once a day at midnight, the patient is counted as being present in unit A only. However, the patient is indicated in unit B's census as a transfer.*

4. Intrahospital transfer

5. 124 patients. *Hospitals include only inpatients in the inpatient census calculations.*

Exercise 3.3

Census = The number of inpatients present in a healthcare facility at any given time

Inpatient census = Same as census

Daily inpatient census = The number of inpatients present at census-taking time each day, plus any inpatients who were both admitted and discharged after the census-taking time the previous day

Inpatient service day = A unit of measure equivalent to the services received by one inpatient during one 24-hour period

The figure representing an inpatient service day will be the same as the figure for the daily inpatient census. (It may be the same as the inpatient census, provided there were no patient admitted/discharged on the same day.)

Students are working with the same data in each case and calculating the same answer. The difference is that an inpatient service day is a unit of measure (of service given).

Therefore, the term inpatient service days is used here as a measuring device for all computations based on census. This may seem merely a trap in terminology, but there is a fine distinction between a term that represents a total (daily census) and one that represents a unit of measure (inpatient service day), even though they are the same numerically.

Exercise 3.5

1. **b.** Consistent
2. **a.** Inpatient service day
3. **d.** 26
4. **c.** Both a and b
5. **c.** Total inpatient service days

Exercise 3.7

	12:01 a.m. Census		Adm		Trf	Total		Dis	Dis	Trf	11:59 p.m. Census			Serv Days	
Day	A/C	NB	A/C	Bir	in	A/C	NB	A/C	NB	out	A/C	NB	A/D	A/C	NB
6/1	230	12	20	4	3	**253**	**16**	19	3	2	**232**	**13**	1	233	13
6/2	**232**	**13**	21	4	1	**254**	**17**	19	4	1	**234**	**13**	0	234	13
6/3	**234**	**13**	23	6	0	**257**	**19**	24	5	0	233	14	3	236	14
6/4	**233**	**14**	25	5	1	**259**	**19**	23	4	1	235	15	1	236	15
6/5	**235**	**15**	24	4	2	**261**	**19**	18	3	2	**241**	**16**	2	243	16

Exercise 3.9

Worksheet No. 1

	12:01 a.m. Census		Adm		Trf	Total		Disch		Trf	11:59 p.m. Census			Serv Days	
Day	A/C	NB	A/C	NB	in	A/C	NB	A/C	NB	out	A/C	NB	A/D	A/C	NB
1	165	3	29	0	8	202	3	10	0	7	185	3	0	**185**	**3**
2	185	3	24	4	7	**216**	**7**	12	3	6	**198**	**4**	1	199	4
3	**198**	**4**	18	3	3	**219**	**7**	16	2	2	**201**	**5**	0	201	5
4	**201**	**5**	17	2	5	**223**	**7**	15	2	4	204	5	0	204	5

(continued on next page)

Day	12:01 a.m. Census A/C	NB	Adm A/C	NB	Trf in	Total A/C	NB	Disch A/C	NB	Trf out	11:59 p.m. Census A/C	NB	A/D	Serv Days A/C	NB
5	204	5	13	0	1	218	5	12	1	3	203	4	0	203	4
6	203	4	20	0	6	229	4	19	2	4	206	2	0	206	2
7	206	2	21	0	14	241	2	17	0	12	212	2	0	212	2
8	212	2	27	1	10	249	3	23	3	8	218	0	3	221	0
9	218	0	23	4	6	247	4	22	3	14	211	1	2	213	1
10	211	1	22	2	8	241	3	15	1	10	216	2	1	217	2
11	216	2	17	3	7	240	5	14	4	5	221	1	3	224	1
12	221	1	19	3	6	246	4	17	2	4	225	2	0	225	2
13	225	2	14	1	4	243	3	12	2	2	229	1	0	229	1
14	229	1	15	4	5	249	5	19	3	7	223	2	0	223	2
15	223	2	20	14	8	251	16	13	0	6	232	16	1	233	16
16	232	16	23	3	6	261	19	15	4	2	244	15	0	244	15
17	244	15	17	1	3	264	16	13	3	1	250	13	1	251	13
18	250	13	15	0	2	267	13	21	1	6	240	12	2	242	12
19	240	12	17	0	7	264	12	25	3	2	237	9	1	238	9
20	237	9	13	2	3	253	11	27	4	4	222	7	0	222	7
21	222	7	12	1	5	239	8	21	2	5	213	6	3	216	6
22	213	6	10	0	1	224	6	17	4	1	206	2	2	208	2
23	206	2	9	2	4	219	4	18	1	4	197	3	0	197	3
24	197	3	23	4	3	223	7	12	3	2	209	4	2	211	4
25	209	4	15	2	4	228	6	22	2	3	203	4	1	204	4
26	203	4	13	3	2	218	7	9	1	4	205	6	0	205	6
27	205	6	21	1	3	229	7	29	1	0	200	6	2	202	6
28	200	6	29	2	5	234	8	22	4	4	208	4	3	211	4
29	208	4	23	4	1	232	8	25	3	2	205	5	1	206	5
30	205	5	15	1	4	224	6	21	2	3	200	4	0	200	4
31	200	4	16	4	2	218	8	18	3	2	198	5	3	201	5
Totals			570	71	153			551	69	139			32	6653	155

Worksheet No. 2

Recap of Monthly Data for Adults and Children: May 20XX (enter numbers from Worksheet No. 1)		
12:01 a.m. Census A/C		165
Admissions Adult and Children	+	570
Transfers in	+	153
Total A/C	=	888
Discharges Adult and Children	–	551
Transfers out	–	139
11:59 p.m. Census A/C on May 31	=	198
Recap of Monthly Data for Newborns:		
12:01 a.m. Census NB		3
Newborn Admissions	+	71
Total NB	=	74
Discharges NB	–	69
11:59 p.m. Census NB on May 31	=	5
Serv Days A/C (total inpatient service days excluding newborns) 6,653		
Serv Days NB (total newborn service days) 155		
Total inpatient service days 6,808		

Chapter 4

Exercise 4.1

1. No.
   Beds set up for temporary and emergency use (for example, cots in the hall) are not included in the hospital's bed count because they are not continually staffed and available for use. Moreover, hospitals are licensed by the state for a certain number of beds, which does not include disaster needs, and so they cannot set up beds indiscriminately. PCUs are staffed (from housekeeping to nursing) according to their number of beds.

2. Bed count: The number of inpatient beds set up and staffed for use on a given day; also called bed complement.

   Bed complement: The same as bed count.

   Bed capacity: The number of beds that a facility has been designed and constructed to house.

Exercise 4.3

Children's Hospital June 20XX			
Unit	Number of Beds	Inpatient Service Days	Percentage of Occupancy
Pediatric Surgical	30	833	$\dfrac{(833 \times 100)}{(30 \times 30)} = \dfrac{83,300}{900} = 92.6\%$
Hematology Oncology	20	566	$\dfrac{(566 \times 100)}{(20 \times 30)} = \dfrac{56,600}{600} = 94.3\%$
Neurology/ Neurosurgical	30	756	$\dfrac{(756 \times 100)}{(30 \times 30)} = \dfrac{75,600}{900} = 84.0\%$
Renal/ Gastroenterology/ Endocrinology	20	555	$\dfrac{(555 \times 100)}{(20 \times 30)} = \dfrac{55,500}{600} = 92.5\%$
Respiratory	30	897	$\dfrac{(897 \times 100)}{(30 \times 30)} = \dfrac{89,700}{900} = 99.7\%$
Cardiac Medicine/ Surgical	20	589	$\dfrac{(589 \times 100)}{(20 \times 30)} = \dfrac{58,900}{600} = 98.2\%$
Infant Care Unit	10	281	$\dfrac{(281 \times 100)}{(10 \times 30)} = \dfrac{28,100}{300} = 93.7\%$
Pediatric Intensive Care	20	540	$\dfrac{(540 \times 100)}{(20 \times 30)} = \dfrac{54,000}{600} = 90.0\%$
Total	**180**	**5,017**	$\dfrac{(5,017 \times 100)}{(180 \times 30)} = \dfrac{501,700}{5,400} = 92.9\%$

Example of unit totals:

For example, the pediatric surgical unit has 30 beds and 833 inpatient service days in the month of June (30 days). The percentage of occupancy is therefore the inpatient service days multiplied by 100 and divided by the product of the number of beds (30) and the number of days (30) to get 92.6%. $\dfrac{(833 \times 100)}{(30 \times 30 \text{ days})} = \dfrac{83,300}{900} = 92.6\%$

Answers: Total = 92.9%

To find the total, add the inpatient service days for each of the units to get 5,017. Multiply that by 100 and divide by the product of the total number of beds (180) and the number of days (30). $\dfrac{(5,017 \times 100)}{(180 \times 30)} = \dfrac{501,700}{5,400} = 92.9\%$

Exercise 4.5

	Inpatient Service Days	Bed Count	Percentage of Occupancy
University Hospital January 20XX			
PCU			
Medicine	3,752	130	$\dfrac{(3,752 \times 100)}{(130 \times 31)} = \dfrac{375,200}{4,030} = 93.1\%$
Rehabilitation/ Neurology	600	35	$\dfrac{(600 \times 100)}{(35 \times 31)} = \dfrac{60,000}{1,085} = 55.3\%$
Orthopedics/Trauma	485	20	$\dfrac{(485 \times 100)}{(20 \times 31)} = \dfrac{48,500}{620} = 78.2\%$
Medicine/ Surgical Oncology	1,803	60	$\dfrac{(1,803 \times 100)}{(60 \times 31)} = \dfrac{180,300}{1,860} = 96.9\%$
Pediatrics	2,142	80	$\dfrac{(2,142 \times 100)}{(80 \times 31)} = \dfrac{214,200}{2,480} = 86.4\%$
Critical Care:			
Medicine ICU	1,603	55	$\dfrac{(1,603 \times 100)}{(55 \times 31)} = \dfrac{160,300}{1,705} = 94.0\%$
Surgical ICU (Adult)	1,584	55	$\dfrac{(1,584 \times 100)}{(55 \times 31)} = \dfrac{158,400}{1,705} = 92.9\%$
Transplant	895	30	$\dfrac{(895 \times 100)}{(30 \times 31)} = \dfrac{89,500}{930} = 96.2\%$
Surgical ICU (Pediatrics)	923	40	$\dfrac{(923 \times 100)}{(40 \times 31)} = \dfrac{92,300}{1,240} = 74.4\%$
Total	**13,787**	**505**	$\dfrac{(13,787 \times 100)}{(505 \times 31)} = \dfrac{1,378,700}{15,655} = 88.1\%$

For example, the medicine unit has 3,752 inpatient service days and 130 beds in the month of January (31 days). The percentage of occupancy is therefore the inpatient service days multiplied by 100 and divided by the product of the number of beds (130) and the number of days (31) to get 93.1%.

$$\frac{(3,752 \times 100)}{(130 \times 31)} = \frac{375,200}{4,030} = 93.1\%$$

Exercise 4.7

1. 35.3
   To use the direct formula, divide patients discharged and died (7,054) by the number of beds (200) to get 35.3.

   $$\frac{7,054}{200} = 35.3$$

2. *To use the indirect formula, multiply the occupancy rate (85%) by the number of days in the year (365) and divide by the average length of stay (9 days) to get 34.5. Note that in the indirect formula the bed occupancy rate must be changed to a decimal. This example shows that during 20XX, each of the hospital's 200 beds changed occupants 34.5 times.* $\dfrac{(0.85 \times 365)}{9} = \dfrac{310.25}{9} = 34.5$

Chapter 5

Exercise 5.1

Date Admitted	Date Discharged	Length of Stay
7/9	7/10	**1**
9/12	9/22	**10**
3/10	3/24	**14**
6/17	7/18	**6/30 – 6/17 = 13 days** **July = 18 days** **Total 31 days**
10/20	11/25	**10/31 – 10/20 = 11 days** **November = 25 days** **Total 36 days**

Exercise 5.3

1.

Patient	Time Admitted	Time Seen by Physician	Time between Checking In at Reception and Being Seen by Physician
Patient 1	8:00 a.m.	8:17 a.m.	**17 minutes**
Patient 2	1:22 p.m.	2:05 p.m.	**43 minutes**

(continued on next page)

Patient	Time Admitted	Time Seen by Physician	Time between Checking In at Reception and Being Seen by Physician
Patient 3	10:30 a.m.	11:43 a.m.	**1 hour and 13 minutes**
Patient 4	1:30 p.m.	3:00 p.m.	**1 hour 30 minutes**
Patient 5	2:15 p.m.	2:56 p.m.	**41 minutes**

Answers:

Patient 1: *Subtract 8:00 from 8:17 = 17 minutes wait time (Same hour)*

Patient 2: *Change 2:05 to 1:65 then subtract 1:22 from 1:65 = 43 minutes wait time (Different hour)*

Patient 3: *Subtract the "arrival" minutes from the "seen" minutes (43 – 30 = 13); then subtract the "arrival" hour from the "seen" hour (11 – 10 + 1) 1 hour 13 minutes wait time. (Different hour)*

Patient 4: *Change 3:00 to 2:60 and subtract 1:30 (2:60 – 1:30 = 1 hour 30 minutes wait time)*

Patient 5: *Subtract 2:15 from 2:56 = 41 minutes wait time (Same hour)*

2.

Patient	Time of Arrival	Time Patient Was Triaged	Wait Time
Patient A	8:00 a.m.	8:23 a.m.	23 minutes
Patient B	8:23 a.m.	8:56 a.m.	33 minutes
Patient C	8:56 a.m.	9:20 a.m.	24 minutes
Patient D	9:45 a.m.	10:46 a.m.	1 hour 1 minute
Patient E	10:20 a.m.	1:45 p.m.	3 hours 25 minutes
Patient F	11:20 a.m.	1:50 p.m.	2 hours 30 minutes
Patient G	12:15 p.m.	2:40 p.m.	2 hours 25 minutes
Patient H	1:05 p.m.	2:56 p.m.	1 hour 51 minutes
Patient I	3:27 p.m.	5:05 p.m.	1 hour 38 minutes
Patient J	4:05 p.m.	4:56 p.m.	51 minutes

a. Patient A: *23 minutes minus 0 minutes = 23 minute wait (within the same hour)*

Patient B: *56 minutes minus 23 minutes = 33 minute wait (within the same hour)*

Patient C: *Change 9:20 to 8:80 and subtract 8:56; 8:80 – 8:56 = 24 minute wait. Change 9:20 to 8:80 and subtract 8:56. (Different hour but time did not cross the noon hour)*

Patient D: *10:46 – 9:45 = 1 hour 1 minute. (46 – 45 minutes = 1 minute; 10 – 9 = 1 hour)*

Patient E: *Add 12 to 1:27 to make 13:27. The arrival minutes (20) are less than the triaged minutes (45) 45 – 20 = 25; Subtract the arrival hour (10) from triaged hour (13) 13 – 10 = 3. The wait time was 3 hours 25 minutes wait. (Time crossed noon.)*

Patient F: *Add 12 to 1:50 to make 13:50. The arrival minutes (22) are less than the triaged minutes (50) 50 – 20 = 30; Subtract arrival hour (11) from triaged hour (13) 13 – 11 = 2. The wait time was 2 hours 30 minutes wait. (Time crossed noon.)*

Patient G: *Add 12 to 2:40 to make 14:40. Subtract the arrival minutes (15) from the triaged minutes (40) 40 – 15 = 25; Then subtract the arrival hour (12) from the triaged hour (14); The wait time was 2 hours 25 minutes. (Time crossed noon.)*

Patient H: *56 minutes minus 05 minutes = 51 minutes 2:00 – 1:00 = 1. 1 hour and 51 minute wait. (Different hour and arrival minutes less than triage minutes.)*

Patient I: *Change 5:05 to 4:65 and subtract 3:27; 65 – 27 = 38 minutes and 4 – 3 = 1. Wait time is 1 hour 38 minutes. (Different hour but time did not cross the noon hour.)*

Patient J: *56 minutes – 05 minutes = 51 minutes wait (within the same hour)*

b. Average wait time = 90.1 minutes or 1 hour 30 minutes average wait time *Change all times to minutes then add together. 23 + 33 + 24 + 61 + 205 + 150 + 145 + 111 + 98 + 51 = 901 total minutes. 901 / 10 = 90.1 minutes or 1 hour 30 minutes.*

c. No, the hospital ESD is not in compliance.

Exercise 5.5

1. 4.8 days

Adults and children: $\frac{923}{192} = 4.8$

2.

a. 20.1 days

$\frac{302}{15} = 20.1$

b. 29.0 days

$\frac{203}{7} = 29.0$

c. 22.8 days

$\frac{91}{4} = 22.75 = 22.8$

d. 2 days

$\frac{8}{4} = 2$

e. 2 days

$$\frac{6}{3}=2$$

f. 29.7 days

$$\frac{89}{3}=29.7$$

g. 17.7 days

$$\frac{53}{3}=17.7$$

h. 22 days

$$\frac{44}{2}=22$$

i. 27.5 days

$$\frac{110}{4}=27.5$$

3.

University Medical Center January–June 20XX			
Clinical Units	**Discharges**	**Discharge Days**	**ALOS**
Medicine	12,280	61,400	$\frac{61,400}{12,280}=5.0$
Surgery	10,320	51,762	$\frac{51,762}{10,320}=5.0$
Neurology	12,464	68,320	$\frac{68,320}{12,464}=5.5$
Oncology	6,228	61,280	$\frac{61,280}{6,228}=9.8$
Orthopedics	4,906	20,624	$\frac{20,624}{4,906}=4.2$
Rehabilitation	1,926	48,250	$\frac{48,250}{1,926}=25.1$

(continued on next page)

University Medical Center January–June 20XX			
Clinical Units	**Discharges**	**Discharge Days**	**ALOS**
Urology	678	2,698	$\dfrac{2,698}{678} = 4.0$
Psychiatry	936	22,400	$\dfrac{22,400}{936} = 23.9$
Ophthalmology	385	804	$\dfrac{804}{385} = 2.1$
Obstetrics/ Gynecology	3,528	8,820	$\dfrac{8,820}{3,528} = 2.5$
Pediatrics	3,148	18,388	$\dfrac{18,388}{3,148} = 5.8$
Total	**56,799**	**364,746**	$\dfrac{364,746}{56,799} = 6.4$

Exercise 5.7

1.

Admitted	Discharged	LOS
1/10	1/31	**1.31 – 1.10 = 21 days**
7/8	7/30	**7/30 – 7/8 = 22 days**
1/1/2012	2/1/2015	**2012 = 365** **2013 = 365** **2014 = 365** **2015 = January – February 1 = 32 days** **Total = 1,127 days**
11/20	11/20	**1 day**
6/19/2011	1/4/2012	**2011 = June = 11 days** **July – December = 184 days** **2014 = 4 days** **Total = 199 days**

2. 21 + 22 + 1,127 + 1 + 199 = 1,370

3. Adults and Children ALOS:
$$\frac{67,392}{15,672} = 4.3$$

4. Newborns ALOS:
$$\frac{3,453}{1,502} = 2.3$$

5. Medicine ALOS:
$$\frac{40,780}{9,455} = 4.3$$

6. Surgery ALOS:
$$\frac{22,957}{4,650} = 4.9$$

7. Obstetrics ALOS:
$$\frac{3,655}{1,567} = 2.3$$

8. Calculate the ALOS for the following Medicare patients. Round to one decimal place.

Community Hospital Medicare Discharge Statistics July 20XX			
Unit	Medicare Discharges	Medicare Discharge Days	ALOS
Medicine	478	3,411	$\frac{3,411}{478} = 7.1$ days
Surgery	253	2,566	$\frac{2,566}{253} = 10.1$ days
Rehabilitation	261	4,507	$\frac{4,507}{261} = 17.3$ days
Skilled Nursing	394	11,132	$\frac{11,132}{394} = 28.3$ days

Chapter 6

Exercise 6.1

1. $\dfrac{(4+1)\times 100}{(645+4+87+1)} = \dfrac{500}{737} = 0.68\%$

2. $\dfrac{(3\times 100)}{58} = \dfrac{300}{58} = 5.17\%$

3. $\dfrac{(3\times 100)}{15} = 20.00\%$

Exercise 6.3

$$\frac{\begin{array}{c}(7 \text{ A/C deaths} + 2 \text{ NB deaths}) - \\ (2 \text{ A/C deaths} < 48 \text{ hours} + \\ 1 \text{ NB death} < 48 \text{ hours}) \times 100\end{array}}{\begin{array}{c}(409 \text{ A/C Discharges} + 7 \text{ A/C deaths}) + \\ (68 \text{ NB discharges} + 2 \text{ NB deaths}) - \\ (2 \text{ A/C deaths} < 48 \text{ hours} + 1 \text{ NB death} < 48 \text{ hours})\end{array}} = \frac{(9-3)\times 100}{(416+70)-3} = \frac{600}{483} = 1.24\%$$

Exercise 6.5

Using the information in the table below, calculate the postoperative death rate for each surgeon at Community Hospital during the semi-annual period of July through December. Round to two decimal places.

Community Hospital July–December 20XX Number of Surgery Patients and Deaths, by Surgeon			
Physician Number	**No. of Surgery Patients**	**No. of Deaths within 10 Days after Surgery**	**Postoperative Death Rate**
Dr. 102	298	6	$\dfrac{(6\times 100)}{298} = \dfrac{600}{298} = 2.01\%$
Dr. 237	247	4	$\dfrac{(4\times 100)}{247} = \dfrac{400}{247} = 1.62\%$
Dr. 391	110	2	$\dfrac{(2\times 100)}{110} = \dfrac{200}{110} = 1.82\%$
Dr. 518	144	2	$\dfrac{(2\times 100)}{144} = \dfrac{200}{144} = 1.39\%$
Dr. 637	206	8	$\dfrac{(8\times 100)}{206} = \dfrac{800}{206} = 3.88\%$

(continued on next page)

Community Hospital July–December 20XX Number of Surgery Patients and Deaths, by Surgeon			
Physician Number	No. of Surgery Patients	No. of Deaths within 10 Days after Surgery	Postoperative Death Rate
Dr. 802	82	3	$\dfrac{(3 \times 100)}{82} = \dfrac{300}{82} = 3.66\%$
Dr. 900	120	3	$\dfrac{(3 \times 100)}{120} = \dfrac{300}{120} = 2.50\%$
Total	1,207	28	$\dfrac{(28 \times 100)}{1,207} = \dfrac{2,800}{1,207} = 2.32\%$

Exercise 6.7

Using the information in the table below, calculate the postoperative death rate at Community Hospital for each MS-DRG listed for January through June and the total for this semiannual period. Round to two decimal places.

Community Hospital January–June 20XX Selected MS-DRGs—Postoperative Deaths Number of Surgery Patients and Deaths Surgery Service				
MS-DRG	MS-DRG Title	No. of Surgery Patients	No. of Deaths within 10 Days after Surgery	Postoperative Death Rate
139	Salivary gland procedures	12	1	$\dfrac{(1 \times 100)}{12} = \dfrac{100}{12} = 8.33\%$
217	Cardiac valve & oth maj cardiothoracic proc w card cath w CC	427	5	$\dfrac{(5 \times 100)}{427} = \dfrac{500}{427} = 1.17\%$
239	Amputation for circ sys disorders exc upper limb & toe w MCC	8	2	$\dfrac{(2 \times 100)}{8} = \dfrac{200}{8} = 25.00\%$
327	Stomach, esophageal & duodenal proc w CC	84	3	$\dfrac{(3 \times 100)}{84} = \dfrac{300}{84} = 3.57\%$
338	Appendectomy w complicated principal diag w MCC	6	1	$\dfrac{(1 \times 100)}{6} = \dfrac{100}{6} = 16.67\%$

(continued on next page)

		No. of Surgery Patients	No. of Deaths within 10 Days after Surgery	
MS-DRG	MS-DRG Title			Postoperative Death Rate
405	Pancreas, liver & shunt procedures w MCC	62	4	$\dfrac{(4 \times 100)}{62} = \dfrac{400}{62} = 6.45\%$
469	Major joint replacement or reattachment of lower extremity w MCC	212	3	$\dfrac{(3 \times 100)}{212} = \dfrac{300}{212} = 1.42\%$
625	Thyroid, parathyroid & thyroglossal procedures w MCC	207	1	$\dfrac{(1 \times 100)}{207} = \dfrac{100}{207} = 0.48\%$
652	Kidney transplant	27	4	$\dfrac{(4 \times 100)}{27} = \dfrac{400}{27} = 14.81\%$
736	Uterine & adnexa proc for ovarian or adnexal malignancy w MCC	143	4	$\dfrac{(4 \times 100)}{143} = \dfrac{400}{143} = 2.80\%$
Total		**1,188**	**28**	$\dfrac{(28 \times 100)}{1,188} = \dfrac{2,800}{1,188} = 2.36\%$

Table caption (above): **Community Hospital / January–June 20XX / Selected MS-DRGs—Postoperative Deaths / Number of Surgery Patients and Deaths / Surgery Service**

Exercise 6.9

General anesthesia:

$$\frac{(4 \times 100)}{1,072} = \frac{400}{1,072} = 0.37\%$$

Regional anesthesia:

$$\frac{(2 \times 100)}{1,107} = 0.20\%$$

Local anesthesia:

$$\frac{(1 \times 100)}{547} = 0.18\%$$

Exercise 6.11

$$\frac{(2 \times 100)}{123} = \frac{200}{123} = 1.63\% \, .$$

The only cases that were direct obstetric deaths were the hemorrhage after C-section due to severed uterine artery and pre-eclampsia.

Exercise 6.13

$$\frac{(825 \times 100,000)}{3,999,386} = \frac{82,500,000}{3,999,386} = 21 \text{ maternal deaths per 100,000 population.}$$

Exercise 6.15

$$\frac{(4+3) \times 100}{(37+4+3)} = \frac{700}{44} = 15.91\%$$

Exercise 6.17

Community Hospital Cancer Registry Annual Report Selected Cancers Reported 20XX			
Type of Cancer	**No. of Discharges and Deaths**	**No. of Deaths**	**Cancer Death Rate**
Breast	311	15	$\frac{(15 \times 100)}{311} = \frac{1,500}{311} = 4.82\%$
Prostate	208	17	$\frac{(17 \times 100)}{208} = \frac{1,700}{208} = 8.17\%$
Digestive System	102	13	$\frac{(13 \times 100)}{102} = \frac{1,300}{102} = 12.75\%$
Lung and bronchus	162	12	$\frac{(12 \times 100)}{162} = \frac{1,200}{162} = 7.41\%$
Urinary System	98	13	$\frac{(13 \times 100)}{98} = \frac{1,300}{98} = 13.27\%$
Female Reproductive	48	3	$\frac{(3 \times 100)}{48} = \frac{300}{48} = 6.25\%$

(continued on next page)

Community Hospital Cancer Registry Annual Report Selected Cancers Reported 20XX			
Type of Cancer	No. of Discharges and Deaths	No. of Deaths	Cancer Death Rate
Melanoma of the skin	21	14	$\frac{(14 \times 100)}{21} = \frac{1,400}{21} = 66.67\%$
All other sites	215	52	$\frac{(52 \times 100)}{215} = \frac{5,200}{215} = 24.19\%$
Total	1,165	139	$\frac{(139 \times 100)}{1,165} = \frac{13,900}{1,165} = 11.93\%$

Exercise 6.19

University Hospital Cancer Registry Annual Report Selected Cancers Reported 20XX			
Type of Cancer	No. of Discharges and Deaths	No. of Deaths	Death Rate
Oral Cavity and Pharynx	24	1	$\frac{(1 \times 100)}{24} = \frac{100}{24} = 4.17\%$
Digestive System	198	5	$\frac{(5 \times 100)}{198} = \frac{500}{198} = 2.53\%$
Respiratory System	242	16	$\frac{(16 \times 100)}{242} = \frac{1,600}{242} = 6.61\%$
Bone and Joint	218	4	$\frac{(4 \times 100)}{218} = \frac{400}{218} = 1.83\%$
Skin (excludes Basal Cell)	34	1	$\frac{(1 \times 100)}{34} = \frac{100}{34} = 2.94\%$
Breast	190	12	$\frac{(12 \times 100)}{190} = \frac{1,200}{190} = 6.32\%$

University Hospital Cancer Registry Annual Report Selected Cancers Reported 20XX			
Type of Cancer	No. of Discharges and Deaths	No. of Deaths	Death Rate
Female Genital System	47	8	$\frac{(8\times100)}{47}=\frac{800}{47}=17.02\%$
Male Genital System	228	25	$\frac{(25\times100)}{228}=\frac{2,500}{228}=10.96\%$
Urinary System	77	7	$\frac{(7\times100)}{77}=\frac{700}{77}=9.09\%$
Brain and Other Nervous System	42	19	$\frac{(19\times100)}{42}=\frac{1,900}{42}=45.24\%$
Endocrine System	28	1	$\frac{(1\times100)}{28}=\frac{100}{28}=3.57\%$
Lymphoma	47	6	$\frac{(6\times100)}{47}=\frac{600}{47}=12.77\%$
Myeloma	25	2	$\frac{(2\times100)}{25}=\frac{200}{25}=8.00\%$
Leukemias	15	4	$\frac{(4\times100)}{15}=\frac{400}{15}=26.67\%$
Total	1,415	111	$\frac{(111\times100)}{1,415}=\frac{11,100}{1,415}=7.84\%$

Chapter 7

Exercise 7.1

1. False. The gross autopsy rate is the six autopsies multiplied by 100 and divided by the 18 inpatient deaths.

$$\frac{(6\times100)}{18}=\frac{600}{18}=33.33\%$$

2. $\frac{(2\times100)}{9}=\frac{200}{9}=22.22\%$

3. $\dfrac{(15 \times 100)}{18} = \dfrac{1,500}{18} = 83.33\%$

Exercise 7.3

Gross death rate: $\dfrac{(267 \times 100)}{18,251} = \dfrac{26,700}{18,251} = 1.46\%$

Gross autopsy rate: $\dfrac{(170 \times 100)}{267} = 63.67\%$

Net autopsy rate: $\dfrac{(170 \times 100)}{(267 - 20)} = \dfrac{17,000}{247} = 68.83\%$

Exercise 7.5

					University Hospital Annual Statistics 20XX		
Month	Discharges	Inpatient Deaths	Autopsies	Coroner's Cases	Gross Death Rate	Gross Autopsy Rate	Net Autopsy Rate
January	598	5	2	1	0.84%	40.00%	50.00%
February	587	6	2	2	1.02%	33.33%	50.00%
March	607	7	5	1	1.15%	71.43%	83.33%
April	624	5	1	0	0.80%	20.00%	20.00%
May	620	6	2	1	0.97%	33.33%	40.00%
June	599	7	3	2	1.17%	42.86%	60.00%
July	609	9	5	2	1.48%	55.56%	71.43%
August	575	5	2	0	0.87%	40.00%	40.00%
September	611	7	3	1	1.15%	42.86%	50.00%
October	578	8	4	1	1.38%	50.00%	57.14%
November	622	6	2	0	0.96%	33.33%	33.33%
December	572	7	2	2	1.22%	28.57%	40.00%
Total	7202	78	33	13	1.08%	42.31%	50.77%

Exercise 7.7

a, b, c, e, f (*d does not apply because the autopsy was done by the medical examiner, and g does not apply because fetal deaths and autopsies are calculated separately.*)

Exercise 7.9

Adjusted hospital autopsy rate: $\dfrac{\begin{array}{c}(3 \text{ IP autopsies} + 2 \text{ ESD autopsies} + \\ 1 \text{ home health autopsy}) \times 100\end{array}}{\begin{array}{c}(12 \text{ IP deaths} + 2 \text{ ESD deaths} + \\ 1 \text{ home health death}) - 2 \text{ coroner's cases}\end{array}} = \dfrac{600}{13} = 46.15\%$

Exercise 7.11

Newborn death rate: $\dfrac{(4 \times 100)}{208} = \dfrac{400}{208} = 1.92\%$

Newborn autopsy rate: $\dfrac{(3 \times 100)}{4} = \dfrac{300}{4} = 75.00\%$

Exercise 7.13

Newborn death rate: $\dfrac{(5 \times 100)}{966} = \dfrac{500}{966} = 0.52\%$

Newborn autopsy rate: $\dfrac{(2 \times 100)}{5} = \dfrac{200}{5} = 40.00\%$

Exercise 7.15

Urban Hospital

Newborn death rate: $\dfrac{(2 \times 100)}{250} = \dfrac{200}{250} = 0.80\%$

Fetal death rate: $\dfrac{(4 \text{ intermediate fetal deaths} + 3 \text{ late fetal deaths}) \times 100}{\begin{array}{c}(252 \text{ live births} + 4 \text{ intermediate fetal deaths} + \\ 3 \text{ late fetal deaths})\end{array}} = \dfrac{700}{259} = 2.70\%$

Newborn autopsy rate: $\dfrac{(1 \times 100)}{2} = \dfrac{100}{2} = 50.00\%$

Fetal autopsy rate: $\dfrac{(2 \times 100)}{(4 \text{ intermediate fetal deaths} + 3 \text{ late fetal deaths})} = \dfrac{200}{7} = 28.57\%$

Suburban Hospital

Newborn death rate: $\dfrac{(2 \times 100)}{245} = \dfrac{200}{245} = 0.82\%$

Fetal death rate: $\dfrac{(4 \text{ intermediate fetal deaths} + 1 \text{ late fetal death}) \times 100}{(247 \text{ live births} + 4 \text{ intermediate fetal deaths} + 1 \text{ late fetal death})} = \dfrac{500}{252} = 1.98\%$

Newborn autopsy rate: $\dfrac{(1 \times 100)}{2} = \dfrac{100}{2} = 50.00\%$

Fetal autopsy rate: $\dfrac{(1 \times 100)}{(4 \text{ intermediate fetal deaths} + 1 \text{ late fetal death})} = \dfrac{100}{5} = 20.00\%$

Rural Hospital

Newborn death rate: $\dfrac{(2 \times 100)}{173} = \dfrac{200}{173} = 1.16\%$

Fetal death rate: $\dfrac{(2 \text{ intermediate fetal deaths} + 1 \text{ late fetal death}) \times 100}{(176 \text{ live births} + 2 \text{ intermediate fetal deaths} + 1 \text{ late fetal death})} = \dfrac{300}{179} = 1.68\%$

Newborn autopsy rate: $\dfrac{(1 \times 100)}{2} = \dfrac{100}{2} = 50.00\%$

Fetal autopsy rate: $\dfrac{(2 \times 100)}{(2 \text{ intermediate fetal deaths} + 1 \text{ late fetal death})} = \dfrac{200}{3} = 66.67\%$

Specialty Hospital

Newborn death rate: $\dfrac{(12 \times 100)}{200} = \dfrac{1,200}{200} = 6.00\%$

Fetal death rate: $\dfrac{(8 \text{ intermediate fetal deaths} + 3 \text{ late fetal deaths}) \times 100}{(201 \text{ live births} + 8 \text{ intermediate fetal deaths} + 3 \text{ late fetal deaths})} = \dfrac{1,100}{212} = 5.19\%$

Newborn autopsy rate: $\dfrac{(8 \times 100)}{12} = \dfrac{800}{12} = 66.67\%$

Fetal autopsy rate: $\dfrac{(8 \times 100)}{(8 \text{ intermediate fetal deaths} + 3 \text{ late fetal deaths})} = \dfrac{800}{11} = 72.73\%$

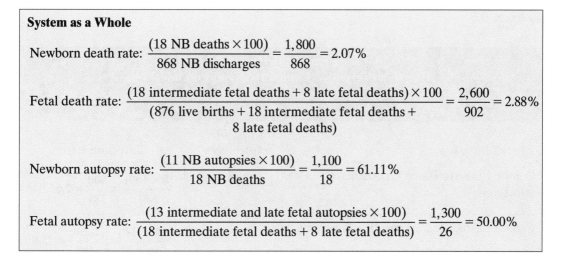

System as a Whole

Newborn death rate: $\dfrac{(18 \text{ NB deaths} \times 100)}{868 \text{ NB discharges}} = \dfrac{1,800}{868} = 2.07\%$

Fetal death rate: $\dfrac{(18 \text{ intermediate fetal deaths} + 8 \text{ late fetal deaths}) \times 100}{(876 \text{ live births} + 18 \text{ intermediate fetal deaths} + 8 \text{ late fetal deaths})} = \dfrac{2,600}{902} = 2.88\%$

Newborn autopsy rate: $\dfrac{(11 \text{ NB autopsies} \times 100)}{18 \text{ NB deaths}} = \dfrac{1,100}{18} = 61.11\%$

Fetal autopsy rate: $\dfrac{(13 \text{ intermediate and late fetal autopsies} \times 100)}{(18 \text{ intermediate fetal deaths} + 8 \text{ late fetal deaths})} = \dfrac{1,300}{26} = 50.00\%$

Chapter 8

Exercise 8.1

Hospital-acquired infection rate for adults and children: $\dfrac{(18 \times 100)}{2,190} = \dfrac{1,800}{2,190} = 0.82\%$

Hospital-acquired infection rate for newborns: $\dfrac{(2 \times 100)}{127} = \dfrac{200}{127} = 1.57\%$

Total Hospital-acquired infection rate for the hosptital: $\dfrac{(18+2) \times 100}{(2,190+127)} = \dfrac{2,000}{2,317} = 0.86\%$

Gross death rate for this annual period: $\dfrac{(13+1) \times 100}{(2,190+127)} = \dfrac{1,400}{2,317} = 0.60\%$

Exercise 8.3

Postoperative infection rate: $\dfrac{(14 \times 100)}{2,176} = \dfrac{1,400}{2,176} = 0.64\%$

Postoperative death rate: $\dfrac{(8 \times 100)}{2,170} = \dfrac{800}{2,170} = 0.37\%$

Exercise 8.5

Community Hospital Infection Prevention Committee Report on Infections January–March 20XX 389 discharges		
Type of Infection	**No. of Infections**	**Infection Rate**
Central Line-associated bloodstream infections	8	$\dfrac{(8 \times 100)}{389} = \dfrac{800}{389} = 2.06\%$
Catheter-associated urinary tract infections	12	$\dfrac{(12 \times 100)}{389} = \dfrac{1,200}{389} = 3.08\%$
Ventilator-associated pneumonia	4	$\dfrac{(4 \times 100)}{389} = \dfrac{400}{389} = 1.03\%$
Surgical-site infections	6	$\dfrac{(6 \times 100)}{389} = \dfrac{600}{389} = 1.54\%$
Cardiovascular system infections	2	$\dfrac{(2 \times 100)}{389} = \dfrac{200}{389} = 0.51\%$
Gastrointestinal tract infections	3	$\dfrac{(3 \times 100)}{389} = \dfrac{300}{389} = 0.77\%$
Skin and soft-tissue infections	1	$\dfrac{(1 \times 100)}{389} = \dfrac{100}{389} = 0.26\%$
Ears, nose, and throat infections	9	$\dfrac{(9 \times 100)}{389} = \dfrac{900}{389} = 2.31\%$
Central nervous system infections	7	$\dfrac{(7 \times 100)}{389} = \dfrac{700}{389} = 1.80\%$
Systemic infections	5	$\dfrac{(5 \times 100)}{389} = \dfrac{500}{389} = 1.29\%$

Exercise 8.7

	Community Hospital Complication Rate by Physician January–June, 20XX		
Physician No.	No. Discharges and Deaths	No. Complications	Complication Rate
102	298	2	$\dfrac{(2 \times 100)}{298} = \dfrac{200}{298} = 0.67\%$
237	247	4	$\dfrac{(4 \times 100)}{247} = \dfrac{400}{247} = 1.62\%$
391	110	3	$\dfrac{(3 \times 100)}{110} = \dfrac{300}{110} = 2.73\%$
518	144	2	$\dfrac{(2 \times 100)}{144} = \dfrac{200}{144} = 1.39\%$
637	206	3	$\dfrac{(3 \times 100)}{206} = \dfrac{300}{206} = 1.46\%$
802	82	1	$\dfrac{(1 \times 100)}{82} = \dfrac{100}{82} = 1.22\%$
900	100	3	$\dfrac{(3 \times 100)}{100} = \dfrac{300}{100} = 3.00\%$
Total	**1,187**	**18**	$\dfrac{(18 \times 100)}{1,187} = \dfrac{1,800}{1,187} = 1.52\%$

Exercise 8.9

C-section rate: $\dfrac{(20 \times 100)}{130} = \dfrac{2,000}{130} = 15.38\%$

Newborn death rate: $\dfrac{(1 \times 100)}{130} = \dfrac{100}{130} = 0.77\%$

Fetal death rate: $\dfrac{(2 + 2) \times 100}{130 + (2 + 2)} = \dfrac{400}{134} = 2.99\%$

Exercise 8.11

Community Hospital
Surgery Service
Annual Statistics 20XX

Month	Discharges including Deaths	Deaths	Consults	Consultation Rate	Gross Death Rate
January	602	18	119	$\dfrac{(119 \times 100)}{602} = \dfrac{11,900}{602} = 19.77\%$	$\dfrac{(18 \times 100)}{602} = \dfrac{1,800}{602} = 2.99\%$
February	675	12	107	$\dfrac{(107 \times 100)}{675} = \dfrac{10,700}{675} = 15.85\%$	$\dfrac{(12 \times 100)}{675} = \dfrac{1,200}{675} = 1.78\%$
March	598	11	92	$\dfrac{(92 \times 100)}{598} = \dfrac{9,200}{598} = 15.38\%$	$\dfrac{(11 \times 100)}{598} = \dfrac{1,100}{598} = 1.84\%$
April	555	14	74	$\dfrac{(74 \times 100)}{555} = \dfrac{7,400}{555} = 13.33\%$	$\dfrac{(14 \times 100)}{555} = \dfrac{1,400}{555} = 2.52\%$
May	630	10	105	$\dfrac{(105 \times 100)}{630} = \dfrac{10,500}{630} = 16.67\%$	$\dfrac{(10 \times 100)}{630} = \dfrac{1,100}{630} = 1.59\%$
June	592	6	96	$\dfrac{(96 \times 100)}{592} = \dfrac{9,600}{592} = 16.22\%$	$\dfrac{(6 \times 100)}{592} = \dfrac{600}{592} = 1.01\%$
July	581	9	85	$\dfrac{(85 \times 100)}{581} = \dfrac{8,500}{581} = 14.63\%$	$\dfrac{(9 \times 100)}{581} = \dfrac{900}{581} = 1.55\%$

August	593	7	72	$\dfrac{(72\times100)}{593}=\dfrac{7{,}200}{593}=12.14\%$	$\dfrac{(7\times100)}{593}=\dfrac{700}{593}=1.18\%$
Sept	621	5	89	$\dfrac{(89\times100)}{621}=\dfrac{8{,}900}{621}=14.33\%$	$\dfrac{(5\times100)}{621}=\dfrac{500}{621}=0.81\%$
October	610	12	56	$\dfrac{(56\times100)}{610}=\dfrac{5{,}600}{610}=9.18\%$	$\dfrac{(12\times100)}{610}=\dfrac{1{,}200}{610}=1.97\%$
November	601	10	95	$\dfrac{(95\times100)}{601}=\dfrac{9{,}500}{601}=15.81\%$	$\dfrac{(10\times100)}{601}=\dfrac{1{,}000}{601}=1.66\%$
December	581	14	82	$\dfrac{(82\times100)}{581}=\dfrac{8{,}200}{581}=14.11\%$	$\dfrac{(14\times100)}{581}=\dfrac{1{,}400}{581}=2.41\%$
Total	7,239	128	1,072	$\dfrac{(1{,}072\times100)}{7{,}239}=\dfrac{107{,}200}{7{,}239}=14.81\%$	$\dfrac{(128\times100)}{7{,}239}=\dfrac{12{,}800}{7{,}239}=1.77\%$

Exercise 8.13

		University Hospital Surgery Service Semiannual Statistics July–December 20XX	
Month	No. of Patients Discharged Alive	No. of Patients Readmitted within 30 Days of the Previous Discharge	Readmission Rate
July	673	38	$\frac{(38 \times 100)}{673} = \frac{3,800}{673} = 5.65\%$
August	765	43	$\frac{(43 \times 100)}{765} = \frac{4,300}{765} = 5.62\%$
September	789	49	$\frac{(49 \times 100)}{789} = \frac{4,900}{789} = 6.21\%$
October	750	32	$\frac{(32 \times 100)}{750} = \frac{3,200}{750} = 4.27\%$
November	769	36	$\frac{(36 \times 100)}{769} = \frac{3,600}{769} = 4.68\%$
December	778	45	$\frac{(45 \times 100)}{778} = \frac{4,500}{778} = 5.78\%$
Total	4,524	243	$\frac{(243 \times 100)}{4,524} = \frac{24,300}{4,524} = 5.37\%$

Exercise 8.15

		Community Hospital Semiannual Statistics, 20XX Readmissions by Physicians	
Physician	No. of Live Discharges	No. of Readmissions within 30 days of Previous Discharge	Readmission Rate
102	298	8	$\frac{(8 \times 100)}{298} = \frac{800}{298} = 2.68\%$

(continued on next page)

		Community Hospital **Semiannual Statistics, 20XX** **Readmissions by Physicians**	
Physician	**No. of Live Discharges**	**No. of Readmissions within 30 days of Previous Discharge**	**Readmission Rate**
237	247	4	$\dfrac{(4 \times 100)}{247} = \dfrac{400}{247} = 1.62\%$
391	110	3	$\dfrac{(3 \times 100)}{110} = \dfrac{300}{110} = 2.73\%$
518	144	2	$\dfrac{(2 \times 100)}{144} = \dfrac{200}{144} = 1.39\%$
637	206	12	$\dfrac{(12 \times 100)}{206} = \dfrac{1,200}{206} = 5.83\%$
802	82	6	$\dfrac{(6 \times 100)}{82} = \dfrac{600}{82} = 7.32\%$
900	100	5	$\dfrac{(5 \times 100)}{100} = \dfrac{500}{100} = 5.00\%$
Total	**1,187**	**40**	$\dfrac{(40 \times 100)}{1,187} = \dfrac{4,000}{1,187} = 3.37\%$

Exercise 8.17

1. 60.61% of the patients were in the Medicine Service.
$$\frac{(5,967 \times 100)}{9,845} = \frac{596,700}{9,845} = 60.61\%$$

2. $\dfrac{(236 \times 100)}{5,967} = \dfrac{23,600}{5,967} = 3.96\%$

3. $\dfrac{(89 \times 100)}{5,967} = \dfrac{8,900}{5,967} = 1.49\%$

4. $\dfrac{(71 \times 100)}{5,967} = \dfrac{7,100}{5,967} = 1.19\%$

5.

a. $\dfrac{(1{,}016 \times 100)}{5{,}967} = \dfrac{101{,}600}{5{,}967} = 17.03\%$

b. $\dfrac{(923 \times 100)}{5{,}967} = \dfrac{92{,}300}{5{,}967} = 15.47\%$

c. $\dfrac{(3{,}237 \times 100)}{5{,}967} = \dfrac{323{,}700}{5{,}967} = 54.25\%$

d. $\dfrac{(791 \times 100)}{5{,}967} = \dfrac{79{,}100}{5{,}967} = 13.26\%$

6.

a. $\dfrac{(370 \times 100)}{5{,}967} = \dfrac{37{,}000}{5{,}967} = 6.20\%$

b. $\dfrac{(875 \times 100)}{5{,}967} = \dfrac{87{,}500}{5{,}967} = 14.66\%$

c. $\dfrac{(736 \times 100)}{5{,}967} = \dfrac{73{,}600}{5{,}967} = 12.33\%$

d. $\dfrac{(92 \times 100)}{5{,}967} = \dfrac{9{,}200}{5{,}967} = 1.54\%$

e. $\dfrac{(701 \times 100)}{5{,}967} = \dfrac{70{,}100}{5{,}967} = 11.75\%$

f. $\dfrac{(561 \times 100)}{5{,}967} = \dfrac{56{,}100}{5{,}967} = 9.40\%$

Chapter 9

Exercise 9.1

1. $\dfrac{\$31{,}200}{312{,}000} = \$0.10$ per line

2. $\dfrac{\$29{,}120}{234{,}000} = \$0.12$ per line

3.

a. The difference in cost per line is: $\$0.11 - \$0.09 = \$0.02$

The transcriptionist who produces 1,000 lines per day at \$14.00/hour:

Salary: \$14.00 × 2,080 = \$29,120 yearly salary

Productivity: 1,000 lines produced each day × 5 days × 52 weeks = 260,000 lines produced each year

$$\frac{\$29,120}{260,000} = \$0.11 \text{ per line}$$

The transcriptionist who produces 1,200 lines per day at $14.00/hour:

Salary: $14.00 × 2,080 = $29,120 yearly salary

Productivity: 1,200 lines produced each day × 5 days × 52 weeks = 312,000

$$\frac{\$29,120}{312,000} = \$0.09 \text{ per line}$$

Students should perform this calculation by multiplying the hourly salary by 2,080

Productivity should be calculated by multiplying the individual transcriptionist's production by 5 workdays per week × 52 weeks.

b. The employees make the same hourly rate, but one produces less than the other, resulting in a higher per line rate for the employee who produces 1,000 lines per day than the employee who produces 1,200 lines per day.

c. The difference in cost per line is: $0.13 – $0.10 = $0.03

The transcriptionist who produces 1,000 lines per day at $16.00/hour:

Salary: $16.00 × 2,080 = $33,280 yearly salary

Productivity: (1,000 lines produced each day × 5 days × 52 weeks) = 260,000 lines produced each year

$$\frac{\$33,280}{260,000} = \$0.13 \text{ per line}$$

The transcriptionist who produces 1,100 lines per day at $14.25/hour:

Salary: $14.25 × 2,080 = $29,640 yearly salary

Productivity: 1,100 lines produced each day × 5 days × 52 weeks = 286,000

$$\frac{\$29,640}{286,000} = \$0.10 \text{ per line}$$

d. Total salaries: Add all salaries and multiply by 2,080 = $248,872

Total productivity: Add all productivity and multiply by 5 days per week and 52 weeks per year = 2,184,000.

$$\frac{\$248,872}{2,184,000} = \$0.11 \text{ per line}$$

4. **a.** Lead coder: Salary = $20.35 × 2,080 = $42,328

Productivity: 7.5 hours per day × 4 records per hour = 30 records per day

30 records × 5 days per week × 52 weeks per year = 7,800

$$\frac{\$42,328}{7,800} = \$5.43 \text{ per record}$$

New graduate: Salary = $15.50 × 2,080 = $32,240

Productivity: 7.5 hours per day × 3 records per hour = 22.5 records per day

22.5 records × 5 days per week × 52 weeks per year = 5,850

$$\frac{\$32,240}{5,850} = \$5.51 \text{ per record}$$

Experienced coder: Salary = $18.90 × 2,080 = $39,312

Productivity: 7.5 hours per day × 6 records per hour = 45 records per day

45 records × 5 days per week × 52 weeks per year = 11,700

$$\frac{\$39,312}{11,700} = \$3.36 \text{ per record}$$

b. Salaries: Add all salaries together = $113,880

Productivity = Add all productivity together = 13 records per hour = 97.5 per day

97.5 × 5 days per week × 52 weeks per year = 25,350 records coded per year

$$\frac{\$113,880}{25,350} = \$4.49 \text{ per record}$$

5.

Coder	Salary	Records Coded per Hour	Salary per Year	Unit Cost
A	$15.00	4	**$31,200**	**7.5 × 4 records = 30** **30 × 5 days per week = 150 records coded per week** **150 × 52 weeks = 7,800 records coded per year** $$\frac{\$31,200}{7,800} = \$4.00 \text{ per record}$$
B	$15.45	5	**$32,136**	**7.5 × 5 records = 37.5** **37.5 × 5 days per week = 187.5 records coded per week** **187.5 × 52 weeks = 9,750 records coded per year** $$\frac{\$32,136}{9,750} = \$3.30 \text{ per record}$$

(continued on next page)

Coder	Salary	Records Coded per Hour	Salary per Year	Unit Cost
C	$15.10	4	$31,408	7.5×4 records = 30 30×5 days per week = 150 coded per week 150×52 weeks = 7,800 records coded per year $\dfrac{\$31,408}{7,800} = \$4.03$ per record
D	$16.79	6	$34,923	7.5×6 records = 45 45×5 days per week = 225 coded per week 225×52 weeks = 11,700 records coded per year $\dfrac{\$34,923}{11,700} = \$2.98$ per record
E	$18.22	6	$37,898	7.5×6 records = 45 45×5 days per week = 225 coded per week 225×52 weeks = 11,700 records coded per year $\dfrac{\$37,898}{11,700} = \$3.24$ per record
F	$22.65	6	$47,112	7.5×6 records = 45 45×5 days per week = 225 coded per week 225×52 weeks = 11,700 records coded per year $\dfrac{\$47,112}{11,700} = \$4.03$ per record
G	$16.03	6	$33,342	7.5×6 records = 45 45×5 days per week = 225 coded per week 225×52 weeks = 11,700 records coded per year $\dfrac{\$33,342}{11,700} = \$2.85$ per record
H	$16.85	6	$35,048	7.5×6 records = 45 45×5 days per week = 225 coded per week 225×52 weeks = 11,700 records coded per year $\dfrac{\$35,048}{11,700} = \$3.00$ per record
I	$21.76	8	$45,261	7.5×8 records = 60 60×5 days per week = 300 coded per week 300×52 weeks = 15,600 records coded per year $\dfrac{\$45,261}{15,600} = \$2.90$ per record

(continued on next page)

Coder	Salary	Records Coded per Hour	Salary per Year	Unit Cost
J	$17.34	6	$36,067	7.5 × 6 records = 45 45 × 5 days per week = 225 coded per week 225 × 52 weeks = 11,700 records coded per year $\dfrac{\$36,067}{11,700} = \$3.08$ per record
Total			$364,395	7.5 × 57 records per day = 427.5 427.5 × 5 days per week = 2,137.5 coded per week 2,137.5 × 52 weeks = 111,150 coded per year $\dfrac{\$364,395}{111,150} = \$3.28$ per record

Exercise 9.3

1. Postage: $\dfrac{\$790}{550} = \$1.44$

   Service contract: $\dfrac{\$265}{550} = \$0.48$

   Equipment: $\dfrac{\$150}{550} = \$0.27$

   Supplies: $\dfrac{\$95}{550} = \$0.17$

   Wages: $\$13.00 \times 2,080 = \$27,040$

   $\dfrac{\$27,040}{12 \text{ months}} = \$2,253$

   $\dfrac{\$2,253}{550} = \$4.10$

2. $\$1.44 + \$0.48 + \$0.27 + \$0.17 + \$4.10 = \$6.46$

   $\$6.46 \times 550$ requests $= \$3,553$

3. $\$3,553 - \$1,800 = \$1,753$ per month in losses

4. Advantages: No financial loss to the facility; possible use of employee in other areas of department.

   Disadvantages: Possible loss of employee; not sure staff is qualified; loss of control of the ROI function.

5.

a. $\dfrac{(6,382 \times 100)}{100,000} = \dfrac{638,200}{100,000} = 6.38\%$

b. $\dfrac{(3,375 \times 100)}{6,382} = \dfrac{337,500}{6,382} = 52.88\%$

Exercise 9.5

a. Telephone appointment: $3.50 \times 250 = \$875.00$

E-mail appointment: $1.75 \times 250 = \$437.50$

Cost Savings: $\$875.00 - \$437.50 = \$437.50$

b. Cost Savings: $\$875.00 - \$437.50 = \$437.50$. This represents a 50% savings.

Exercise 9.7

1.

		Community Hospital Health Information Services Unapproved Abbreviations List November 20XX	
Physician No.	No. Discharges	No. of Unapproved Abbreviations	Rate of Unapproved Abbreviations
102	298	34	$\dfrac{(34 \times 100)}{298} = \dfrac{3,400}{298} = 11.41\%$
237	247	21	$\dfrac{(21 \times 100)}{247} = \dfrac{2,100}{247} = 8.50\%$
391	110	26	$\dfrac{(26 \times 100)}{110} = \dfrac{2,600}{110} = 23.64\%$
518	144	22	$\dfrac{(22 \times 100)}{144} = \dfrac{2,200}{144} = 15.28\%$
637	206	4	$\dfrac{(4 \times 100)}{206} = \dfrac{400}{206} = 1.94\%$
802	82	21	$\dfrac{(21 \times 100)}{82} = \dfrac{2,100}{82} = 25.61\%$
900	100	12	$\dfrac{(12 \times 100)}{100} = \dfrac{1,200}{100} = 12.00\%$
Total	1,187	140	$\dfrac{(140 \times 100)}{1,187} = \dfrac{14,000}{1,187} = 11.79\%$

2.

Community Hospital **Health Information Services** **Physician Documentation Deficiencies** **January 20XX**			
Physician No.	**No. Admissions**	**No. H&Ps Not Completed Within 24 Hours of Admission**	**Rate of Deficiency**
102	189	5	$\dfrac{(5 \times 100)}{189} = \dfrac{500}{189} = 2.64$
237	234	4	$\dfrac{(4 \times 100)}{234} = \dfrac{400}{234} = 1.71$
391	98	8	$\dfrac{(8 \times 100)}{98} = \dfrac{800}{98} = 8.16$
518	122	5	$\dfrac{(5 \times 100)}{122} = 4.10$
637	178	3	$\dfrac{(3 \times 100)}{178} = 1.69$
802	92	7	$\dfrac{(7 \times 100)}{92} = 7.61$
900	99	2	$\dfrac{(2 \times 100)}{99} = 2.02$
Total	**1,012**	**34**	$\dfrac{(34 \times 100)}{1,012} = \dfrac{3,400}{1,012} = 3.36$

Exercise 9.9

1. *The number of days to complete the transition is the total number of pages divided by the number of pages that can be scanned per day.*

    7,500 inpatient records × 30 pages = 225,000 pages

    3,000 outpatient records × 4 pages = 12,000 pages

    2,500 ED records × 4 pages = 10,000

    Total pages = 225,000 + 12,000 + 10,000 = 247,000

    $\dfrac{247,000 \text{ total pages}}{7,500 \text{ pages that can be scanned}} = 32.93 \text{ days}$

2. $\dfrac{32.93 \text{ days to complete}}{10 \text{ days}} = 3.3 \text{ FTEs}$

OR

$\dfrac{247{,}000}{10 \text{ days}} = 24{,}700 \text{ pages needing to be scanned each day}$

$\dfrac{24{,}700}{7{,}500} = 3.3 \text{ FTEs}$

3.

  a. Coder A:

    $\dfrac{(450 \times 100)}{1{,}345} = \dfrac{45{,}000}{1{,}345} = 33.46\%$

    Coder B:

    $\dfrac{(510 \times 100)}{1{,}345} = \dfrac{51{,}000}{1{,}345} = 37.92\%$

    Coder C:

    $\dfrac{(385 \times 100)}{1{,}345} = \dfrac{38{,}500}{1{,}345} = 28.62\%$

  b.

    Coder A:

    $\dfrac{450}{21} = 21.43$

    Coder B:

    $\dfrac{510}{21} = 24.29$

    Coder C:

    $\dfrac{385}{21} = 18.33$

  c.

    Coder A:

    $\dfrac{21.43}{7.5} = 2.86$

    Coder B:

    $\dfrac{24.29}{7.5} = 3.24$

    Coder C:

    $\dfrac{18.33}{7.5} = 2.44$

d.

Coder A:

$$\frac{60}{2.86} = 20.98$$

Coder B:

$$\frac{60}{3.24} = 18.52$$

Coder C:

$$\frac{60}{2.44} = 24.59$$

e.

Coder A:

450 records coded – 4 not passing the quality screen = 446 passing the quality screen

$$\frac{(466 \times 100)}{450} = \frac{44,600}{450} = 99.11\%$$

Coder B:

510 records coded – 4 not passing the quality screen = 506 passing the quality screen

$$\frac{(506 \times 100)}{510} = \frac{50,600}{510} = 99.22\%$$

Coder C:

385 records coded – 11 not passing the quality screen = 374 passing the quality screen

$$\frac{(374 \times 100)}{385} = \frac{37,400}{385} = 97.14\%$$

Exercise 9.11

1. $\dfrac{\$32,000}{4,500} = 7.1\ \text{years}$

   The department should purchase the equipment if it will pay back its cost in savings within three years. To find the number of years it will take to pay back the cost, divide the cost by the annual savings. $\frac{\$32,000}{\$4,500} = 7.1\ \text{years}$. In this case, the department should not purchase this equipment because the savings do not justify its purchase.

2. *The budget variance is the difference between actual cost and expected cost, multiplied by 100 and then divided by the expected cost.*

   $\$76,000 - \$72,000 = \$4,000$

   $\dfrac{(\$4,000 \times 100)}{\$72,000} = 5.6\%$

3. $\dfrac{\$2,750,000}{\$575,000} = 4.78\ \text{years}$

4.

Community Hospital HIM Department Budget Variance Annual Report 20XX			
Line Item	**Budgeted Amount**	**Actual Amount**	**Percentage of Variance**
Service Contracts	$2,000	$2,500	$2,500 – $2,000 = $500 over budget $$\frac{(\$500 \times 100)}{2,000} = \frac{50,000}{2,000} = 25.00\% \text{ over budget}$$
Education/ Conferences	$4,500	$2,400	4,500 × $2,400 = $2,100 under budget $$\frac{(\$2,100 \times 100)}{\$4,500} = \frac{210,000}{4,500} = 46.67\% \text{ under budget}$$
Travel	$2,000	$1,750	$2,000 – $1,750 = $250 under budget $$\frac{(\$250 \times 100)}{\$2,000} = \frac{25,000}{2,000} = 12.50\% \text{ under budget}$$
Dues/ Memberships	$720	$545	$720 – $545 = $175 $$\frac{(\$175 \times 100)}{\$720} = \frac{17,500}{720} = 24.31\% \text{ under budget}$$
Subscriptions/ Books	$600	$250	$600 – $250 = $350 under budget $$\frac{(\$350 \times 100)}{\$600} = \frac{35,000}{600} = 58.33\% \text{ under budget}$$
Supplies	$600	$725	$725 – $600 = $125 over budget $$\frac{(\$125 \times 100)}{\$600} = \frac{12,500}{600} = 20.83\% \text{ over budget}$$
Total	**$10,420**	**$8,170**	$10,420 – $8,170 = $2,250 under budget $$\frac{(\$2,250 \times 100)}{\$10,420} = \frac{225,100}{10,420} = 21.59\% \text{ under budget}$$

5. 247.13 total hours with 61.78 hours of overtime for each coder.

Add all the salaries together, then multiply by 1.5 (for time-and-a-half payment). Then take the new budgeted amount and divide by the time-and-a-half payment ($101.16). This is 247.13 total hours that can be worked. If you wanted to determine how many hours each coder could work individually, divide the total hours by $ (number of coders).

($15.75 + $16.00 + $18.40 + $17.29) = $67.44 per hour for all coders.

$67.44 × 1.5 = $101.16

$$\frac{\$25,000 \text{ added to the budget}}{\$101.16} = 247.13 \text{ hours total hours can be worked}$$

$$\frac{247.13 \text{ hours}}{4 \text{ coders}} = 61.78 \text{ hours could be worked by each coder}$$

Exercise 9.13

1.

	Census		Adm		Transfer	Total		Dis		Transfer	Census		A/D	Service Days	
	A/c	NB	A/C	NB	In	a/c	NB	A/C	NB	Out	A/c	NB		AC	NB
1	165	3	29	0	8	202	3	10	0	7	185	3	0	185	3
2	185	3	24	4	7	216	7	12	3	6	198	4	1	199	4
3	198	4	18	3	3	219	7	16	2	2	201	5	0	201	5
4	201	5	17	2	5	223	7	15	2	4	204	5	0	204	5
5	204	5	13	0	1	218	5	12	1	3	203	4	0	203	4
6	203	4	20	0	6	229	4	19	2	4	206	2	0	206	2
7	206	2	21	0	14	241	2	17	0	12	212	2	0	212	2
8	212	2	27	1	10	249	3	23	3	8	218	0	3	221	0
9	218	0	23	4	6	247	4	22	3	14	211	1	2	213	1
10	211	1	22	2	8	241	3	15	1	10	216	2	1	217	2
11	216	2	17	3	7	240	5	14	4	5	221	1	3	224	1
12	221	1	19	3	6	246	4	17	2	4	225	2	0	225	2
13	225	2	14	1	4	243	3	12	2	2	229	1	0	229	1
14	229	1	15	4	5	249	5	19	3	7	223	2	0	223	2
15	223	2	20	2	8	251	16	13	0	6	232	16	1	233	16

(continued on next page)

	Census		Adm		Transfer	Total		Dis		Transfer	Census			Service Days	
16	232	16	23	3	6	261	19	15	4	2	244	15	0	244	15
17	244	15	17	1	3	264	16	13	3	1	250	13	1	251	13
18	250	13	15	0	2	267	13	21	1	6	240	12	2	242	12
19	240	12	17	0	7	264	12	25	3	2	237	9	1	238	9
20	237	9	13	2	3	253	11	27	4	4	222	7	0	222	7
21	222	7	12	1	5	239	8	21	2	5	213	6	3	216	6
22	213	6	10	0	1	224	6	17	4	1	206	2	2	208	2
23	206	2	9	2	4	219	4	18	1	4	197	3	0	197	3
24	197	3	23	4	3	223	7	12	3	2	209	4	2	211	4
25	209	4	15	2	4	228	6	22	2	3	203	4	1	204	4
26	203	4	13	3	2	218	7	9	1	4	205	6	0	205	6
27	205	6	21	1	3	229	7	29	1	0	200	6	2	202	6
28	200	6	29	2	5	234	8	22	4	4	208	4	3	211	4
29	208	4	23	4	1	232	8	25	3	2	205	5	1	206	5
30	205	5	15	1	4	224	6	21	2	3	200	4	0	200	4
31	200	4	16	4	2	218	8	18	3	2	198	5	3	201	5

2.

	EXERCISE 5.4			
	COMMUNITY HOSPITAL			
	Discharge List			
	October 20, 20XX			
Pt. Name	**Age**	**Clinical Service**	**Admission Date**	**Length of Stay**
Schulman	71	Surgery	18-Sep	32
Hubbard	40	Medicine	12-Sep	38
Miraboto	35	Obstetrics	18-Oct	2
Tatum	23	Obstetrics	18-Oct	2
Rankins	71	Medicine	28-Sep	22
Lampton	90	Medicine	4-Sep	46
Hruska	45	Surgery	5-Oct	15
Adman	17	Obstetrics	19-Oct	1
Savage	37	Medicine	1-Sep	49
Beachton	46	Medicine	1-Oct	19
Sanders	14	Obstetrics	17-Oct	3
Pavalchik	62	Surgery	26-Sep	24
Walters	57	Surgery	30-Sep	20
Harding	51	Medicine	1-Oct	19
Clay	82	Medicine	10-Oct	10
Total				302
			ALOS =	**20.1**

Chapter 10

Exercise 10.1

1. True

2. *Find your percentile by putting all of the scores in order and determining the rank of your score. Multiply that rank by 100 and divide by the total number of scores to get your percentile.*

27, 35, 54, 56, 65, 74, 75, 76, 77, 84, 86, 88, 89, 91, 92, 93, 94, 95, 96, 97, 99, 100

$$\frac{(11 \times 100)}{22} = 50\text{th percentile}$$

3.

    a. *List the number of C-sections in order:*

    1, 2, 3, 4, 5, 7, 8, 9, 12, 15, 18, 20, 22, 27, 33

    To determine what percentile Dr. 975 falls in take the number of C-sections he performed (20) and see where it falls in the list which is the 12th place, then divide 12 by 15 (the N) and multiply by 100.

$$\frac{12}{15} = 0.8$$

    $0.8 \times 100 = 80\text{th percentile}$

    b. *To find the 60th percentile:*

    Multiply 60% by 15 (the N) = 9

    Find the 9th score (12)

    The 60th percentile is 12

4.

    a. *Put the weights in order:*

    147, 150, 155, 165, 172, 175, 180, 185, 186, 189, 192, 195, 196, 207, 209, 222, 232, 242, 245, 307

    Multiply 85% by 20 (the N) = 17

    Find the 17th score = 232 lbs. Any patients who weigh 232 lbs. or more would be included in the free diet counseling.

    b. 172 is in the 5th place. $\frac{5}{20} \times 100 = 25\text{th percentile}$

5.

    a. *All patients who had an A1C of 6.7 or above would be included in the weight-loss clinic.*

    Place the A1C results in order:

    5.5, 5.7, 5.7, 5.8, 6.0, 6.1, 6.2, 6.7, 6.7, 6.8, 6.8, 6.9, 7.2, 8.4, 8.5, 9.2, 9.6, 10.4, 10,7,11.4

    Multiply 40% by 20 (the N) = 8

    Find the 8th score = 6.7

Exercise 10.3

1. The range for the data may be expressed as 18 (the difference) or as 1 to 19 (quoting the smallest and largest values); however, keep in mind that in mathematics, the range is usually expressed as one value.

2. **a.** 2 to 20 or 18

   b. 0 to 20 or 20

   c. 35 to 132 or 97

3. $2 + 20 = 22$

4. $109 - 45 = 64$

5. $245 - 125 = 120$

Chapter 11

Exercise 11.1

1. This is an example of the nominal data or scale.

   In the nominal scale of measurement, you are only allowed to examine whether the data are equal to some particular value or to count the number of occurrences of each value. For example, gender is a nominal scale variable. You can examine whether the gender of a person is female or to count the number of males in a sample.

2. No.

   Temperature is an interval scale of measurement and the zero on the scale does not represent the absence of the thing being measured. Interval measurement ratios do not make sense: 80 degrees is not twice as hot as 40 degrees (although the attribute value is twice as large).

3. Yes.

   This is an example of ratio scale of measurement. There is a zero point; that is you can have zero patients.

4. This is an example of ordinal scale.

   Ordinal data are types of data where the values are in ordered categories. On the ordinal scale, the order of the labels is meaningful, not the label itself. This is because the intervals or distance between categories are not necessarily equal.

5. This is an example of an ordinal scale of measurement.

   Measurements with ordinal scales are ordered in the sense that higher numbers represent higher values. However, the intervals between the numbers are not necessarily equal. For example, on the five-point rating scale measuring correct information given by the clerk, the difference between a rating of 2 and a rating of 3 may not represent the same difference as the difference between a rating of 4 and a rating of 5.

Exercise 11.3

Community Hospital Ages of Patients with Colon Cancer Annual Statistics 20XX		
Age	No. of Patients	Proportion
≤30	3	$\dfrac{3}{206} = 0.01$
31–40	12	$\dfrac{12}{206} = 0.06$
41–50	18	$\dfrac{18}{206} = 0.09$
51–60	60	$\dfrac{60}{206} = 0.29$
61–70	65	$\dfrac{65}{206} = 0.32$
71+	48	$\dfrac{48}{206} = 0.23$

Exercise 11.5

1. Create a histogram to display the distribution of total discharge days by age.

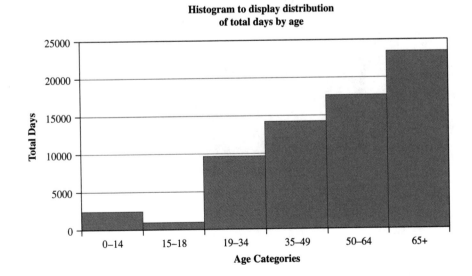

Histogram to display distribution of total days by age

2. Create a bar graph to display the admission by day of week for Medicare patients in comparison to the admission by day of week for all patients.

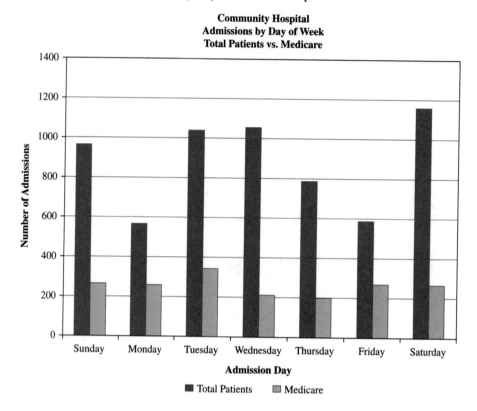

Community Hospital
Admissions by Day of Week
Total Patients vs. Medicare

3. Create a pie chart to display the percentage of patients discharged by major service category.

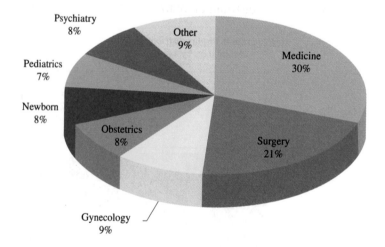

4. Create a table for length of stay distribution.

Length of Stay Distribution		
	Patients	**% Cases**
Same day	114	1.7
1 day	755	11.3
2–4 days	1,343	20.2
5–7 days	1,555	23.3
8–14 days	1,469	22.0
15–42 days	1,217	18.3
43+ days	210	3.2
Total	6,663	100.0

Exercise 11.7

University Hospital reported the following incidence of lung and bronchus cancer patients treated at the hospital during the past 10 years. Construct a line graph of the data.

University Hospital Cancer Registry Data Lung and Bronchus Cancer by Year and Gender		
Year	**Males**	**Females**
2006	172	48
2007	175	47
2008	169	49
2009	165	50
2010	168	54
2011	121	93
2012	123	101
2013	130	118
2014	121	121
2015	112	123

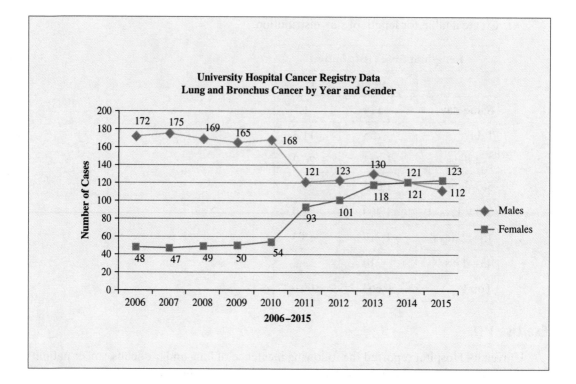

Chapter 12

Exercise 12.1

1. __a__ Researcher often has an inside perspective.

2. __b__ Uses controlled measurements.

3. __b__ Uses numbers to describe the results.

4. __a__ The sample is purposefully selected.

5. __a__ The study is process oriented.

6. __b__ Structured interviews are used.

Exercise 12.3

1. __g__ A health information professional is gathering information for a study from the coding professionals in her department.

2. __f__ The marketing department of your facility will choose 50 patient satisfaction surveys from patients age 35 to 45.

3. __d__ A researcher will study the incidence of cancer in your state. First he selects the city, then the hospitals, and finally the patients to study.

4. __h__ A researcher would like to study nurse practitioners who treat diabetic children in your state. He finds the first nurse practitioner to interview, then asks her to identify two others for him to interview. He intends to ask those two for two additional names and so on.

5. _c_ Your college is conducting a study on study habits of students. The first thing they do is divide the study body into undergraduate and graduate students. Then, they select a random sample of each group to interview.

6. _b_ You were asked by the health information committee to evaluate the discharge summaries on every 10th patient discharged last quarter.

7. _a_ A health information researcher wants to report on the salary of professionals over the last year. She uses a database from the American Health Information Management Association in which every person has the same chance of being selected for the study.

8. _e_ A health information researcher wants to study the effects of the Health Insurance Portability and Accountability Act (HIPAA) regulations on employees so she selects privacy officers with at least 5-years of experience to interview.

Chapter 13

Exercise 13.1

$\bar{x} = 14$, $sd = 2$, $n = 30$, $SE_m = 0.4$

68% C.I. = 13.6 to 14.4

95% C.I. = 13.2 to 14.8

99.7% C.I. = 12.8 to 15.2

To calculate these, take the mean (14) + and – the standard error of the mean for 68% C.I., and the standard error of the mean × 2 for the 95% C.I. and standard error of the mean × 3 for the 99.7% C.I.

For 68% confidence interval: 14 – 0.4 = 13.6 and 14 + 0.4 = 14.4

For 95% confidence interval: 14 – (0.4 × 2) = 14 – 0.8 = 13.2 and 14 + (0.4 × 2) = 14 + 0.8 = 14.8

For 99.7 % confidence interval: 14 – (0.4 × 3) = 14 – 1.2 = 12.8 and 14 + (0.4 × 3) = 14 + 1.2 = 15.2

Exercise 13.3

Type I Error: The null hypothesis is rejected, but it is true. It is determined that there is a difference between the effectiveness of the placebo and the medication, but in fact there is no difference between their effectiveness in lowering cholesterol.

Type II Error: The null hypothesis is not rejected, yet it is false. It is determined that there is no difference between the effectiveness of the placebo and the medication, but there is in fact a difference between their effectiveness in lowering cholesterol.

Index

A

Accreditation agencies, use of statistics, 8
Adjusted hospital autopsy rate, 128–131, 335
    example, 128
Admission date, 72
Agency for Healthcare Research and Quality (AHRQ), 3
Alternative hypothesis, 290
Ambulatory care facility, definition, 5
American Statistical Association (ASA), Ethical
        Guidelines for Statistical Practice, 303–304
Analysis of variance (ANOVA), 316–317
Anesthesia death rate, 100–102, 335
    example, 100
Applied research, definition, 284
Autopsy, definition, 121
Autopsy rate, 122–126
    calculation of, 134
    fetal, 133–138
    gross, 121–123
    net, 123–126
    newborn, 132–133
Average, 25–26, 335
Average daily inpatient census, 45–46, 335
Average daily newborn census, 46–47, 336
Average duration of hospitalization. *See* Average length
    of stay (ALOS)
Average length of stay (ALOS), 72, 78–79, 336
    newborn, 79–80, 336

B

Bar charts. *See* Bar graphs
Bar graphs, 257–258
Baseline, ignoring, 297
Basic research, definition, 284
Bed capacity, 54
Bed count, 54
    change in, 59–61
Bed count day, 55
    example, 55
Bed occupancy ratio, 56, 336
Bed turnover rate, 64–65, 336
Big data, definition, 321–322

B (continued)

Bimodal distribution curve, 234–235
Budget, 193–196
    capital, 194–195
    definition, 193
    operational, 193–194
Bureau of Labor Statistics, 2

C

Cancer mortality rate, 112–115, 336
    example, 112–113
Cancer registrar, 113
Cancer registries, use of statistics, 7
Cancer registry, 113
Capital budget, 194–195
Case fatality rate, 93, 336
Case-mix index, 336
Case-mix index (CMI) reports, 200–204
    definition, 200
Categorical data, 246
Causal research, 288
Census, 4–5. *See also* Inpatient census
    patient, 31–52
    real-world example, 6
Census day, 36
Centers for Disease Control and Prevention (CDC), 2
    infection reporting system, 146
Centers for Medicare and Medicaid Services (CMS), 2, 92
Certificate of need (CON), 53
Cesarean section, definition, 155
Cesarean section rate, 155–158, 337
    example, 156
Chi-square, definition, 317–318
Clinical and biomedical research, privacy considerations
        in, 300–303
Clinical data warehouse, 324
Cluster sampling, 292
Complete master census, 32–34
Complication
    definition, 153
    maternal death rate and, 102
Complication rate, 153–155, 337
    definition, 153
    example, 154

Computerized discharge reports, 197–200
    definition, 197
    example, 197–200
Computerized financial reports, 200–204
Computerized readmission rate reports, 200–204
Conclusions, in research, 296
Conclusive research, 287
Concomitant (chronic) conditions, 146
Confidence interval (CI), 310–311
Consultation, definition, 158
Consultation rates, 158–161, 337
    example, 159
Content analysis, in data analysis, 295
Continuous data, definition, 248
Convenience sampling, 293
Coroner, definition, 124
Correlation
    definition, 236
    example, 236–238
Correlational research, 288
Crude death rate, 113

D
Daily inpatient census, 34–35
Dashboard, definition, 326
Data
    analysis of, 295–296, 322
    display, 249–275
    importance of, 3
    presentation of, 245–281
    types, 245–248 (See also specific type)
Data analytics, 321–330
    introduction, 321–323
    types, 323–327
    using for decision-making, 325–327
Data collection, 290–291
Data interpretation issues, 296–304
    graphical misrepresentations, 297
    ignoring the baseline, 297
    misleading presentation of numbers, 297
    sabotage, 298
    selection bias, 297
Data mining, 324
Data validation, importance of, 298
Days of stay. See Length of stay (LOS)
Dead on arrival (DOA), 92
Death rates, 91–120
    guidelines for calculation of, 92–93
Decile, 216
Decimals
    changing a percentage to, 19
    changing to a percentage, 18
    definition, 15
    rounding of, 16
Delivery, definition, 155
Denominator, definition, 14
Department of Health and Human Services (HHS), 2
    Office of Research Integrity (ORI), 296

Descriptive analytics, 322, 323
Descriptive research, 287
Descriptive statistics, 213–243, 310
    in data analysis, 295
    definition, 3, 214
Dialysis Surveillance Network (DSN), 146
Discharge date, 72
Discharge days, definition, 72
Discrete data, definition, 248
Disposition, 92
Drug and alcohol facilities, use of statistics, 8
Duration of inpatient hospitalization. See Length of
    stay (LOS)

E
Early fetal death, 109
Electronic signature, 179
Emergency services department (ESD)
    beds, 55
    hospital autopsies, 127
Employee compensation, 174–177
Encounters, definition, 5
Ethical guidelines, in statistical practice, 303–304
Ethnography, 291
Evaluation research, 288
Evidence-based medicine, 322
Experimental research, 288
Experimental study, 291
Exploratory research, 287

F
Fabrication, 296
Falsification, 296
Federal government, use of statistics, 8
Fetal autopsy rate, 133–138, 337
    example, 134
Fetal death, definition, 93
Fetal death rate, 109–112, 337
    calculation of hospital-based mortality rates, 110
    classification of, 109
    example, 109
Fractions, 13–14
    changing a percentage to, 19
    changing to a percentage, 18
    definition, 13
Frequency distribution, 214
    example, 214
Frequency distribution tables, 251–256
    example, 251
Frequency polygon, 261
F test. See Analysis of variance (ANOVA)
Full-time equivalent employee (FTE), 186–192

G
Graphical misrepresentations, 297–298
Graphs, 257–275

Gross autopsy rate, 122–123, 337
    example, 122
    net, 123–126
Gross (hospital) death rate, 93–95, 337
    example, 93–94
Grounded theory, in data analysis, 295

H
Healthcare administration, use of statistics, 6–7
Healthcare data, types, 322–323
Healthcare department managers, use of statistics, 7
Healthcare-related infections (HAIs), 146
Healthcare researchers, use of statistics, 8
Health data analysts, 322
Health informatics, 321
Health information management (HIM)
    inferential statistics in, 309
    statistic computed within the department, 173–212
    use of statistics, 8
Health Insurance Portability and Accountability Act
    (HIPAA), 177, 302
Histograms, 260–261
Historical research, 287
Home health care, patients for hospital autopsies, 127
Home health (HH), use of statistics, 7
Hospice
    patients for hospital autopsies, 127
    use of statistics, 7
Hospital-acquired infection. See Nosocomial infection
Hospital autopsies, 127–138
    definition, 127
    example, 128
    inpatient, 127
    patients available for, 128
Hospital death rate. See Gross (hospital) death rates
Hospital inpatient autopsy, definition, 127
Hospital inpatient beds, 54
Hospitalization, 36
Hospital live birth, 104
Hospital newborn bassinets, 55
Hypothesis
    definition, 289
    statement of, 289–290

I
Individually identifiable health information, 300
Infant death, 106
    computing populations statistics for, 107
Infection rate, 146–149, 337
    postoperative, 150–153
Inferential statistics, 309–320
    in data analysis, 295
    definition, 3–4, 310
Information governance (IG), 327
Informed consent, definition, 299
Inpatient, definition, 5
Inpatient admission, 35
Inpatient autopsy, 122, 127

Inpatient bed count, 54
Inpatient bed occupancy ratio/percentage, 56–59
    example, 56
Inpatient census, 5
    admission and discharge on same day, 40
    average daily, 45–46
        for PCU, 47–48
    average daily newborn, 46–47
    census day, 36
    complete master census, 32–33
    daily, 34–35
    definition, 32
    hospitalization, 36
    inpatient admission, 35
    inpatient service days, 35–36
    leave of absence, 35
    patient day, 36
Inpatient days of stay. See Length of stay (LOS)
Inpatient hospitalization duration. See Length of stay
    (LOS)
Inpatient service days, 35
    calculation of, 37–40
    total, 36
Institutional death rate. See Net death rate
Institutional Review Board (IRB), 298–300
Instrument
    definition, 291
    selection of, 291–292
Intermediate fetal death, 109
Interval data, definition, 247
Intrahospital transfers, 34

J
J-shaped curve, 234–235
Judgment sampling, 293

L
Labor productivity, 185, 337
Labor room beds, 54–55
Late fetal death, 109
Leave of absence, 35, 80
    days, 80–81
Length of stay (LOS), 71–90
    average (See Average length of stay [ALOS])
    calculating in an outpatient setting, 74–75
    definition, 71
    median used for, 223–224
    total, 76–77
Line graphs, 260
Literature review, 287
Long-term care facilities (LTC), use of statistics, 7

M
Managed care organizations (MCOs), use of statistics, 8
Maternal death rate, 102–106, 338
    computing population statistics for, 103–104
    definition, 102
    example, 103, 104

Mathematics, 13–30
Mean, 221–222, 338
    example, 221
Measurement, scales of, 246
Measurements, normal distribution, 231
Measures of central tendency, 220–227
Measures of variation, 227–238
Median, 222, 223
    to describe LOS, 223–224
    example, 223
Medical examiner, definition, 124
Medicare severity diagnosis-related groups (MS-DRGs),
        72
Mental health facilities, use of statistics, 7
Military time, 74
Mode, 224–226
    example, 224–225
Morbidity, definition, 146
Morbidity rates, 146–171
Morgue, 122
Mortality rates. *See also* Death rates and Cancer
        mortality rate
    definition, 112
Multimodal distribution curve, 234–235

N
National Center for Health Statistics (NCHS), 4
National Healthcare Anti-Fraud Association (NHCAA),
        324
National Healthcare Safety Network (NHSN), 146
National Nosocomial Infections Surveillance (NNIS)
        System, 146
National Surveillance System for Healthcare Workers
        (NaSH), 146
National Vital Statistics System (NVSS), 4
Naturalistic inquiry, 291
Necropsy. *See* Autopsy
Neonatal death, 106
    computing populations statistics for, 107
Neonatal period, 106
Net autopsy rate, 123–126, 338
    example, 124
Net death rate, 95–97, 338
    example, 96
Newborn autopsy rate, 132–133, 338
    example, 132
Newborn bassinet occupancy ratio/percentage, 61–64, 338
    example, 62
Newborn bassinets, 54–55
Newborn death rate, 106–108, 338
    definitions, 106
    example, 107
    guidelines for calculation of, 92
Nominal data, 246
    definition, 246
Normal distribution of data
    definition, 231
    example, 232

Nosocomial infection
    definition, 146
    example, 147
    rate, 146–149, 338
Null hypothesis, 290, 312–313
    definition, 312
Numbers, misleading presentation of, 297
Numerator, definition, 14
Numerical data, 248
Nursing facilities, use of statistics, 7

O
Observation, 291
Observational research, 288
Observation patient, 55
Occupancy percent, 56
Occupancy rate, 56
Occupancy ratio, 56
Open-ended questions. *See* Questions
Operational budget, 193–194
Ordinal data, 246–247
    definition, 246
Other rates formula, 161–162, 339
Outliers, 222
Outpatient facilities, use of statistics, 8

P
Patient care unit (PCU), 32
    average daily inpatient census for, 47–48
Patient day, 36
Payback period, 195, 339
Payment categories, 246
Percentage
    calculation of, 24
    changing a decimal to, 18
    changing a fraction to, 18
    changing to a decimal, 19
    changing to a fraction, 19
    definition, 18
Percentage of occupancy, 54–64
Percentile, 216–220
    examples, 217
Percent of occupancy, 56
Perinatal death, 106
Physician reports, 204–207
Pictogram, 261–262
Pie charts, 258–259
Pie graph. *See* Pie charts
Plagiarism, 296
Postmortem examination. *See* Autopsy
Postneonatal death, 106
Postoperative death rate, 97–99, 339
Postoperative infection rate, 150–153, 339
    definition, 150
    example, 150
Postpartum, 102
Predictive analytics, 322, 323–324

Predictive modeling, 324–325
Prepartum, 102
Prescriptive analytics, 322, 325
Primary data source, 4–5
Primary research, 287
Privacy consideration, clinical and biomedical research,
    300–303
Privacy Rule, 301
Problem definition, 286
Productivity, 185–186
    definition, 185
    real-world example, 185
Profiling, definition, 204
Proportion
    calculation of, 24
    definition, 22
Public health, need for statistics, 2–3

Q
Qualitative data, 322
Qualitative research, 284–286
    definition, 284
Quantitative data, 322
Quantitative research, 284–286
    definition, 284
Quartile, 215
Questionnaires, 288
Questions, unrestricted or unstructured, 291
Quasi-experimental research, 288
Quota sampling, 293
Quotient, definition, 15

R
Random sampling, 292
Range, definition, 228
Rank, 215
Rate, 24, 339
    calculation of, 24
    definition, 23
Ratio
    calculation of, 21–22, 24
    definition, 21
Ratio data
    definition, 247
    example, 247
Real-time analytics, 325
Recapitulation, 40
    census data, 41
Release of information (ROI)
    definition, 177
    unit costs for, 177–184
Reliability, 290
Reports, preparation of, 275–277
Research. *See also* specific type
    analyzing the data, 295–296
    basic principles, 283–307
    data interpretation issues, 296–304
    data validation in, 298
    definition, 284

    drawing conclusions, 296
    primary, 287
    privacy considerations, 300–303
    secondary, 287
Research design, 287–295
Research methodology, 284–286
Research process, 286–296
Return on investment, 195, 339
Reverse J-shaped curve, 234–235
Rounding numbers, 15–18
    definition, 15
Run charts. *See* Line graphs

S
Sabotage, in research, 298
Samples
    selection of, 292–294
    size, 294–295
Scales of measurement, 246
Scatter diagram, 266–269
Secondary data sources, 5–6
Secondary research, 287
Selection bias, 297
Skewness, 234
Snowball sampling, 293
Spreadsheets, 208
Staffing levels, 186–192, 339
    example, 187, 188
Standard deviation (SD), 231–234, 339
    example, 231–233
Standard error of the mean (SE_m), 310
Statistical reports
    case-mix index reports, 200
    computerized discharge reports, 197
    computerized financial reports, 200
    computerized readmission reports, 200
    physician reports, 204–207
    verification of, 197–207
Statistical research. *See* Descriptive research
Statistics, 1–12
    computed within HIM department, 173–212
    definition, 1–2
    descriptive, 213–243 (*See* Descriptive statistics)
    ethical guidelines in, 303–304
    in healthcare, 2
        sources of, 4–6
    health information, 174–177
    inferential, 309–320 (*See* Inferential statistics)
    public health needs, 2–3
    reason for studying, 2–3
    software packages, 295–296
    users of, 6–8
Stillbirth, 109
Stratified random sampling, 292
Structured interview, 291
Surgical death rate, 97
Surgical operation, definition, 97, 150
Surgical procedure, definition, 97, 150
Surveys, 290–291

Swing bed hospital, 63
Systematic random sampling, 292

T
Tables, 249–256
    components of, 250
    definition, 249
Total bed count days, 55
Total length of stay. *See* Length of stay (LOS)
Transfer, definition, 34
t test, 314–316
Type I error, 313–314
Type II error, 313–314

U
Unit labor costs, 174–177, 339
    definition, 174
    example, 174–175
    loose papers, 180
    performance improvement activities, 180

    provider-patient e-mail, 180
    scanning of records, 179
Utilization management, 72

V
Validity, 290
Variability, definition, 228
Variable, 214
Variance, 229, 340
    definition, 193
Visits, definition, 5
Vital statistics, 4
    infant mortality rate, 107, 340
    maternal mortality rate, 103, 340
    neonatal mortality rate, 107, 340

W
Whole number, 15
World Health Organization (WHO), 3
    maternal death statistics, 106, 340